THE BIOLOGICAL BASIS OF CANCER

Introducing the biology of neoplastic disorders, this accessible book looks at how cancer damages the body, and how the treatments work. Updated with the most recent research evidence, this unique text explains the basic biology of neoplastic disease; discusses the biology of the wide range of common cancers, now including neurological disorders; identifies and explains the biological causes of cancer, with a focus on genetics, hormones, and environmental factors; explains drug action in chemotherapy and analgesia; discusses the role of nutrition in neoplastic disorders and their treatment. Presenting the essential knowledge for working with cancer patients and their families, this textbook is an important read for those working in cancer care or undertaking study in this area.

William T. Blows was formerly a lecturer at City University of London, UK, where he taught biology to nurses.

THE BIOLOGICAL BASIS OF CANCER

Second Edition

William T. Blows

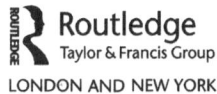

Routledge
Taylor & Francis Group

LONDON AND NEW YORK

Designed cover image: Getty images

Second edition published 2025
by Routledge
4 Park Square, Milton Park, Abingdon, Oxon, OX14 4RN

and by Routledge
605 Third Avenue, New York, NY 10158

Routledge is an imprint of the Taylor & Francis Group, an informa business

First edition published by Routledge 2005

British Library Cataloguing-in-Publication Data
A catalogue record for this book is available from the British Library

ISBN: 978-1-032-48448-8 (hbk)
ISBN: 978-1-032-48447-1 (pbk)
ISBN: 978-1-003-38912-5 (ebk)

DOI: 10.4324/9781003389125

Typeset in Times New Roman
by Apex CoVantage, LLC

CONTENTS

FIGURES

Chromosomes

TABLES

1

CELL BIOLOGY AND CANCER

- Introduction
- The cell
- The cell cycle and growth
- Tissues of the body
- The malignant cell
- A classification of malignancy
- A revolution in multiomics
- Key points

Introduction

Life is built from cells, and cells are the functional unit of life. In single-cell animals, for example, amoeba, one cell does everything the animal needs to live. In humans, and in other multicellular life forms, individual cells provide a contribution towards existence. Cells become specialised in their function. A multicellular life form can achieve so much more than a single-cell animal can, in both activity and growth. It is not possible to pack the sophisticated biochemistry of a human's complex life into just one cell. The work must be shared between all the cells that constitute a human body. The downside to this structure is that failure of just a few specialised and critical cells can jeopardise the very existence of all the others, and this is partly what happens in cancer.

The cell

Humans and animals have a type of cell called **eukaryotic** cells, whilst bacteria are **prokaryotic** cells (Figure 1.1). Eukaryotic cells have more membranes than prokaryotes, including organelles,[1] surrounded by membranes. Bacteria have complex cell walls but no fully formed nucleus. Eukaryotic cells do not have a cell wall but do have a fully formed nucleus with chromosomes.

DOI: 10.4324/9781003389125-1

Humans are made from an estimated 10^{14} cells, that is, 100,000,000,000,000 cells. All these are derived from a single fertilised ovum. From this ovum the earliest cell divisions create a collection of cells that are all the same, but later growth in cell numbers allows the start of another process, called **differentiation**. Cells begin to take on specific specialised roles so that they will become tissues, such as blood, bone, and brain. Every cell that has a nucleus also has the entire set of genes needed to make the whole body, but not all cells need every gene. Most genes will be 'switched off' in those cells that do not need them, and only those genes needed for survival and their specialist function will remain active.

Cells are made from **protoplasm**, which is mostly water with proteins; amino acids, that is, the components that make up proteins; minerals; and other nutrients. Surrounding this protoplasm is a **cell membrane** (or **plasma membrane**), which is semi-permeable, that is, it allows passage of some things through, but not others. Those that pass through include water and nutrients that enter the cell and wastes that leave the cell. **Oxygen (O_2)** enters the cell, and **carbon**

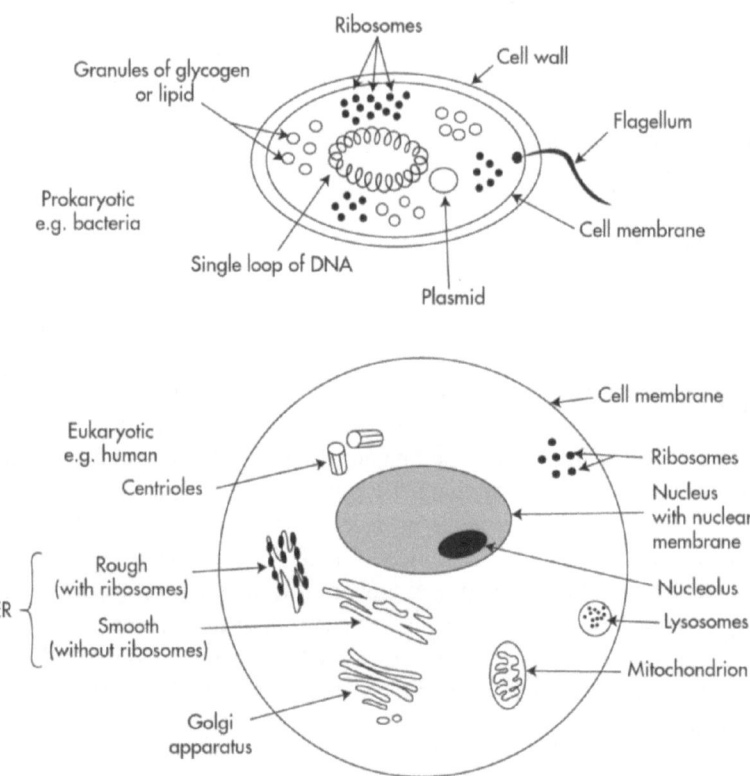

FIGURE 1.1   Two different cell types. The prokaryote (top) and eukaryote cell (bottom). The prokaryote cell is usually smaller, with no definite nucleus, that is, no nuclear membrane and no nucleolus. There is a cell wall in prokaryotes that eukaryotes do not have. The DNA of prokaryotes comes in a single loop, unlike the complex chromosomes found in eukaryotes. Some prokaryotes have a small additional loop of DNA called a plasmid, and some have a tail-like flagellum to aid movement, both structures not found in eukaryotes. Mitochondria, endoplasmic reticulum (ER) and Golgi apparatus are features of eukaryotes (Table 1.1).

dioxide (CO_2) leaves the cell (Figure 1.2). Most cells also have a nucleus, surrounded by a membrane (the **nuclear membrane**), which is also semi-permeable, with holes of a size that allows only the passage of molecules small enough to enter or leave the nucleus, for example, **messenger ribonucleic acid (mRNA)** (see 'Genes and protein synthesis', Chapter 2, p. 25).

Cells have a series of **organelles** which carry out the various processes needed for life. Organelles are '*mini-organs*', hence the term *organelle*. A definition of an *organelle* is 'a membrane-bound protein structure which carries out a specific function inside a cell'. Most of the organelles exist within the **cytoplasm**, that is, the protoplasm between the cell membrane and the nuclear membrane. One important organelle occurs inside the nucleus, the nucleolus. Table 1.1 is a list of the organelles found in a cell and their functions.

The nucleus, genes, and chromosomes

The nucleus has a key central control over all cellular activities. This is because the nucleus houses the **genes** that code for the proteins involved in most cellular functions. Genes are stretches of the molecule **deoxyribonucleic acid (DNA)** (Figure 1.4). Genes determine which amino acids will be in the finished protein, and in what sequence these amino acids will occur (see 'Genes and protein synthesis', Chapter 2, p. 25). DNA has four **bases** mounted on a **sugar–phosphate** molecule, the sugar being **deoxyribose**. Two strands of DNA twist round each other in a double-helix form, and the bases are linked across from one strand to the other (Figure 1.4). The four bases are **adenine**, **thymine**, **cytosine**, and

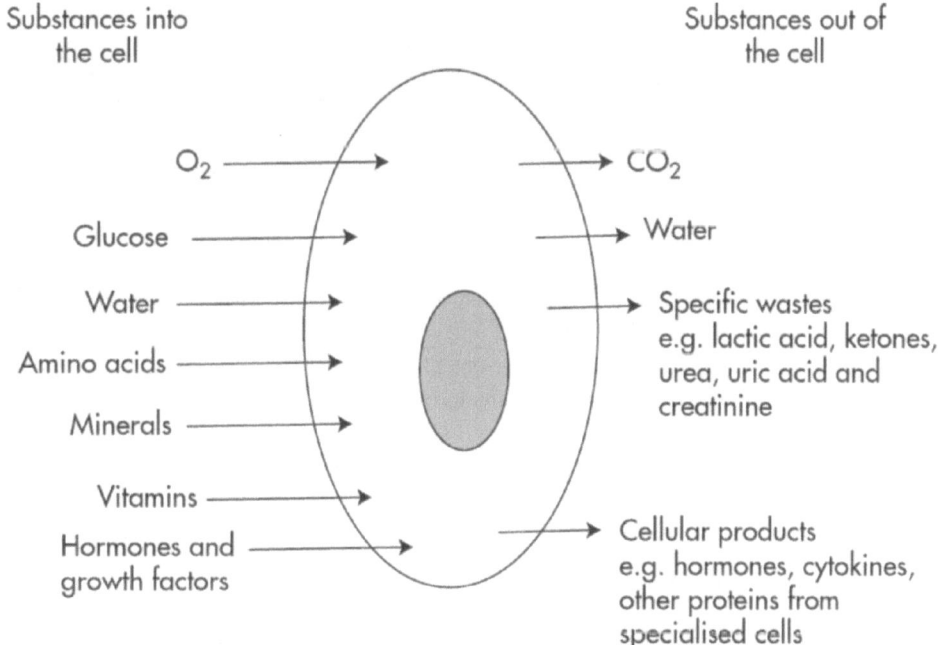

FIGURE 1.2   Movement across the cell membranes. The input is shown on the left, and the output is shown on the right.

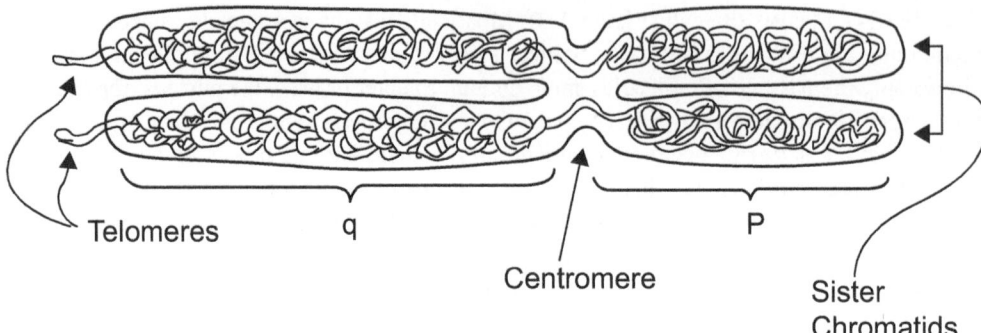

Telomeres q

Centromere

P

Sister Chromatids

FIGURE 1.3 The structure of a chromosome. The chromosome consists of two sister chromatid strands made from chromatin and joined at the centromere. In each strand there are coils of DNA wrapped around histones (see 'Epigenetics', 'Histone modification', Chapter 2, p. 37). The centromere is placed either in the middle of the chromosome or more towards one end, creating a longer 'q' arm and a shorter 'p' arm (see 'Chromosomes', Addendum, starting on p. 342). Telomeres extend from the end (see 'Tissue invasion', 'Telomeres', Chapter 6, p. 124)

guanine, where adenine and thymine link together and cytosine and guanine link together across the strands. The linkage is in the form of **hydrogen bonds**, two such bonds between the adenine and the thymine, three between the cytosine and the guanine. Hydrogen bonds are weak links that can be separated when the two strands come apart and reformed when the molecule joins up again. This happens for protein synthesis and during replication of DNA (see 'The cell cycle and growth', p. 4).

Chromosomes are made from two strands of **chromatin**. Chromatin is made from DNA and its packaging proteins, called **histones** (see 'Histone modification', Chapter 2, p. 37). Long chromatin threads of DNA and histones are coiled to form **chromatid** strands. Chromosomes consist of two identical chromatid strands, called **sister chromatids**, joined at a single point, the **centromere** (Figure 1.3).

The nucleus of human cells has 46 chromosomes, which make up the **karyotype** (Figure 1.5).

The karyotype is a complete assemblage of the chromosomes which consists of 22 pairs of **autosomes** (44 autosomes) and 1 pair of sex chromosomes. Chromosomes are paired because we inherit one set of 23 chromosomes from one parent and one set of 23 chromosomes from the other parent. As an example, the number one chromosome from the father is 'the same' as the number one chromosome from the mother, and so on. The term used is **homologous**, which means 'the same'. Each chromosome of a homologous pair has the same genes. This means that the cell has two versions of every gene, one version from each parent. These alternative versions of the same gene are called **alleles**.

The cell cycle and growth

Cells grow in two ways: they grow in size, that is, **auxetic growth**, and they grow in numbers, that is, **multiplicative growth**. Size growth is limited because the volume of a cell, the cytoplasm, grows faster than the surface area, the cell membrane. It is through the membrane that the nutrients and oxygen needed for growth must pass (Figure 1.2). Another way of putting this is to say that the volume grows by the *radius cubed* (radius^3), whilst the surface area grows

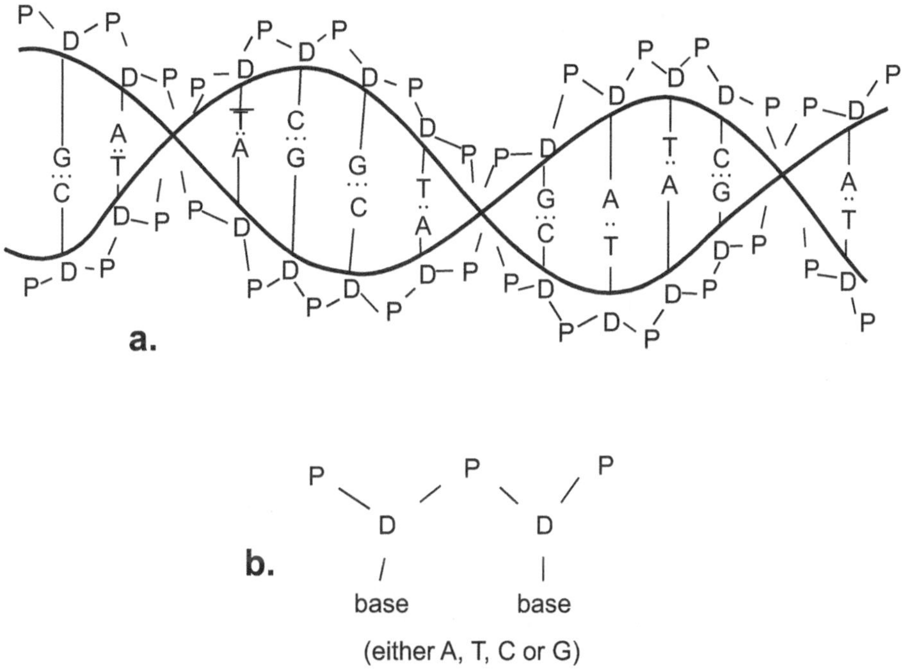

FIGURE 1.4 A simplified DNA molecule: (a) Short section of DNA showing four possible bases – adenine (A) linking with thymine (T) with two hydrogen bonds (two dots), and guanine (G) linking with cytosine (C) with three hydrogen bonds (three dots). The molecule is incredibly long and twisted into a double helix. (b) DNA is made of nucleotides. Each nucleotide has a sugar (D = deoxyribose), a phosphate (P), and one of the bases (either A, T, C, or G) attached to the sugar.

TABLE 1.1 The cellular organelles

Organelle	Description/function
Cytoplasmic	
Mitochondria	Produce energy in the form of adenosine triphosphate (ATP)
Ribosomes	Produce proteins from amino acids according to instructions from the genes (deoxyribonucleic acid, or DNA)
Vacuoles	Storage spaces within the cytoplasm
Lysosomes	Specialised vacuoles containing digestive enzymes
Rough endoplasmic reticulum (ER) is ER with ribosomes;	Cytoplasmic spaces bound by a continuous membrane within which proteins are produced, modified, and packaged
Smooth endoplasmic reticulum (ER) (ER without ribosomes)	Cytoplasmic spaces bound by a continuous membrane within which fat-based products are modified and packaged
Golgi apparatus	Cytoplasmic spaces bound by a separate membrane system within which products from ER are further modified, packaged, and distributed or secreted from the cell
Centrioles	Structures outside the nucleus that form the nuclear spindle during cell division (called mitosis)
Nucleic	
Nucleolus	Produces the components of ribosomes

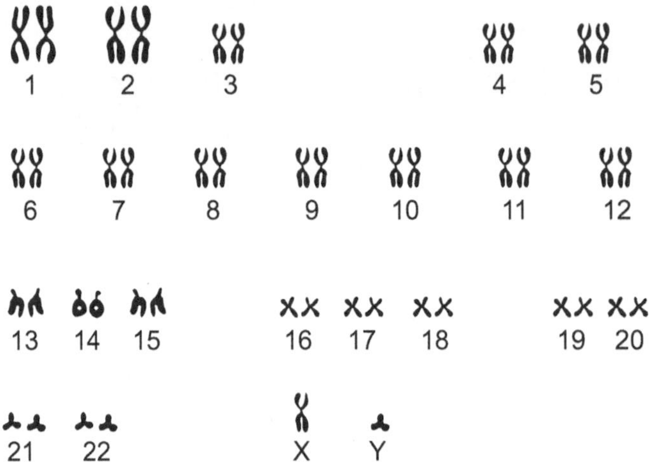

FIGURE 1.5 The human karyotype. This is an artificial presentation of the 46 chromosomes that are found in the nucleus of the cell. Matching pairs are numbered 1 to 22 (the autosomes) and X + Y (the sex chromosomes). One chromosome from each pair is from the father; the other is from the mother. This is a male karyotype because it contains both X and Y. The female karyotype would contain X and X. Normally, in the nucleus, the chromosomes are jumbled and not visible, except during mitosis.

Source: From Blows (2022).

by only the *square of the radius* (radius²). Therefore, metabolism in the volume outstrips the nutrient supply available through the surface area, and before that happens, the cell must divide into two **daughter cells** in order to reduce the volume. The overall size of any multicellular life form is dependent on the limits of multiplicative growth rather than on auxetic growth, which is already limited. This also explains why single-cell organisms, like amoeba, are always so small.

Cells undergo a **cell cycle** (Figure 1.6) which involves both cell division (called **mitosis**) and the period between two successive divisions (called the **interphase**). *Mitosis* is the division of most cells, that is, all cells except for the **gametes**, which are the female **ova** ('egg' cell) and the male **sperm**. These divide by a different process, called **meiosis**.

Mitosis and cytokinesis

Mitosis, as seen in most tissue cells, is the division of the cell nucleus. It consists of a sequence of phases, namely (in order), **prophase**, **metaphase**, **anaphase**, and **telophase**. **Cytokinesis** follows on from mitosis and is the division of the cytoplasm (Figure 1.7).

Prophase

This is the earliest and longest period of mitosis, during which preparations for division occur. During prophase, the chromatin strands, which were previously invisible, coil up and condense to form visible chromosomes, each chromosome consisting of a pair of sister chromatids joined

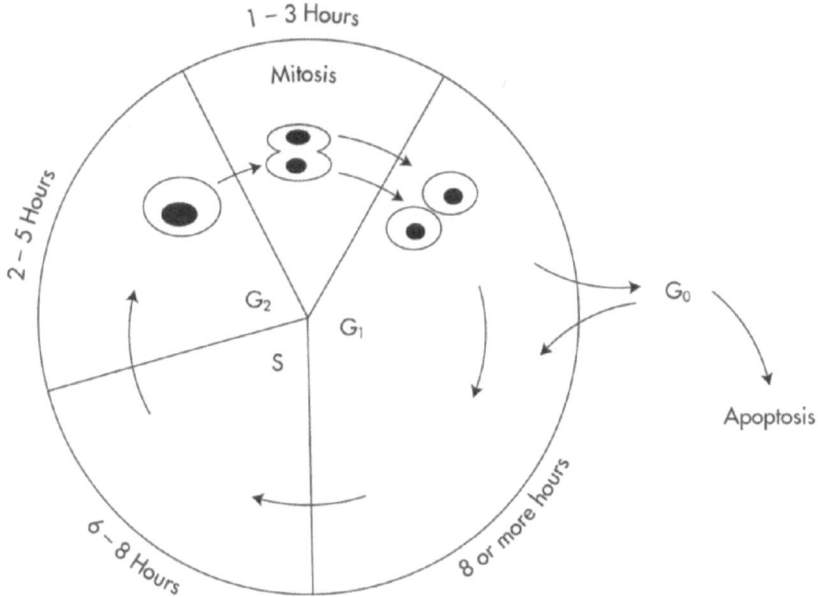

FIGURE 1.6 The cell cycle. After mitosis, the daughter cells arrive in G_1, the first and the longer of the two growth phases. From here, if there is any problem with the DNA, the cell may go to G_0 and return to G_1 if the DNA is recoverable. If not, the cell may die (apoptosis). The S phase is a period of DNA replication, followed by a shorter growth phase, G_2, which prepares the cell for mitosis (cell division) again.

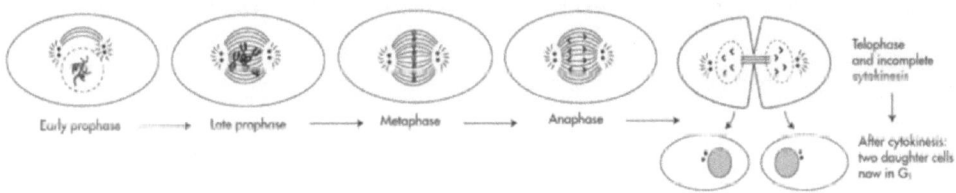

FIGURE 1.7 Mitosis and cytokinesis. The four phases of mitosis are prophase, metaphase, anaphase, and telophase, followed by the division of the cytoplasm, called cytokinesis.

at a centromere (Figure 1.3). The nucleolus becomes invisible and may be dispersed throughout the nucleus. Then the nuclear membrane breaks down and can no longer be seen. At this point, because the nuclear boundary has gone, the cell has no recognisable nucleus – a condition retained until the later stages of mitosis. The **centrioles** (Table 1.1 and Figure 1.7) duplicate, and these pairs migrate to positions at the opposing pole to each other. From these structures the mitotic spindle develops on both sides. The *spindle* is a protein framework of **microtubules** which grows outward and crosses the space previously occupied by the nucleus. The two halves of the spindle do not quite meet in the middle, leaving a gap for the chromosomes to come between them and attach to both halves of the spindle via the chromosomal centromeres (Figure 1.7).

Metaphase

This is much shorter than prophase and consists of the chromosomes adopting a central position along the equatorial plane of the spindle, in the spindle gaps. There are 46 chromosomes in the human cell, and these must be divided between the two new cells, so each will receive 46 single separate chromatid strands.

Anaphase

This is the brief phase of chromosomal movement, when the spindles on both sides retract, pulling the chromosomes apart into their separate chromatid strands, that is, they separate at the centromere. One chromatid strand will be pulled to one side of the cell; the other chromatid strand is pulled to the other side of the cell (Figure 1.7).

Telophase

This is almost the reverse of prophase. The chromatid strands disappear by uncoiling and becoming thread-like again as the two new nuclear membranes surrounding the chromatids are restored. This means that, for a brief moment, before the rest of the cell divides, the cell has two nuclei. The nucleolus is also restored within each of these nuclei.

Cytokinesis

This is not part of mitosis but is the division of the remaining cytoplasm, completing the process of producing two separate daughter cells (Figure 1.7). The plasma membrane is produced in sufficient quantities by both cells to span completely between them, cutting the cytoplasm in half. The division of the cytoplasm also involves the equal distribution of the organelles between the two new cells.

Interphase

This is the period between one mitotic event and the next. The cell is very active during all stages of interphase. The stages of interphase are, in order of sequence from mitosis, G_0, G_1, S, and G_2 (Figure 1.6).

G_0 stage

This is an indefinite period, during which the cell is carrying out its normal metabolic functions but is not preparing for further division. Some cells, like most **neurons** (nerve cells), remain in G_0 and never divide. Others, such as bone marrow stem cells, divide so quickly that they spend little time, if any, in G_0. G_0 is also important to getting the cell out of the cycle if the DNA is damaged, to allow time for repair, or to pass the cell on to apoptosis (cell death) (see 'G_0 and cell cycle control', p. 9).

G_1 stage

This is the first of two growth phases (G for 'growth') in preparation for further cell division. Having grown in numbers from one cell to two cells during mitosis (multiplicative growth), the cells undergo some auxetic growth, with a corresponding increase in organelle numbers which must meet the needs of the two further daughter cells produced at the next mitosis. All the new components must be synthesised from proteins and lipids, using glucose as an energy source, and these components must all be imported into the cells through the cell membrane. This is a major metabolic exercise, and the enzymes that drive this metabolism must all be produced in sufficient quantities. By the end of G_1, both cells should be ready to proceed to the next phase, the S phase.

The S (or synthesis) stage

This involves the replication and production of new DNA and the proteins (called **histones**) that are used for packaging the DNA. This provides enough DNA by duplicating the missing chromatin strands, for the future daughter cells after the next mitosis.

G_2 stage

This is the second of the two growth phases. At this point, final preparations for mitosis take place, including further essential protein synthesis and completion of centriole replication.

G_0 and cell cycle control

G_0 is the stationary phase of the cell cycle, when the cell is not preparing for division. During its stay in G_0, the cell undergoes certain checks that are made by the cell repair enzymes to assess the integrity of the DNA following mitosis. With chromosomes being pulled in two different directions during anaphase (Figure 1.7), it is possible that DNA was damaged, and this damage needs repair. Failure to do this could result in the damage being duplicated in the S stage of interphase, ready to be incorporated into each new daughter cell. The damage, that is, gene errors, not only affects the current cell but will also be passed onto the future generations of daughter cells, a situation that occurs in cancer. Chapter 2 discusses the genetic control of G_0 in more detail (see 'G_0 and DNA repair', Chapter 2, p. 30).

Tissues of the body

Cells are grouped into **tissues**, and there are two major categories of structural tissues in the body, the **epithelial** and **connective** tissues, plus tissues of specialist function, such as the nervous system; blood formation tissue, that is, bone marrow; muscle; and the lymphatic system.

Epithelial tissues

Epithelial tissues are the simplest tissues, and they line surfaces, for example, cavities or tubes. They are made from a single layer of cells, called **simple**, or multiple layers of cells, called **stratified**, resting on a **basement membrane**. The cells may be **squamous**, that is, flat; **cuboid**, that is, blocks; or **columnar**, that is, tall (Figure 1.8).

  Simple squamous epithelium is a single flat layer of smooth, pavement-like cells that provides a smooth surface *inside* blood vessels, the **endothelium**, and *inside* the heart, the **endocardium**, and forms the walls of lymphatic vessels and air sacs in the lungs, called **alveoli**. It is also found in other membranes, for example, the membrane around the heart, called the

pericardium. **Simple cuboid epithelium** lines the glands and ducts leading from the glands and is also found in the **renal tubules**, that is, part of the **nephron**, the functional unit of the kidney (see Figure 10.1, Chapter 10, p. 194). **Simple columnar epithelium** is found lining the gall bladder, the stomach, and the intestines. It is also found in digestive glands and the respiratory tract. In many of these sites, it forms a **mucous membrane**. In mucous membranes, some cells are called **goblet cells** because they have a cup-like shape, and these secrete mucus. Respiratory mucous columnar cells also have **cilia**, that is, tiny hair-like projections which can perform a sweeping action to filter the air we breathe in (see 'Tobacco smoking', 'mucociliary escalator', Chapter 3, p. 48).

Stratified (multilayered) squamous epithelium covers the surface of the body as **epidermis**, the outer layer of the skin (see 'Structure and function of skin', Chapter 13, p. 241). The living cells of the epidermis are roughly square and occur at the base of the layers, where they are constantly dividing. The new cells created migrate upward through the various layers, and during this process, they produce a protein called **keratin**. As this fills the cytoplasm, the cell flattens and dies. In the upper (outer) layers, these dead flat cells flake off and are lost (on the scalp, this is **dandruff**). This tissue forms a tough outer layer to the body, where erosion of the body surface is likely and constant replacement from the basal layers is necessary. It is also found in the mouth, oesophagus, and vagina.

Stratified cuboidal epithelium consists of multiple layers of square cells found in **sweat glands**, that is, glands in the skin secreting sweat, and **sebaceous glands**, that is, tiny glands attached to the base of hairs in the skin that secrete **sebum**, an oily fluid which lubricates the hair. Stratified cuboidal epithelium is also found in the **ovaries** and **testes**, that is, the **gonads**.

Stratified columnar epithelium comprises a superficial layer of columnar cells on top of several layers of cuboidal cells. This forms moist surfaces, such as inside the larynx, parts of the pharynx and the urethra, and lines the ducts of both the **salivary glands** and **mammary glands**. This tissue allows the movement of substances over its surface, like saliva and breast milk, along the ducts.

Pseudostratified columnar epithelium (*pseudo* means 'false') is a single layer of cells with nuclei at different heights, giving a false impression of several layers. Careful examination reveals that all the cells are in contact with a basement membrane, but they do not all reach the free, superficial surface (Figure 1.9). This is found in large excretory ducts of the male reproductive system, the nasal cavity, and other parts of the respiratory tract. Like stratified columnar epithelium, this tissue allows the movement of substances over its surface and secretes fluid.

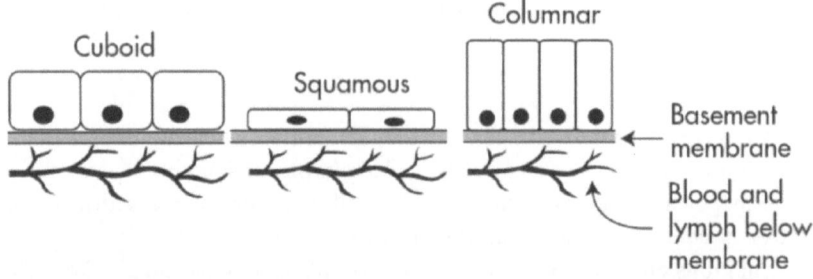

FIGURE 1.8 Simple epithelial tissues. Cuboid, squamous, and columnar epithelium on basement membrane. Beneath the basement membrane are blood and lymph vessels.

Transitional epithelium consists of cells which change shape, from cuboid to flat and back again, when stretching is required, for example, it lines the urinary bladder and stretches during bladder filling.

Connective tissues

These are tissues that give structure and support to the body whilst connecting parts together and filling spaces. They include areolar, collagen, cartilage, muscle, fat, and bone.

Areolar connective tissue is the most common connective tissue in the body. It is made from a loose collection of two different fibres interwoven together in a mesh with scattered cells throughout. The first of these fibres is **collagen**, a very common structural protein found in many sites around the body. These fibres are tough and give strength to the tissue. The second is **elastic fibres**, and as the name suggests, these are stretchy and provide some elasticity to the tissue. Among the cells are those of the immune system, that is, **macrophages**, and those that help produce the tissue, that is, **fibroblasts**. Areolar tissue is ubiquitous, that is, it is almost everywhere, and in most places, areolar tissue is used as packaging around blood vessels, nerves, skin, and organs.

Dense, collagenous tissue is similar to areolar, except it is packed with collagen but with no elastic fibres. This is a very tough tissue in either of its two forms: *regular* or *irregular*. In regular collagenous tissue, the collagen fibres all lay parallel in bundles, allowing the tissue to have a great tensile strength. Such strength is needed in tendons and ligaments that pull on bones. Irregular tissue has the fibres all mixed up and lying at many different angles. The dermis of the skin is one good example of this type.

Elastic connective tissue has many yellow elastic fibres which are extensively branched, forming a network. The spaces in this net contain fibroblasts and small amounts of collagen. Elastic tissue allows stretching with recoil plus support and suspension of other structures. It is found in the stomach wall, the largest arteries, and parts of the trachea, vocal cords, bronchi, and the heart.

Adipose connective tissue is made from fat cells, called **adipocytes**. The cytoplasm of adipocytes is packed with lipid, displacing the nucleus to one side. About 10% of the average adult body weight is adipose tissue. Adipose tissue forms under the dermis of the skin, where it helps

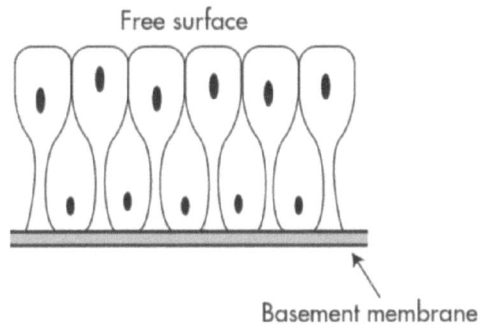

FIGURE 1.9 Pseudostratified epithelium. It appears as two layers but is, in fact, only one layer of cells, with each cell touching the basement membrane and with varying heights of the nuclei.

insulate against excessive heat loss. It is also found around internal organs, where it helps provide a protective cushion against potential injury. Adipose tissue is also a valuable food reserve, since fat is the body's second-line energy source after glucose.

Reticular connective tissue is a latticework of fine multibranching interwoven fibres forming a web-like structure with **reticular cells** in the spaces. This is found inside the liver, spleen, lymph nodes, tonsils, stomach, and intestinal wall, and it supports adipose tissue.

Cartilage

Cartilage is the toughest of the connective soft tissues and is mostly associated with the skeleton and bone function. The three cartilage types are very similar to areolar, dense collagenous, and elastic connective tissues, the difference being the tough, dense, gel-like matrix within which the fibres and cartilage cells (called **chondrocytes**) are set.

Hyaline cartilage is a network of collagen fibres in a gel-like matrix. The joint ends of long bones, where it is called **articular cartilage**, are a good example of hyaline cartilage. Here, it needs to be tough to withstand erosion from joint movements and, in the case of the legs, weight-bearing pressures. Other sites include the tracheal and laryngeal cartilages, the bronchial cartilages, the nose (below the bridge), and the **costal cartilages**, which link the ends of the ribs to the **sternum** (or breastbone). Toughness at the joint ends is tempered with flexibility in places like the nose and ribs.

Fibrocartilage consists of bundles of collagen fibres packed together in a tough gel-like matrix. The addition of collagen to the matrix gives fibrocartilage the quality of being the toughest soft tissue in the body. As such, it is found in places like the **intervertebral discs** (cartilaginous pads between the vertebrae of the spine), where weight-bearing and spinal movements put great strain on soft tissues. A supportive role for fibrocartilage is found in the **meniscus** (specialised stabilising cartilages within the knee joints) and surrounding the rims of joint sockets.

Elastic cartilage is a concentration of dense elastic fibres in matrix. Flexibility, coupled with the ability to retain the original shape, is important for this tissue. It is found in the external ear, the nasopharynx, the larynx, and the **epiglottis**, the flap in the larynx that guards the entrance to the trachea, preventing inhalation of food and drink during swallowing (Martini et al. 2023).

Bone tissue

Bone is the second hardest tissue in the body – only tooth enamel is harder than bone. Bone tissue makes up the skeleton, which provides shape and support for the body; protects vital organs, for example, the skull protects the brain; coordinates movement through a system of joints; and creates anchorage for muscles and critical storage for calcium (Martini et al. 2023) (see 'The skeleton', Chapter 14, p. 253). Bone is made from organic and inorganic components (Figure 1.10). The organic components are the cells, called **osteocytes**, and the cellular products, notably proteins, such as collagen. The inorganic components are the minerals, mostly calcium compounds, such as **calcium phosphate** and **calcium carbonate**. The inorganic minerals form crystals along the protein framework, with the cells living in spaces. There are two types of bone tissue: **compact** bone and **cancellous** (or **spongy**) bone. The 200 bones in the skeleton (plus 6 in the ears) have an outer casing of compact bone with the spongy bone inside. This cancellous spongy bone has many spaces in it, like honeycomb, and these spaces are filled with **bone marrow**. Unlike the skeletons seen in museums and biology laboratories, living bone is not a dry material. In life, it has a rich blood supply and contains about 20% water. It also has many living,

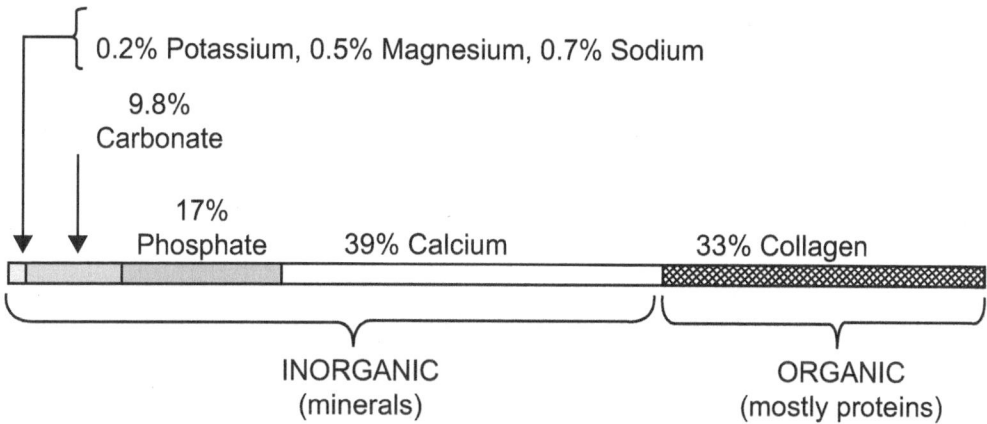

0.2% Potassium, 0.5% Magnesium, 0.7% Sodium

9.8%
Carbonate

17%
Phosphate   39% Calcium   33% Collagen

INORGANIC   ORGANIC
(minerals)   (mostly proteins)

FIGURE 1.10   The composition of bone. The organic material (cells and cellular proteins, such as collagen) occupies about 33% of the content. The inorganic material (minerals, mostly calcium) occupies the remainder.

reproducing cells, and it can grow and heal if injured. Bone has an outer membrane, called the **periosteum**, which houses another type of cells (**osteogenic** cells) vital in the healing process and can become new osteocytes.

The skeleton consists of 206 bones. These are divided into 80 bones of the **axial skeleton**, that is, the skull, spine, and ribcage, and 126 bones of the **appendicular skeleton**, that is, the upper limb and shoulder bones and the lower limbs and pelvis (see 'The skeleton', Chapter 14, p. 253).

Muscle tissue

There are three muscle types in the body (Figure 1.11) (Martini et al. 2023). **Skeletal muscle** is the type we are all aware of, that is, that of the trunk, neck, and limbs. It is attached to bones and works by voluntary control. Under the microscope, it appears as very long, thin, cylindrical cells, called **myocytes**. These cells are striated (which means 'striped') or banded in appearance. Their role is voluntary movement, controlled by the brain via the **motor nervous system**. **Smooth muscle** is involuntary muscle, that is, we have no control or awareness of its function. It is found in the walls of the digestive tract, the blood vessels, and the respiratory tract. Under the microscope, the cells are spindle-shaped and have no stripes. It is controlled by the **sympathetic** component of the **autonomic nervous system**. **Cardiac muscle** is a specialised heart muscle found only in the **myocardium**, the middle layer of the heart wall. It is involuntary in function, controlled by both the autonomic nervous system and its own internal conduction system. Under the microscope, it consists of long, cylindrical, branched cells which, like skeletal muscle, have stripes (or bands).

Blood tissue

Blood is a tissue in fluid form. This is because blood must circulate around the body and supply all the other tissues with oxygen and nutrients and remove waste. We have about 5 L (5,000 ml) of blood in the adult body, and of this, about 55% is the fluid component, called **plasma**. The

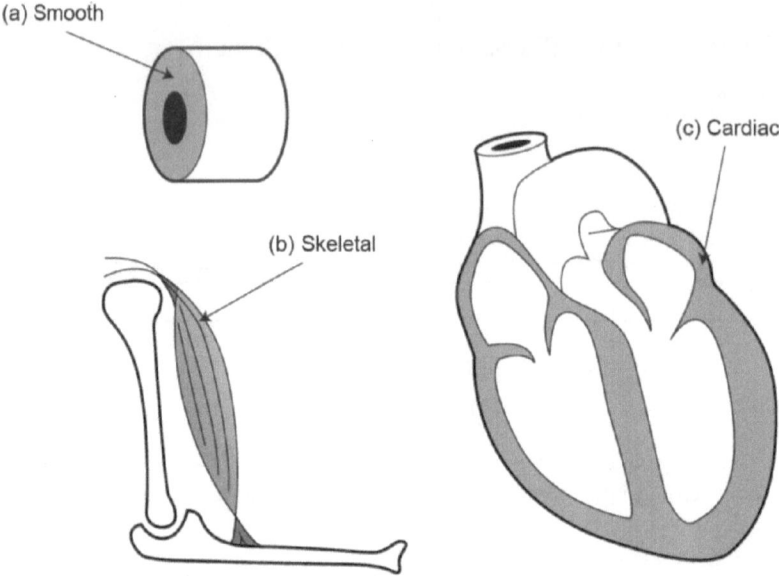

FIGURE 1.11 Three types of muscle: (a) smooth muscle is found in the walls of tubes, such as blood vessels and the gut wall; (b) skeletal muscle is found in the muscles attached to bones; (c) cardiac muscle is only found in the myocardium of the heart.

other 45% is the **formed elements**, a collective term which means the various cells of the blood (Figure 1.12). The plasma is about 92% water, with a wide range of other substances dissolved in it. These substances include many kinds of proteins, such as **albumin** and **globulin**, clotting factors, hormones, and antibodies. Other substances present in plasma are amino acids, glucose, minerals, vitamins, steroidal hormones, the gases oxygen and carbon dioxide, and waste of various kinds, particularly **urea** (nitrogenous waste from proteins). Plasma is also the mechanism for the distribution of heat around the body.

The cells in the plasma fall into three main categories, that is, the erythrocytes, the leukocytes, and the thrombocytes (platelets). The **erythrocytes** (**red blood cells**, or **RBC**) account for almost 99.9% of the blood cells, and they carry much of the blood gases, oxygen and carbon dioxide. These gases are mostly transported by the molecule **haemoglobin** (**Hb**), which fills the erythrocytes. One haemoglobin molecule has four **globin** proteins, each containing a **haeme** component, and at the core of the haeme is an iron atom. One haemoglobin molecule can carry four oxygen molecules ($4 \times O_2$). Each RBC contains about 250 million Hb molecules and can therefore carry 1 billion oxygen molecules when fully saturated. The globin component carries around 20% of the carbon dioxide transported in the blood.

The remaining 0.1% of the blood cells are **leucocytes** (**white blood cells**, or **WBC**) and **thrombocytes** (or **platelets**). The role of WBCs is to fight infection; they are a major component of our immune system (see 'Adaptive (acquired or specific) immunity', Chapter 5, p. 81). Platelets prevent blood loss in several ways, especially by activating the blood clotting process, creating a blood clot (or **thrombus**). Blood cells are derived from stem cells in bone marrow, in a process called **haemopoiesis** (or **haematopoiesis**), which means 'blood forming' (see 'Blood cell formation', Chapter 7, p. 130).

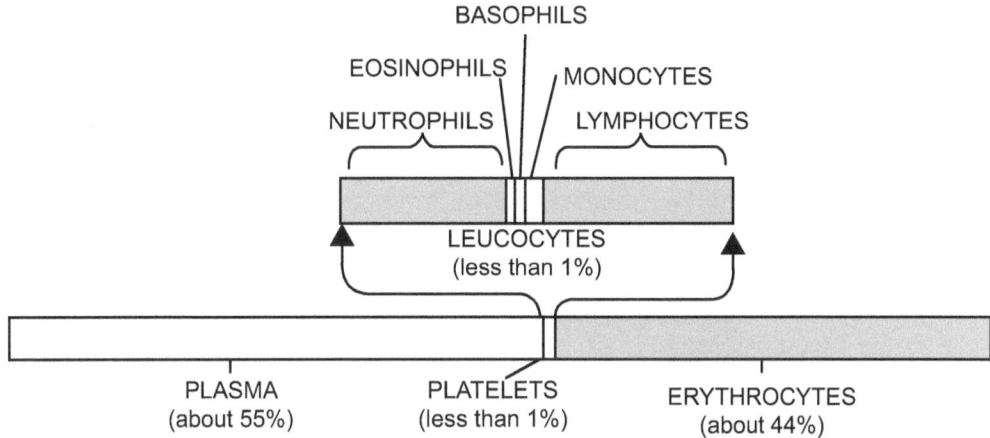

FIGURE 1.12   The composition of whole blood. Plasma, at about 55% of the volume, and red cells (erythrocytes), at about 44% of the volume, leave very little (less than 1%) for the white cells (leucocytes) and platelets (thrombocytes).

Lymphatic tissue

The **lymphatic system** is a key component of the immune system of the body. Lymph, like blood, is mostly water, and it is derived from, and returns to, blood plasma. Lymphatic vessels drain excess fluid from the tissues, and this fluid is filtered in **lymphatic glands** (or **nodes**), where unwanted and potentially harmful foreign substances (called **antigens**) are removed and destroyed by **lymphocytes**. The lymphatic system is described in more detail in Chapters 6 and 7 because the system is involved in both the fight against cancer and its spread.

Nerve tissue

Nervous tissue makes up the brain and the spinal cord (collectively called the **central nervous system**, or **CNS**) and the nerves (called the **peripheral nervous system**, or **PNS**). The functional cell of nerve impulse conduction is the **neuron** (Figure 1.13). These are highly specialised cells which have mostly lost the ability for replication, that is, they remain in G_0 of the cell cycle. They create impulses, known as **action potentials**, which pass down long fibres (**axons**) extending from the cell body (Martini et al. 2023). These fibres link up with either other neurons or other cells, for example, muscular or glandular cells, and the impulses increase (or reduce) activity in those cells, thus having some control over the function of many cells. Supportive cells of the nervous system (**neuroglia**, or **glial cells**, or **glia**) do not produce or convey impulses, but they play a vital role in maintaining neuron function (see 'The brain', Chapter 14, p. 258).

The malignant cell

The major difference between a normal cell and a malignant cell is **genetic instability**. This means that the malignant cell has increased susceptibility towards DNA damage and genetic mutations. DNA and RNA can fracture and leak into the environment and the blood.[2] This

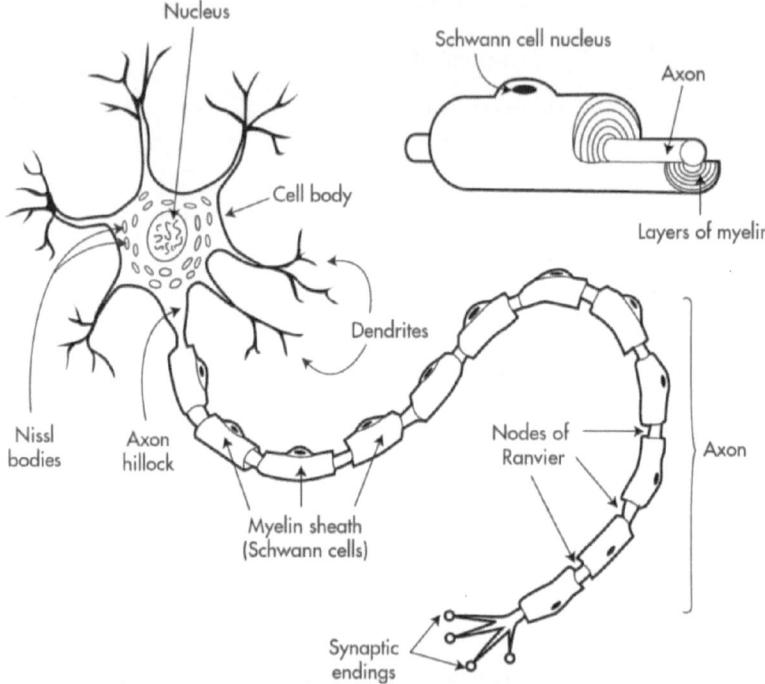

FIGURE 1.13 The neuron (or nerve cell). It consists of a cell body with dendrites and a long axon, usually covered with a myelin sheath (shown in detail).

Source: From Blows (2024).

leakage and the production of chemokines[3] into the cellular environment usually triggers the immune system to attack and kill malignant cells. But some cancer cells survive by overcoming this immune response.

Six changes must take place for a normal cell to become a malignant cancer cell (Table 1.2).

Tumours are either **benign** or **malignant** (Kumar et al. 2022). Benign tumours are more common than malignant tumours, and they are potentially less dangerous (Table 1.3). The word 'cancer' describes a tumour that infiltrates and grows into the surrounding tissues and organs. Only malignant tumours do this. Most non-malignant (i.e. benign) tumours do not infiltrate in this manner, only doing so after they have turned malignant. Therefore, the word *cancer* should *only be used in the context of malignant infiltrative tumours* but not used for tumours that are non-malignant and non-infiltrative.

When a liquid or solid **biopsy**[5] is taken, it will be examined in the laboratory for abnormalities, a process known as **histopathology**. This means cutting a thin section through the tissue for microscopic examination. Close detailed examination of this kind reveals if the tissues and the cells are normal or not, and it is therefore a key step in the diagnosis of the problem. Normal epithelial cells appear regular in shape and size, and they are well-organised. They also have regular-shaped nuclei and small round nucleoli. Most normal epithelial cells will be positioned along a **basement membrane** which acts as a flat surface along which the cells are anchored in place (see 'Cellular adhesion molecules (CAMs)', Chapter 6, p. 114). Basement membranes are

TABLE 1.2 Normal versus malignant cell

	Normal cell	Cancer cell
1	Growth occurs in response to growth factors and in accordance with body needs.	Growth becomes independent of growth factors and ignores body needs.
2	Growth stops when signalled to do so by stop signals from the body.	Growth continues despite growth stop signals.
3	Internal autodestruct mechanisms lead to cell death (apoptosis) when things go wrong.	Autodestruct mechanisms are bypassed even when things inside the cell go wrong.
4	Tissues only construct new blood vessels to sustain normal tissue growth.	Produces new blood vessels abnormally to support the tumour.
5	Cells divide about 70 times, that is, 70 cell cycles, before apoptosis kills the cell.	No limit to the number of cancer cell divisions, so the malignant cell becomes immortal.
6	Most cells remain in fixed positions and die from apoptosis if they become dislodged.	Cancer cells can survive after breaking free from the main tumour and migrate to other parts of the body.

TABLE 1.3 Benign versus malignant tumours

Benign tumours	Malignant tumours (cancers)
Common.	Rarer, becoming more common in the elderly.
Cells of the tumour are the same as the tissue of origin.	Cells of the tumour are usually very unlike the tissue of origin, that is, they are atypical.
Growth is slow. The tumour is encapsulated and grows by expansion, not infiltration.	Growth is usually fast. The tumour has no capsule and grows by infiltration.
Does *not* produce metastases.	Can (and often does) produce metastases.
Does cause complications by obstructing tubes, blocking blood flow, putting pressure on surrounding structures, producing excess hormones, and other problems.	Dangerous. Can spread to other parts of the body, cause tissue erosion, bleeding, obstruction, anaemia, necrosis, cachexia,[4] and death.

a vital component in the understanding of how cancers spread. Below the basement membrane are blood and lymph vessels supplying the tissue.

Cancer cells are different in appearance, having variable shapes for both the cell and the nucleus, large nucleoli, and a loss, or disruption, of the basement membrane. This last feature allows the malignant cells to gain access to the blood and lymph for the purposes of spreading to other parts of the body. Malignant tissues also show a disturbance to the tissue **architecture**, that is, the way the tissue is structured. Normally, there is a set ratio between the number of epithelial cells and the number of **stromal** cells in the extracellular fluid. Think of the epithelial cells as being the ones that are carrying out the tissue function, while stromal cells form the matrix, or packaging, around the epithelial cells. Disruption of the architecture may well mean an increase in the ratio of epithelial to stromal cells, for example, in a carcinoma, due to excessive epithelial growth. It may also mean disruption to the structure, as in the loss of the basement membrane, so the tissue looks abnormal.

Hyperplasia (Figure 1.14) is the term used to describe an increase in auxetic growth in a tissue (see 'The cell cycle and growth', p. 4), that is, the cells have grown in larger than expected numbers, causing the tissue to thicken and become a mass. Hyperplasia is normal in some parts of the body, but unexpected (and therefore suspicious) in other parts of the body. Consider two areas of the skin, the sole of the foot and the back of the hand. They are very different; the sole of the foot has undergone hyperplasia, causing thickening of the epidermis of the skin due to the stress of weight bearing. The back of the hand is not subject to such stresses. The hyperplasia on the foot is specifically to protect the foot against weight bearing. Hyperplasia is the natural body response to such problems, but it becomes suspicious when it occurs at sites that do not have a need for it. Here, the hyperplasia is not a response to stresses but is caused by something else, and this could be the early stages of malignancy. It is important to recognise that cells in hyperplasia still look normal, but they have developed a tendency to speed up their cell cycle and reproduce faster. This may well be due to a genetic mutation (see 'Mutation of genes', Chapter 2, p. 27).

Eventually, some cells from the hyperplasia may undergo further genetic change, and this not only increases further the rate of cell division but also causes the cell appearance and its orientation within the tissue to change abnormally. This is then called a **dysplasia**, otherwise known as **atypical hyperplasia**, because the cells have changed appearance (Figure 1.14), and it potentially marks a stage towards malignancy, called **pre-malignancy**. So far, the growth has remained within the basement membrane, and there are, at this stage, no cells which have left the cell mass. The discovery of dysplasia would require urgent attention, possibly excision of the affected tissues. This would be even more important if the dysplasia was classified as *high grade*, that is, more advanced.

As the tissues become more abnormal and grow faster, the mass becomes malignant. This means that growth in these cells becomes **autonomous**, that is, growth is self-sustaining and has no bearing on the needs of the body. It no longer responds to the normal signals or controls of growth, such as the **hormones** and **cytokines** (see Table 5.2, Chapter 5, p. 94). If this mass has not yet broken through the basement membrane, nor has it yet shed any loose malignant cells, that is, **metastases**, the mass is called **carcinoma *in situ*** (Figure 1.14). Once the tumour has breached the basement membrane, it becomes an **invasive carcinoma** (Figure 1.14). At this point, it will be

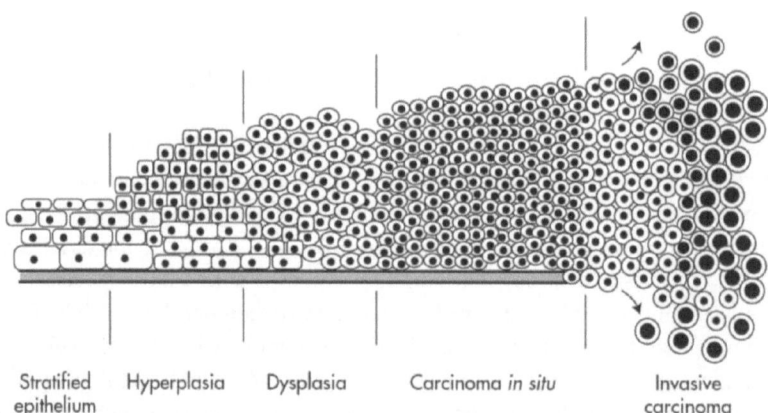

| Stratified epithelium | Hyperplasia | Dysplasia | Carcinoma *in situ* | Invasive carcinoma |

FIGURE 1.14 The stages of cancer development. Here, a stratified epithelium passes through hyperplasia (overgrowth of normal cells), through dysplasia (disorganised tissue structure), through carcinoma *in situ* (changes to a malignant cell type), to invasive carcinoma, which has breached the basement membrane and released metastases.

shedding metastases, which now have access to the blood and lymph vessels below the basement membrane, and these can now be transported around the body. Metastatic cells in the lymph will populate the local lymph nodes (always a sign of cancer spread), and malignant cells in the blood will be delivered to other organs and could form secondary growths there.

In any malignant mass, many cells are dividing at the same time to form different cell lines (Figure 1.15). **Cell lines** are colonies of cells which have the same (or very similar) characteristics because they are all derived from the same parent cell. But the presence of many different parent cells in the original mass due to different genetic mutations results in many different cell lines within the same tumour (Figure 1.15). It is possible that any two cells from the same tumour may be significantly different to each other. This has a bearing on the management of the cancer, as some treatments, for example, hormonal therapy (Chapter 4), may act well on certain cell lines but not on others. The treatment may therefore only shrink the tumour by killing some cell lines but not destroy the tumour completely, as other cell lines survive.

A classification of malignancy

New growths in the body can be classified in a manner based on the type of tissue the tumour arises from, even though the transformation from normal cell to tumour cell may involve varying degrees of changes in the tissue (Figure 1.16). The two major basic tissue classes found in the body are **epithelium** and **connective** tissues, and these form the basis of a classification for tumour

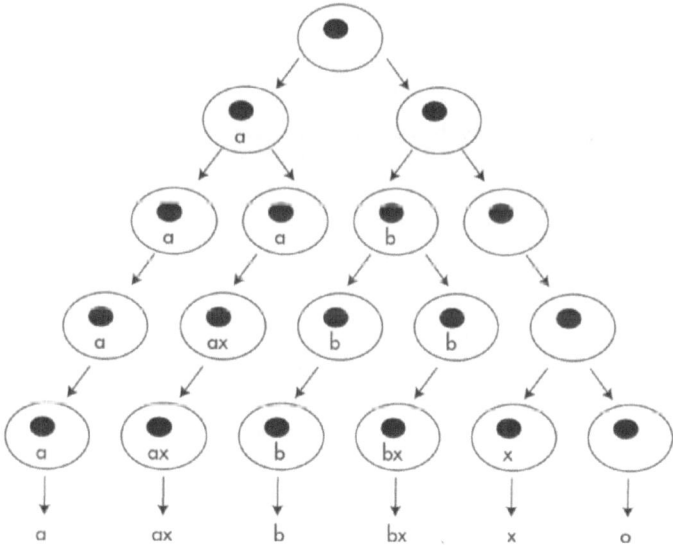

FIGURE 1.15   An example of cell lineage in a tumour. The original cell at the top has no mutations. Of the two daughter cells from this original cell, one has developed a gene mutation (a); the other has not. The daughter cells from the 'a' mutated cell both carry the 'a' mutation, whilst the non-mutated cell has one daughter cell that has developed another mutation (b); the other does not. And so various combinations of cell divisions and genetic mutations in this simple example result in cell lines with 'a', 'ax', 'b', 'bx', 'x', and 'o' ('o' = no mutations), all within the same tumour. It can be seen from this that some treatments may affect a few cell lines more than others within the same tumour.

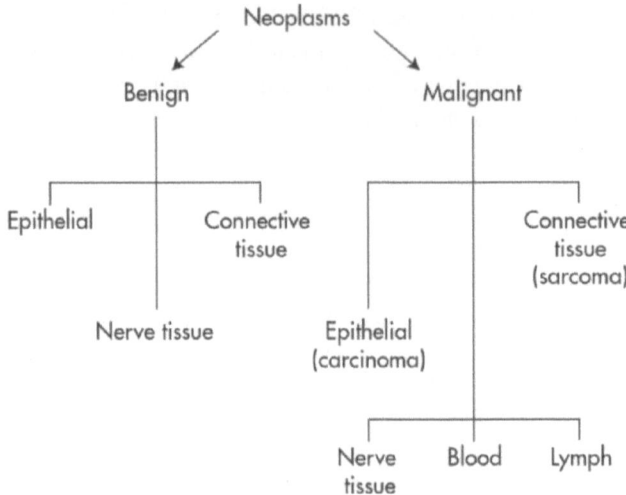

FIGURE 1.16 A classification of neoplasms (new growths). The benign and malignant divisions are both further divided according to their tissue of origin, that is, epithelial and connective tissue, with some specialised tissues included.

growth. Epithelial-derived tumours are called **carcinomas**, and connective tissue–derived tumours are **sarcomas**. Any tumour that arises from tissues other than epithelial or connective tissue, for example, nerve tissue or blood, is added on as an extension of the classification (Figure 1.16). Another consideration is the division of tumours into benign and malignant forms, the characteristics of which can be seen in Table 1.2. A complete classification, therefore, must consider both benign and malignant tumour types in epithelial, connective, and other tissue origins (Figure 1.16).

A revolution in multiomics

The study of diseases such as cancer requires an integration approach where data from various levels of research are combined for analytic purposes. From genes, as part of the chromosomes, through to whole organ/body systems, the information must be linked in a manner that allows events at one level to be followed through the various layers of complexity. The important factors that contribute to multiomics are shown in Figure 1.17.

Multiomics is the integrated biological analysis of data sets, called 'omes', as follows:

- **Genome.** Data from genetics becomes *genomics* (see 'The genome and genomics', Chapter 2, p. 34).
- **Epigenome.** Data from epigenetics becomes *epigenomics* (see 'Epigenetics', Chapter 2, p. 36).
- **Proteome.** Data from protein studies becomes *proteomics*.[6]
- **Transcriptome.** Data from gene transcription analysis becomes *transcriptomics*.
- **Metabolome.** Data from cellular metabolic studies becomes *metabolomics*.
- **Microbiome.** Data from natural colonies of microorganisms present in, or on, the body becomes *microbiomics*.
- **Fragmentome.** Data from DNA/RNA fragments in circulation becomes *fragmentomics*.

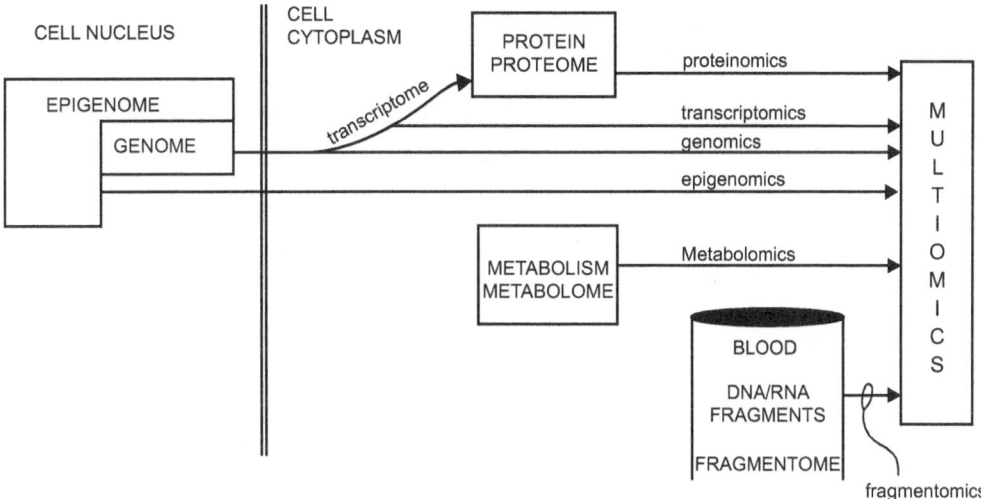

FIGURE 1.17 Factors contributing to multiomics.

And even combinations of these:

• **Proteogenomics**, combining data from protein and gene studies.

Another word sometimes used is **panomics**, which encompasses data processing from the wide range of data sets available from across all '-omic' studies. This is now driven by advances in **artificial intelligence (AI)** (see 'Artificial intelligence (AI) in cancer management', Chapter 17, p. 320), which allows processing of large data sets in a reduced time than before, and advanced computer software for the integration of the data processing results. Several computer software programs, and data sets from every '-omic' level, are available online for comparison with the results obtained.

Single-cell multiomics is where the various levels of data studied are concentrated on one single cell. This isolates the cell from the bulk mass cell approach and provides unprecedented information on what is happening at every level, from genes to whole cell events. This prevents the confounding factors seen in mass cell analysis, where every cell in a tumour is slightly different to all the others (Figure 1.15). Mass cellular tumours are studied by **spatial analysis** (sometimes called **spatial biology**), where the many cellular details and their extracellular environment are studied within a three-dimensional (3D) structure, maintaining their spatial distribution within the tumour sample. This especially applies to **spatial transcriptomics** (see 'Spatial transcriptomics', Chapter 6, p. 120).

Key points

Cells

• Cells are the functional unit of life.
• Cells have organelles, which carry out the metabolic processes of life.

- Cells form tissues, and there are two main structural tissues in the body, epithelial and connective tissues, plus tissues of the nervous system, the blood, the bone, and the lymphatic system.
- Many cells have a cycle of events, the cell cycle, which involves cell division (mitosis) and the period between two successive divisions (interphase).

Mitosis

- *Mitosis* is the division of the cell nucleus and consists of prophase, metaphase, anaphase, and telophase.
- Cytokinesis follows on from mitosis and is the division of the cytoplasm.

Cell cycle

- The stages of interphase are G_0, G_1, S, G_2, and mitosis.

Tissues

- The tissues of the body are classified as epithelial, connective, cartilage, bone, muscular, blood, lymphatic, and nerve.
- There are five types of epithelial tissue and five types of connective tissue.
- There are three types of cartilage: hyaline, fibrocartilage, and elastic cartilage.
- Bone is the second hardest tissue (after tooth enamel), and bone cells are osteocytes.
- There are three kinds of muscle tissue: smooth, skeletal, and cardiac.
- Blood plasma is water with minerals, nutrients, and different proteins, including clotting factors, hormones, antibodies, albumin, and globulin dissolved in it.
- The cells in blood are erythrocytes (red blood cells), leukocytes (white blood cells), and thrombocytes (platelets).
- The functional cell of the nervous system is the *neuron*, with supportive cells called *neuroglia* (glial cells).

Cancer

- *Hyperplasia* means an increase in cell growth, leading to increased tissue mass.
- *Dysplasia* (atypical hyperplasia) means the cells have changed appearance and orientation and the tissues have disrupted architecture. It is called pre-malignancy.
- When the mass is within the basement membrane, with no metastases, it is called carcinoma *in situ*.
- If the tumour breaks through the basement membrane and sheds metastases, it becomes an invasive carcinoma.
- Many cells in a tumour are dividing to form different cell lines, that is, cell colonies all derived from the same parent cell.
- Benign tumours are common; the cells are the same as the tissue of origin, they grow slowly by expansion, and the tumour is encapsulated and does not produce metastases.
- Malignant tumours are rarer, but more common in the elderly. The cells are different from the tissue of origin; they grow fast by infiltration and metastases, and the tumour has no capsule.

Multiomics

- *Multiomics* is the integration and study of information from various data sets covering all aspects of the cancer cell.
- These data sets, obtained from research, are genomics, epigenomics, proteomics, transcriptomics, metabolomics, and microbiomics.

Notes

1 *Organelles* are intracellular 'miniature organs' which carry out specific functions within the cell (Table 1.1, p. 5).
2 See 'Fragmentome', p. 20.
3 See 'Cytokines and chemokines', Chapter 5, p. 94.
4 See 'Kwashiorkor and cachexia', Chapter 18, p. 327.
5 A small sample of fluid or tissue removed from a growth or collected from blood or lymph.
6 Linked to proteomics is the subject of glycoproteomics, that is, small sugar molecules attached to proteins which change in disease and, therefore, can be used to find disease biomarkers.

2

THE CAUSES OF CANCER 1

Genes and epigenetics

- **Introduction**
- **Genes and protein synthesis**
- **Genes and tumour development**
- **Mutation of genes**
- **Major genes linked to cancer**
- **G$_0$ and DNA repair**
- **Gene inheritance**
- **Chromosomal abnormalities**
- **The genome and genomics**
- **Epigenetics**
- **Key points**

Introduction

The root cause of cancer lies at the molecular genetic level. However, it appears that genetic errors (mutations) may not be enough to turn a cell malignant. It appears that it requires a combination of genetic errors and other disruptive factors. These include chromosomal losses, or gaining additional chromosomes, or parts of chromosomes duplicated or damaged, or genes and their local environment blocked by chemical additions. The picture is one of intracellular disruption apart from purely genetic mutations. This is partly the reason that cancers are more common in the elderly than in the young, that is, older cells have had longer to sustain this disruption and collect genetic mutations. But it appears to be random, partly because of lifestyle and the environmental insults our cells are subjected to, because most elderly people do not die from cancer (Gibbs 2004). This chapter looks at the gene mutations and chromosomal abnormalities that are a major part of this disruptive intracellular environment. Chapter 3 will look at the environment factors that contribute towards this disruption of our cells.

Chapter 1 introduced the topic of genetics by defining *genes* as stretches of deoxyribonucleic acid (DNA) that code for specific proteins, and how genes are located on chromosomes. The

DOI: 10.4324/9781003389125-2

normal human karyotype (see 'The nucleus, genes, and chromosomes', Figure 1.5, Chapter 1, p. 3 to 6) has 46 chromosomes; 22 pairs are autosomes (44), plus 1 pair of sex chromosomes, X and Y. Chapter 1 also described the structure of DNA, with the four bases, **adenine (A)**, **thymine (T)**, **cytosine (C)**, and **guanine (G)**, attached to a sugar–phosphate molecule (see Figure 1.4, Chapter 1, p. 5). DNA has two strands coiled into a double helix. Within the DNA, adenine binds to thymine, and cytosine binds to guanine.

Genes and protein synthesis

On the DNA molecule, specific units of *three bases*, that is, **codons**, code for a single amino acid. A *gene* can be defined as the number and sequence of codons on the DNA that are required to produce a complete protein. Some proteins are large, with many amino acids; others can be much smaller. The DNA remains in the nucleus, but the proteins are produced by ribosomes, which are outside the nucleus in the cytoplasm. First, the DNA is copied in the form of **messenger RNA (mRNA)**. The mRNA copy uses the same bases, except it has **uracil (U)** in place of thymine (T). mRNA copy leaves the nucleus and passes to a ribosome within the cytoplasm. The ribosome reads the mRNA codon sequence, and using **transfer RNA (tRNA)**, the ribosome slots into place an appropriate amino acid for each codon. Repeated numerous times, this process creates an amino acid chain, that is, a protein. In this way, the mRNA chain of codons and tRNA ensures that the correct amino acids are delivered to the ribosome and placed in the correct order within the developing protein (Figure 2.1).

The mRNA codons for each amino acid are shown in Table 2.1.

Genes and tumour development

Two types of genes control growth:

1. **Proto-oncogenes**, sometimes called '**c-onc**', a shorthand for the normal version of the gene (see 'V-onc, provirus, and viral replication', Chapter 4, p. 63–64).
2. **Tumour suppressor (TS)** genes.

Proto oncogenes

The normal proto-oncogenes code for proteins that are essential for transmitting the growth signal, a growth hormone, or a cytokine, from the activated cell surface receptor to the nucleus (Figure 2.2). The hormone-bound receptor activates the proteins inside the cell membrane, notably the **G protein**, which then binds **guanosine triphosphate (GTP)**, a high-energy molecule similar to ATP (adenosine triphosphate). Proto-oncogenes, and their protein products, are therefore responsible for activating other genes in the nucleus that are needed for growth when the external hormone or cytokine signal binds (Figure 2.2).

Tumour suppressor genes

Tumour suppressor genes code for proteins responsible for sending signals to the nucleus which block growth gene activation, thus preventing growth from getting out of control. Tumour suppressor gene proteins convey signals from surface receptors activated by growth inhibitor hormones or cytokines.

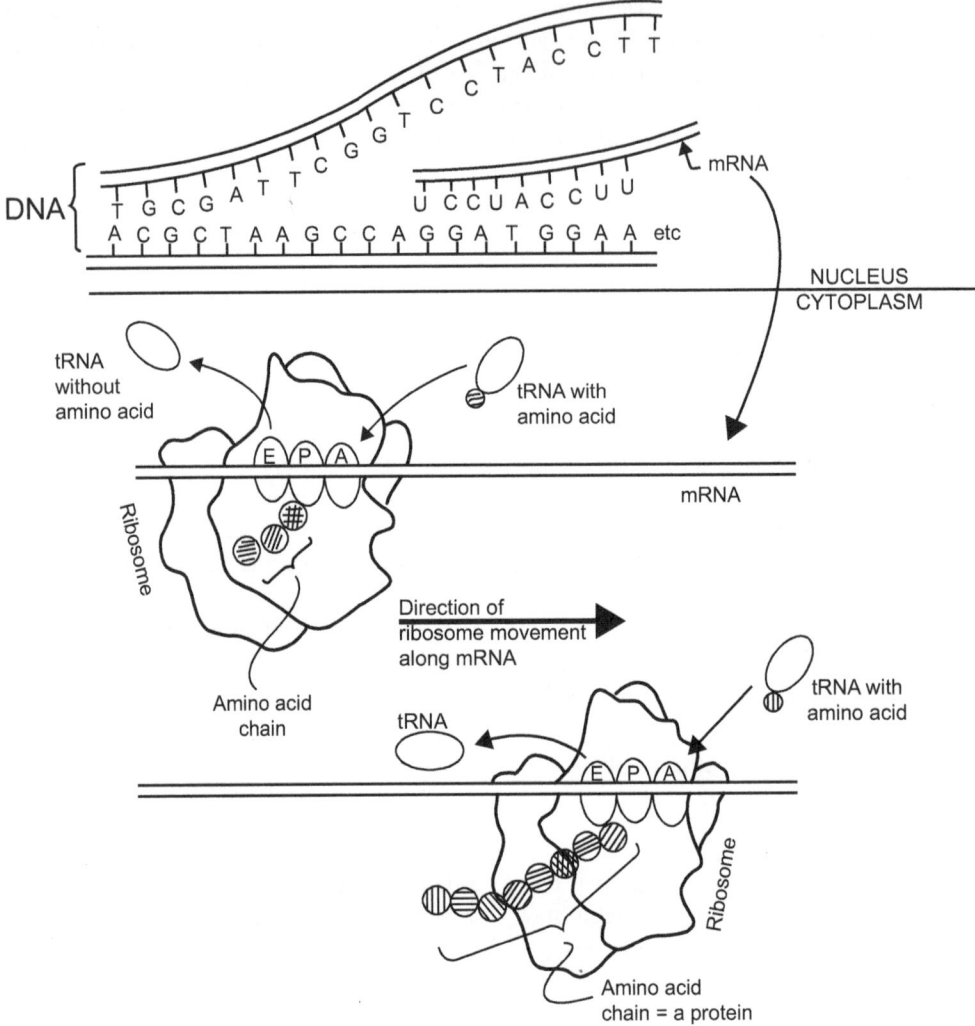

FIGURE 2.1 Protein synthesis. The double strand of DNA has split to allow for the formation of messenger RNA (mRNA). Notice that mRNA uses uracil (U). When finished copying a gene, the mRNA splits from the DNA, which then reforms. The mRNA leaves the nucleus and enters the cytoplasm of the cell. The mRNA slots into a ribosome, which then moves along the mRNA in the direction shown to process the full length of the gene copy. The ribosome has three sites: an acceptance site (A), a peptide bonding site (P), and an exit site (E). The required amino acids arrive one by one, in the correct order, carried by transfer RNA (tRNA). The tRNA binds to the A site and delivers the amino acid. This binds onto the amino acid chain to form a peptide (or small protein) in the P site as the ribosome moves on. The empty tRNA arrives in the E site, then leaves the ribosome. The action is repeated until the gene is fully processed and the final protein is released. Empty tRNAs carry the three-base code for specific amino acids which they will recharge with from dietary sources.

Source: Garrett and Grisham (2023).

TABLE 2.1 The mRNA *three-base* codons for each amino acid

mRNA base codons	Amino acid
GCU, GCC, GCA, GCG	Alanine
CGU, CGC, CGA, CGG, AGA, AGG	Arginine
AAU, AAC	Asparagine
GAU, GAC	Aspartic acid
UGU, UGC	Cysteine
CAA, CAG	Glutamine
GAA, GAG	Glutamic acid
GGU, GGC, GGA, GGG	Glycine
CAU, CAC	Histidine
AUU, AUC, AUA	Isoleucine
CUU, CUC, CUA, CUG, UUA, UUG	Leucine
AAA, AAG	Lysine
AUG	Methionine
UUU, UUC	Phenylalanine
CCU, CCC, CCA, CCG	Proline
UAG	Pyrrolysine
UGA	Selenocysteine
UCU, UCC, UCA, UCG, AGU, AGC	Serine
ACU, ACC, ACA, ACG	Threonine
UGG	Tryptophan
UAU, UAC	Tyrosine
GUU, GUC, GUA, GUG	Valine

Note: The bases are A = adenine, U = uracil, C = cytosine, and G = guanine.

RNA uses uracil instead of thymine. Thymine is only used in the DNA *bases*.

Some use only one codon to code for the amino acid; others can be coded by up to six codons, any one of which can code for the amino *acid.*

Between proto-oncogenes, that is, growth accelerator genes, and tumour suppressor genes, that is, growth-inhibiting genes, the growth of a cell can be controlled and fine-tuned by the hormones and cytokines to meet the demands of the body. Cancer cells grow beyond the limitations set for normal cells because of changes that have occurred in these two gene systems. Genes are prone to DNA damage and disruption, and they may then code for abnormal proteins that do not function properly.

Mutation of genes

DNA changes are **mutations**, many of which still allow the gene to function, albeit in an abnormal or different manner. *Mutations* are usually errors occurring during mitosis (Chapter 1, p. 6) or caused by factors from the environment called **mutagens** (or **mutagenic factors**), which promote the mutations of genes. Such factors are likely to affect the two types of genes-controlling growth and therefore promote cellular changes leading to cancer. Mutations within proto-oncogenes can create highly active genes, called **oncogenes**, which accelerate growth in that cell beyond anything the body requires. Mutations within tumour suppressor genes can cause these genes to fail, and thus, their control over growth is lost.

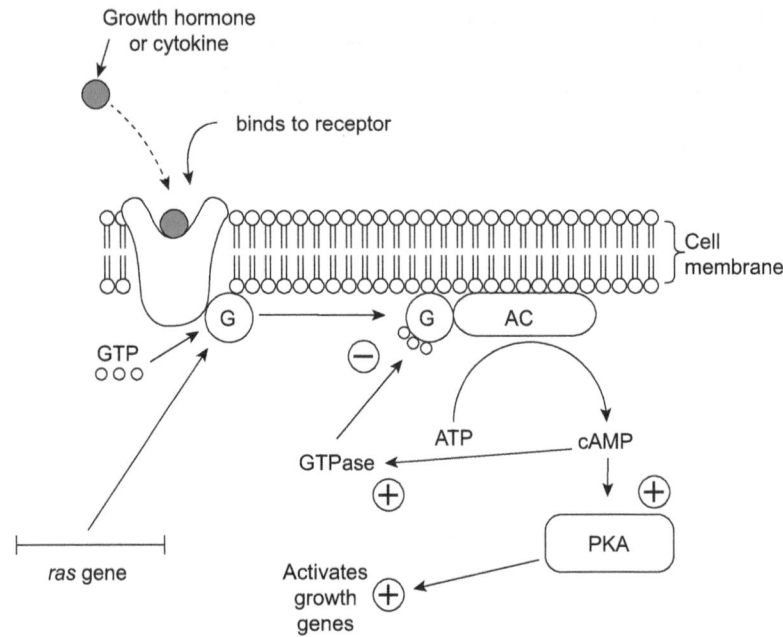

FIGURE 2.2   Growth hormone binding to a receptor. On the cell surface, the growth hormone binds to the receptor, and that activates a G protein on the inside of the membrane. The G protein binds GTP, and moving along the membrane, it activates the membrane-bound enzyme adenylyl cyclase (AC). This enzyme creates the secondary messenger cyclic adenosine monophosphate (cAMP) from adenosine triphosphate (ATP). cAMP activates (+) GTPase, an enzyme that removes GTP from the G protein, thus deactivating (−) the G protein. cAMP also activates (+) PKA (phosphokinase A), which can cause growth by activating (+) growth genes. The *ras* proto-oncogene acts as a switch to turn this process on or off. If *ras* binds GTP, the process is active, but if it binds GDP (guanosine diphosphate), the process is switched off. Mutations of *ras* are involved in 20% to 30% of human cancers.

Mutation results in changes in the structure of the proteins that the genes code for, and these proteins will therefore either malfunction or fail altogether. The simplest mutation that can occur is a **point mutation** (Figure 2.3a), where one base on the DNA is lost and replaced by a different base. As an example, if the DNA base sequence was normally AAT, that is, adenine, adenine, and thymine, coding for **leucine**, then a point mutation may cause the same sequence to become AAA, that is, three adenines, coding for **phenylalanine**. The point mutation was the exchange of thymine for the third adenine. This is often called a **missense mutation**, or **missense substitution**, because the original 'sense' of the codon has been altered to code for a different amino acid. The presence of this different amino acid in the final protein causes the protein to malfunction or fail.

Other mutations include:

1. **Frame shifts** (Figure 2.3b), where a gene is read one or more bases out of normal sequence. The causes of this are additional insertions or deletions of one or two bases[1] (as **nucleotides**[2])

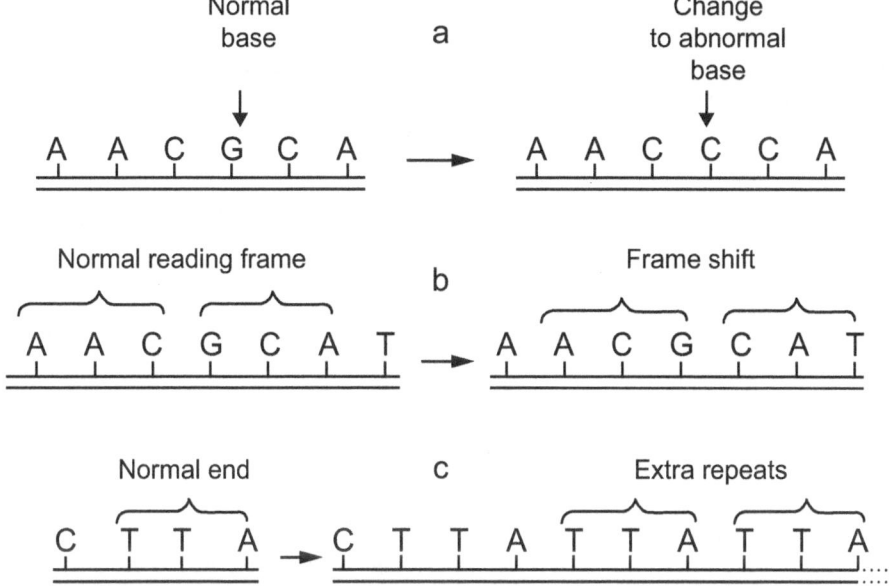

FIGURE 2.3   Gene mutations. In each case, the left figure shows a strand of DNA with bases before the mutation, and the right figure shows the same after the mutation. They are: (a) Point mutation, that is, one base replaced by another. In this case, G is replaced by C. (b) Frame shift. In this case, the normal reading frame of AAC followed by GCA has become, after an extra base insertion somewhere in the sequence, ACG followed by CAT. This would place the wrong amino acids into the protein. (c) Base sequence repeat, that is, the same base sequence repeated over again. In this case, the normal ending of TTA is repeated multiple times, resulting in a long sequence of the same amino acids on the end of the protein.

into (insertion) or out of (deletion) the normal sequence. These bases, added or lost, are called **indels (insertions or deletions)**. They force the reading sequence to be moved one or two places. For example, a sequence such as AACGTTCGGA may normally be read, from left to right, as the codons AAC, then GTT, then CGG, and so on. In a one nucleotide insertion, the frame shift may be read ACG, TTC, GGA, and so on. This would mean that each codon is different from the original, and since each codon codes for a specific amino acid, the resulting protein would have all the wrong amino acids and would therefore fail.

2. **Base sequence repeats** (known as a **stuttering gene**; Figure 2.3c), where the same sequence of three bases (i.e. each codon) is repeated many times, perhaps in some cases more than 100 times (e.g. CTT, CTT, CTT, CTT, etc.). The result is a protein with a long chain of the same amino acids in place. There is significant importance attached to this error in some disorders (Blows 2022).

Some mutations can, and are, repaired, whilst cells with irreparable damage die by a process called **apoptosis**. If a cell survives when the DNA damage persists, it continues to pass around the cell cycle, including mitosis, and all the future daughter cells derived from this original cell will then carry copies of the mutation. This is even more likely to happen if the gene mutation occurs in any of the major tumour suppressor genes that help control the cell cycle, especially ***TP53*** gene (chromosome 17), ***RB1*** gene (chromosome 13), and ***CDKN2A*** gene (chromosome 9) (see 'Chromosomes and the major genes linked to cancer', Addendum, p. 342). It is necessary for at least two of these genes to be inactivated before the cell grows out of control.

DNA mismatch repair (MMR) describes the mechanism for identifying and repairing DNA errors and damage that can happen during cell replication. The errors that are repaired are mostly base to base mismatches (see 'The nucleus, chromosomes, and genes', Chapter 1, p. 3) and insertion and deletion of incorrectly paired bases created during cell replication (see 'Mitosis and cytokinesis', Chapter 1, p. 6). This is important for genome stability. Errors in MMR cause genomic instability that can lead to cancers, chemotherapy resistance, and errors in reproductive cell development that could result in sterility.

G_0 and DNA repair

As discussed in Chapter 1, the cell cycle is identified as having several phases, G_1, S, G_2, and mitosis (see 'Cell cycle and growth', Chapter 1, Figure 1.6, p. 4–7). G_1 is the phase where the cell does not normally progress if the DNA was damaged or faulty. Errors (or mutations) of DNA will require repair before the cell can progress around the cell cycle. DNA repair involves:

- Genes that stop the cell in G_1 and prevent it from progressing
- Genes that code for proteins which carry out the repair
- Genes that control apoptosis, that is, the mechanism by which cells with irreparable damage to the DNA will die

Examples of each of these are present on the list of chromosomes (see Addendum, p. 342).

If the mutations occur on any of these genes, especially if the mutations happen to multiple genes, then the cell may progress beyond G_1 and go on around the cycle with the gene errors, producing new colonies of cells that carry the same mutations. This creates the scenario for the development of new tumours, because cell growth then spirals out of control. Cells have the means to prevent this from happening. Figure 2.4 shows the cell cycle (see also Figure 1.6, Chapter 1, p. 7) with the main genes that control the cycle.

Gene inheritance

Genes are inherited from one generation to the next through either a dominant or a recessive mechanism. New offspring carry 50% of their genes from their mother, and 50% of their genes from their father. This is why the karyotype (see Figure 1.5, Chapter 1, p. 6) has chromosome *pairs*, one chromosome in each pair from the female parent, the other from the male parent. The offspring, therefore, has two copies of each gene, known as **alleles**. Which copy will be used to provide the characteristics of the offspring – the mother's or the father's? Or put in genetic terms, which alleles will be expressed into the **phenotype**? First, *phenotype* means the body. When you look at another person, you see their phenotype, that is, their bodily characteristics, such as hair colour, eye colour, etc. These characteristics are called **traits**. The difference between *genes* and *traits* is best explained with an example. Both parents will have genes that control eye colour, but one may have blue eyes whilst the other has brown eyes. The actual colour of the eyes is the trait and differs between individuals. We all have our own individual

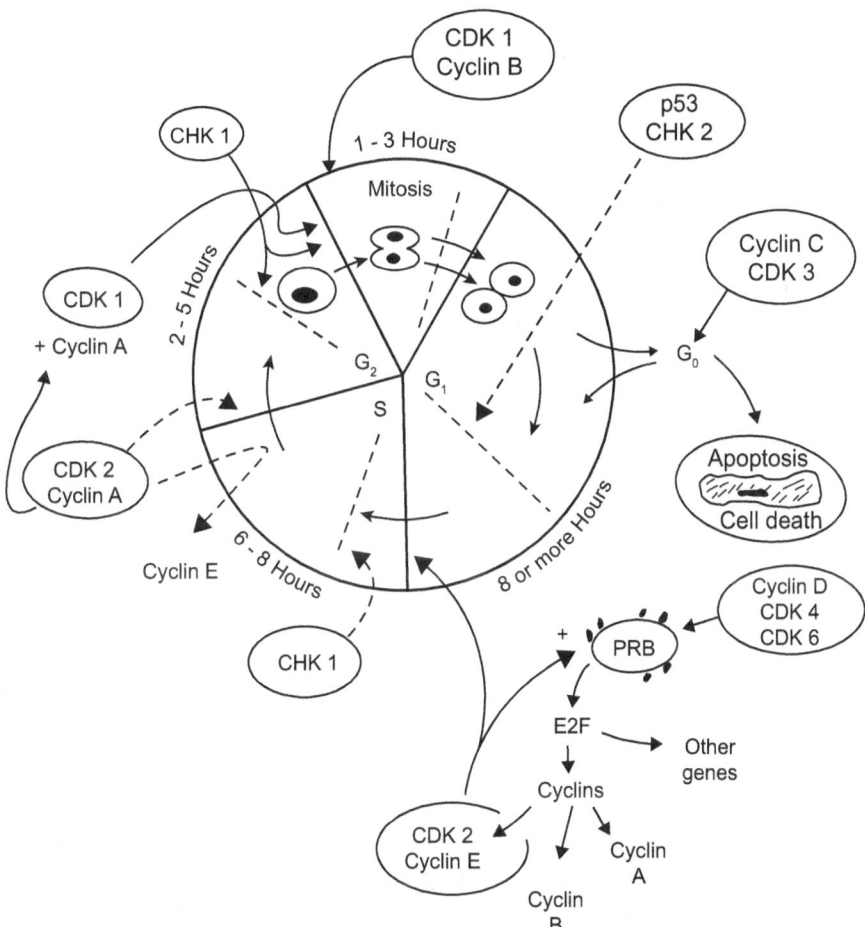

FIGURE 2.4 The genetic control of the cell cycle. The cell with normal DNA. The protein pRB (the protein product of gene *RB1*) would stop the cell cycle in G_1 but is phosphorylated. *Phosphorylation* (shown as black dots on pRB) is the attachment of phosphoryl groups (PO_3) to pRB, and this deactivates the pRB protein. Phosphorylation is carried out by a complex formed from CDK4, CDK6, and cyclin D. The deactivation of pRB allows E2F, a family of transcription factors, to activate genes that produce cyclin A, cyclin B, cyclin E, and other genes. Cyclin E combines with CDK2 to promote passage of the cell from G_1 to the S phase of the cell cycle. The CDK2/cyclin E complex also further promotes (+) pRB phosphorylation. The cycle has various checkpoints, shown as broken lines in S, G_1, and mitosis (M phase), where DNA can be assessed for damage. These are controlled by checkpoint proteins (CHK). CHK1 controls S and G_2 checkpoints, and CHK2 with protein p53 (from the *TP53* gene) can halt the cell cycle in G_1 to repair the damage or initiate apoptosis (cell death). Cyclin A removes cyclin E at the end of the S phase, and cyclin A forms a complex with CDK2 to end the S phase and start the G_2 phase. Cyclin A also promotes the activity of CDK1, which drives the cell on to mitosis. During mitosis, the cell is moved further forward by CDK1 combining with cyclin B. Mutations of some of the genes that encode for these proteins may become mutated and cause a loss of control of the cell cycle, as in cancer.

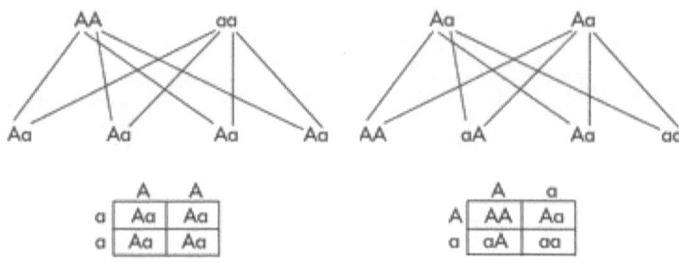

FIGURE 2.5   Gene inheritance patterns. Left: Dominant gene inheritance pattern in crossover and punnet square. One parent has both dominant genes (AA), the other has both recessive genes (aa), and all the four possible offspring have at least one dominant gene (Aa). They will all show the dominant trait. Right: Recessive gene inheritance pattern in crossover and punnet square. The parents are both mixed dominant and recessive genes (Aa). The four offspring are split, three with at least one dominant gene, but one with both recessive genes (aa). It is only this last individual who will express into the phenotype any recessive traits present in this gene.

traits. The genes that are responsible for the traits that present in the phenotype are decided by which genes are **dominant**, that is, always contribute to the phenotype when present at *one or both* alleles (mother or father alleles), or **recessive**, that is, they only contribute to the phenotype when present at *both* mother's and father's alleles, meaning, there is no dominant gene present. The inheritance patterns for dominant and recessive genes, and therefore genetic disorders like some cancers, can be seen in Figure 2.5.

Approximately between 3% and 10% of all cancers are inherited, that is, **familial** – meaning, they are passed from one generation to the next within the same families. These cancers are often part of a **cancer syndrome**, that is, a collection of the same, or similar, cancers that consistently go together because of the same inherited gene mutations.

Chromosomal abnormalities

Chromosomes contain all the genetic material, the DNA, within the cell nucleus (see 'The nucleus, chromosomes, and genes', Chapter 1, p. 3). Abnormalities occurring in malignant cells are not confined to the genetic level. Chromosomes can also become abnormal, and when this happens, many genes are involved. The normal **karyotype** (see Figure 1.5, Chapter 1, p. 6) consists of 46 chromosomes, that is, 23 pairs of chromosomes, one of each pair inherited from the mother, the other pair from the father. Malignant cells can have very different and grossly abnormal karyotypes, that is, the numbers and types of chromosomes can be abnormal. **Aneuploidy** means an abnormal number of chromosomes, either too many (47 or more) or, rarely, too few (45 or less). Too many chromosomes is usually caused by a **trisomy**, that is, three chromosomes instead of the two in a 'pair', and too few chromosomes is usually caused by a **monosomy**, that is, one chromosome instead of the two in a 'pair'. **Euploidy** means that the karyotype number is exactly a multiple of the normal 46 chromosomes. These 46 chromosomes are known as the **diploid** condition, also abbreviated to **2*n***, where *n* is the normal **haploid** state of 23 chromosomes found in ova and sperm. Multiples of *n* would be **3*n*** (**triploid**, with 69 chromosomes) or **4*n*** (**tetraploid**, with 92 chromosomes). Triploid and tetraploid are grossly abnormal states and are often associated with malignancy in a cell. These high numbers of chromosomes indicate a general instability of the chromosomes occurring as part of the onset of malignancy so that chromosome division during mitosis is unpredictable and results in these gross errors, including excessive DNA production. In addition, aneuploidy causes malignant cells to grow faster.

As an example, Table 2.2 lists the grossly abnormal karyotype seen in one cervical cancer cell (only chromosomes 8 to 18 are shown) (Weinberg 1996).

Apart from aneuploidy, individual chromosomes are sometimes subject to structural errors occurring during cell division. Such changes in structure disrupt many genes in the sequence. In these errors, the karyotype chromosome number remains normal. Examples are:

1. **Translocations**, where parts of two chromosomes are dislodged and swapped to each other's place (Figure 2.6a), the resulting unions possibly creating an oncogene.
2. **Deletions** (Figure 2.6b), where some DNA is lost entirely, causing an incomplete chromosome and incomplete or absent protein synthesis related to the missing genes.
3. **Inversions** (Figure 2.6c), where a section of DNA is turned upside down and, therefore, coded and read backwards, causing disruption of the protein.
4. **Duplications** (Figure 2.6d), where some DNA is copied and added on the end of a chromosome, or **amplification**, where there are many additional copies of the same DNA stretch. Amplification is particularly important as a cause of several human cancers because it often involves extra copies of proto-oncogenes, which stimulate cell growth beyond normal or prevent apoptosis.

Chromothripsis

Chromothripsis is a phenomenon where between a few tens and several thousand chromosomal rearrangements happen in a single chromosomal catastrophic event prior to, or often during, early tumour development. The chromosome first shatters into many pieces and is then rejoined with some errors, either by the cell's normal DNA repair mechanisms or by the abnormal cancer replication and repair mechanisms. The result is a rearrangement of the chromosome that transforms the cell by the presence of gene mutations, such as amplifications, loss of tumour suppressor genes, and the creation of active oncogenes. Cells with mutations of the gene *TP53* (see 'Chromosome 17', Addendum, p. 356) show a higher frequency of chromothripsis.

TABLE 2.2 An example of chromosomal (8 to 18) abnormalities in one cancer cell

Chromosome number	Normal cell chromosomes	Chromosomes in one particular cancer cell
8	2	5
9	2	5
10	2	2
11	2	2
12	2	4
13	2	1
14	2	3
15	2	3
16	2	3
17	2	4
18	2	4
Total	22 chromosomes	36 chromosomes

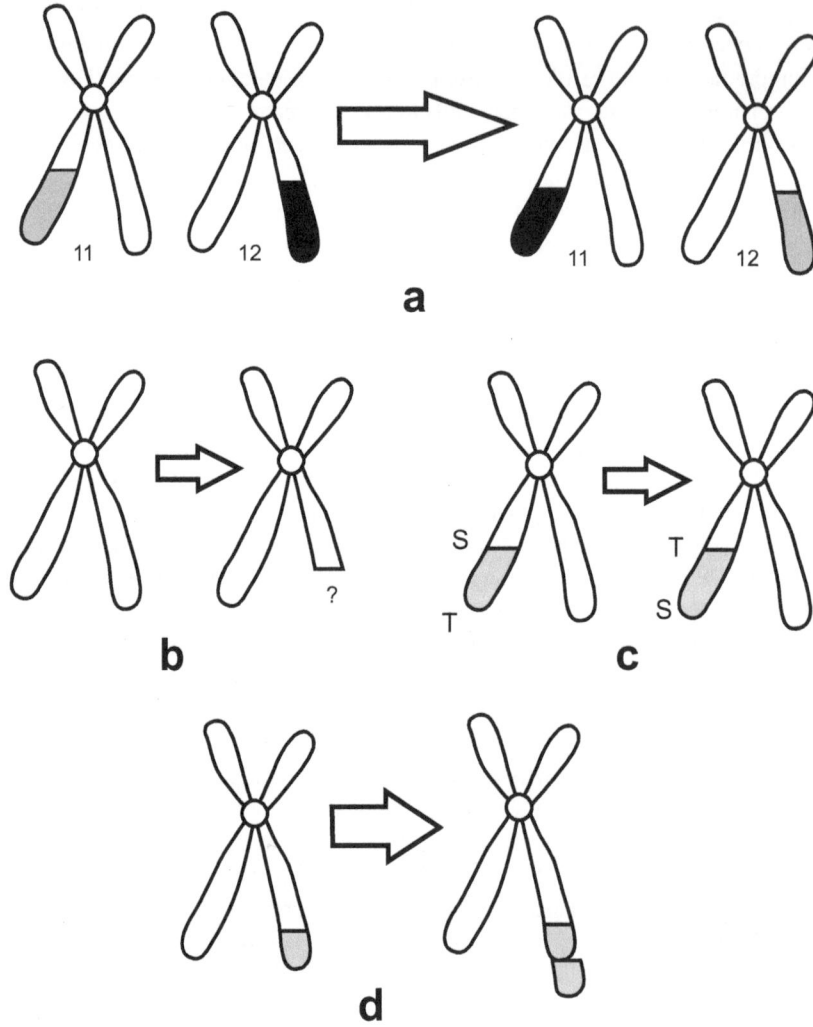

FIGURE 2.6 Chromosome structural errors. The left figure shows before the mutation; the right figure shows after the mutation. They are: (a) translocation, that is, swapping parts of a chromosome, containing many genes, between two chromosomes, in this case, between chromosomes 11 and 12; (b) deletion of part of a chromosome, resulting in loss of many genes (in this case, the loss occurs at the question mark); (c) inversion, or reversing part of a chromosome so the genes are backwards (in this case, genes S to T become T to S); (d) duplication, that is, copying a chromosome sequence and adding in on the end, resulting in an amplification, that is, over-expression of the same duplicated gene sequence.

The genome and genomics

The *genome* is the complete set of genes required to make a human. Since all[3] the genes are housed on the chromosomes within the nucleus, the genome is contained within the karyotype (see Figure 1.5, Chapter 1, p. 6). Many of these genes encode for proteins which will be part of the phenotype, that is, the body structure. The sequence from genome to phenotype is shown in Figure 2.7.

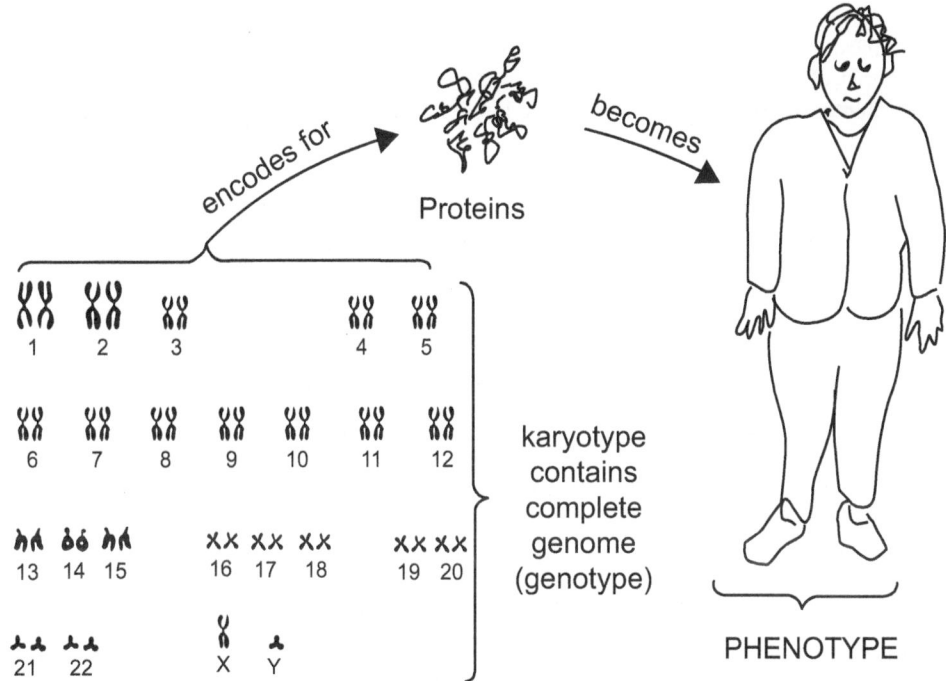

FIGURE 2.7   The sequence of events from genome (or genotype) to phenotype. The *genome* is the complete genetic material housed on chromosomes in the nucleus of cells (as shown, left). These code for proteins (centre) which contribute towards the structure or function of the body (right). The body is therefore the outward expression of the genes in the form of traits, that is, characteristics that vary between individuals, such as eye colour or hair colour. The *genotype* is the actual genetic information conferred by the whole genome, or a subset of genes within the genome.

Genomics is the study of the entire genome in total (see 'A revolution in multiomics', Chapter 1, p. 20). Most cells (except mature erythrocytes) in the human body contain the entire karyotype, and therefore the entire genome. The study of the entire genome provides better information than studying single genes. It concerns how genes interact with each other, how they interreact with environmental factors (see Chapter 3, p. 41), and how these interactions change in disease. In the case of cancer, several genes, both oncogenes and tumour suppressor genes, are involved in the reason a cell becomes malignant. Understanding exactly how these genes each contributes to the cause can lead to greater understanding of prevention and breakthroughs in cancer treatment.

There are four main types of genomic testing:

1. Diagnostic testing helps establish if a patient has a specific disorder and is used to distinguish between two closely related disorders.
2. Predictive testing is carried out to determine if any members of a particular family are carrying a specific gene which is inherited. It may be a targeted test if the gene is already known, or an entire genome test if the gene is unknown.
3. Pharmacogenetic testing is studying how the genome responds to specific drugs. This may provide evidence when trying to find out why some patients respond to treatment better than others. It provides information useful in determining which drug to use and the dosage.

4. Tumour testing is a way of discovering the mutations present in a specific tumour, often using a biopsy, that is, a small sample of the tumour. A comparison of the tumour genetic profile with that of normal tissues will highlight the errors present in the tumour. There may be a treatment available for those specific mutations within the tumour whilst avoiding the normal cells as much as possible.

Epigenetics

Throughout the genome, there are factors, called **epigenetic factors**, that influence and change the activation of genes. They are not part of the protein coding DNA – the genes. Instead, they include DNA sequences that were once called 'junk DNA', that is, they were thought to be of no value. Now they are known to regulate the transcription of genes. In addition, other structures outside the DNA can have an influence over gene transcription.

Mutations occurring in the DNA regulatory sequences and changes on the support structure can have profound effects on how genes are expressed, possibly leading to gene control errors and disease.

Epigenetics includes:

- DNA sequences that start and stop gene activation, called **transcription sequences**. DNA start sequences are called '**promoters**'. They are short segments of DNA positioned next to the gene they can activate. If the promoter is triggered by an outside agent, for example, a hormone, they will begin the activation of the specific gene they are linked to.
- Gene '**enhancer**' sequences that regulate gene promotion. They are often called the second *code of life* and are positioned either close to promoters or some distance away on the DNA strand. They determine the overall pattern of gene expression, and as with all DNA, they may be subject to mutations which seriously affect gene expression.
- Other epigenetic factors include **histones**, that is, proteins that form the framework that supports DNA.
- A wide range of chemical factors.

The three most important ways that epigenetic factors can themselves be influenced are:

- **DNA methylation.** Methyl groups (CH_3), often derived from the diet, can tag DNA (called DNA markers) and influence how genes are expressed, that is, accelerating or repressing gene activation. Methylation of **CpG islands** is frequently involved in carcinogenesis. *CpG* stands for cytosine-phosphate-guanine, that is, tiny patches, or islands, of the two DNA bases cytosine and guanine separated by a phosphate (H_3PO_4). These occur regularly in promoter sequences, and they are areas where methylation occurs. **Hypermethylation** (excessive methylation) of CpG islands represses and *silences* genes, that is, prevents gene activation. If that deactivated gene was a tumour suppressor gene or a DNA repair gene, then that would increase the chance of cancer formation.

Some examples where DNA hypermethylation is involved in carcinogenesis are:

1. *BRCA1* gene, where hypermethylation silences the oestrogen receptor promoter sequence in 30% of breast cancer patients (see 'Chromosome 17', Addendum, p. 356)
2. *RB* (retinoblastoma) gene (see 'Chromosome 13', Addendum, p. 354)

3. *APC* gene (see 'Chromosome 5', Addendum, p. 346)
4. *CDKN2A* gene (see 'Chromosome 9', Addendum, p. 350)
5. *DAPK1* gene (see 'Chromosome 9', Addendum, p. 351)

The same epigenetic DNA methylation changes have been found in the cheek cells of smokers and those using e-cigarettes, as are seen in lung cancers (see 'Tobacco smoking', Chapter 3, p. 48). Seventeen cancers are known to have a lack of one or more DNA repair genes due to hypermethylation (Pecorino 2021).

- **Histone modification.** These are factors that bind to **histones**, that is, the proteins around which DNA is wrapped for packaging within the chromatin (see 'The nucleus, chromosomes, and genes', Chapter 1, p. 3). There are five types of histones, four *core* histones (H2A, H2B,[4] H3, and H4) and two *linker* histones (H1 and H5). Histone modification influences the unwrapping of DNA, the first stage of gene activation. The factors involved, such as **acetylation**, that is, the addition or removal of acetyl groups (-$COCH_3$) to histones, affect gene expression. Mechanisms exist for the adding and removal of such chemical groups, and their eradication (see also 'KDM5D, chromosome Y', Addendum, p. 363).

- **Non-coding RNA (ncRNA) silencing.** These pieces of RNA are transcribed from genes but do not themselves translate into proteins. Silencing ncRNAs will significantly affect the pattern of gene expression throughout the genome. Two groups of ncRNA exist: *short* ncRNAs and *long* ncRNAs. *Short ncRNAs* include microRNA (miRNA), short interfering RNA (siRNA), and piwi-interacting RNA (piRNA). MicroRNAs (miRNAs) are important for down-regulating, that is, reducing activity, of specific targeted mRNA. Approximately 60% of human genes are regulated by miRNA down-regulation of the mRNA. Short interfering RNAs (siRNAs) down-regulate less-targeted mRNA, and piwi-interacting RNAs (piRNAs) regulate chromatin and prevent **transposon** – that is, chromosomal translocation – activity, which means preventing DNA movement within the genome (for example, Figure 2.4a).

  Long ncRNAs are a large group of RNAs with important links to cancer. Many influence the state of chromatin (chromatin remodelling) and gene expression (transcriptional and post-transcriptional regulation).

DNA tangles can occur as it winds around the histones, and the pattern of tangles can affect how genes are expressed. This is a very important influence on the way cancers behave.

Epigenetic factors that promote cancer formation and spread are replicated during every cell division and passed on to the new daughter cells. This enhances the ability for a tumour to survive and proliferate. Lifestyle strongly influences what epigenetic factors are acting on the genome. These lifestyle choices include diet (e.g. methylation), environmental pollutants, obesity, age, physical exercise, smoking tobacco, alcohol consumption, stress, and working night shifts (affecting the normal 24-hour circadian biorhythms).

In addition, aspects of these epigenetic factors are passed on from parent to child. Inheriting epigenetic factors from their parents means that not only does the lifestyle of the individual affect their gene expression but so does their parents', and even their grandparents', lifestyle.

Targeted therapy is the future of cancer management, and that requires testing tumour cells to acquire the knowledge of what genetic and epigenetic factors are involved.

Telomere

At the end of each chromosome, there is a stretch of non-coding, repeating DNA sequences called a **telomere** (see 'Tissue invasion: telomeres', Chapter 6, p. 124).

Key points

Genes and protein synthesis

- A *gene* is a stretch of DNA that encodes for a protein.
- A *codon* is a series of three bases that encodes for a specific amino acid.
- *Protein synthesis* is the production of proteins from the gene in the nucleus of the cell to the ribosome in the cytoplasm.

Genes and tumour development

- *Mutations* are errors in genes that cause abnormal proteins to form, which then malfunction.
- Cellular growth should satisfy the body's needs and no more.
- Two types of genes control growth: the proto-oncogenes and tumour suppressor (TS) genes.
- Proto-oncogenes code for proteins essential for transmitting the growth signal to the nucleus.
- Tumour suppressor genes code for proteins that send signals to the nucleus to block excessive growth.
- Mutations in proto-oncogenes create oncogenes, which accelerate growth in that cell.
- *RAS*, *ERB*, *MYC*, and *ABL* are all proto-oncogenes that mutate in various cancers.
- The gene mutation may also occur in any of the tumour suppressor genes that control the cell cycle, that is, the *TP53* gene, the *RB1* gene, and the *CDKN2A* gene.
- The more the genes that become mutated, the greater the risk of tumour formation.
- Both initiation and promotion are necessary to cause cancerous changes in a cell.

Chromosomal abnormalities

- *Aneuploidy* is an abnormal number of chromosomes often seen in cancer cells.
- This is usually caused by a trisomy (three chromosomes replace two) or by a monosomy (one chromosome replaces two), but larger chromosome numbers are seen in some cancers.

Gene inheritance

- Dominant gene inheritance requires only one copy of a gene from either parent to be present in order to be expressed into the phenotype.
- Recessive gene inheritance requires both copies of a gene, one from each parent, to be present in order to be expressed into the phenotype.

The genome and genomics

- The *genome* is the entire set of genes in a nucleus.
- *Genomics* is the study of the entire genome or a subset of genes.
- The *phenotype* is the ultimate expression of the genome.
- *Traits* are characteristics of a phenotype.

Epigenetics

• *Epigenetic* factors are non-genetic factors that affect gene expression and may be inherited.

Notes

1 Three bases inserted or deleted would result in the normal sequence being read, but with one extra (inserted) amino acid or one missing (deleted) amino acid in the final protein.
2 *Nucleotides* are bases attached to their sugar–phosphate frame (see Figure 1.4, Chapter 1, p. 4).
3 All within the nucleus, that is, excluding mitochondrial genes.
4 H2A and H2B count as subtypes of the H2 type.

3

THE CAUSES OF CANCER 2

Chemical and radiation

- **Introduction**
- **Environmental factors: chemical carcinogens**
- **Environmental factors: radiation**
- **Background radiation**
- **Artificial sources of radiation**
- **Key points**

Introduction

Genetic mutations are a very important cause of cancer, and these can occur naturally through mitosis, when cells are more vulnerable to damage. Most damage and errors are repaired. **Carcinogens** are external environmental agents that enter the cells, where they interact with the genome, causing genetic errors. Carcinogens include a wide range of chemicals that initiate and promote cancer formation. **Mutagens** are substances that promote the formation of mutations in genes. **Mitogens** are substances that promote mitosis, that is, accelerating cell growth, and **teratogens** are substances that cross the placenta from mother to child during pregnancy and harm the foetus.

In Chapter 1 we discussed two types of cellular growth (see 'The cell cycle and growth', Chapter 1, p. 4). These are **auxetic** growth, that is, growth in cell *size*, known as **hypertrophy**, and **multiplicative** growth, that is, growth in cell *numbers*, known as **hyperplasia**. Whilst hypertrophy is limited, due to cell size limitations, hyperplasia is, in theory, unlimited, except by what the body can sustain before vital functions fail. The overriding consideration is that cellular growth must satisfy the body's needs, and no more. This requires sophisticated signalling to instruct cells when growth is needed and when it is not.

The body needs two periods of growth:

1. Growth from child to adult, that is, growing in both body size and sophistication. This is limited to childhood and ceases when final adult size is reached.

DOI: 10.4324/9781003389125-3

2. Growth for replacing old dead cells, that is, making good the cells lost from wear and tear, or through aging, but not involving size or developmental changes. This continues throughout life but gradually declines with increasing age.

Outside of these areas, any further forms of growth are not going to be required and will need to be *switched off* by genes. Cancer is a process where the growth is not only unwanted, that is, it is not related to the body's needs, but also cannot be switched off, that is, growth of the tumour has gotten out of control. It has become **autonomous**.

Environmental factors: chemical carcinogens

Carcinogens are anything from outside the body that both initiates and promotes changes in the cells leading to cancer. Both **initiation** and **promotion** are necessary to cause abnormal **neoplastic growth** (new growth) to occur. Initiation is the starting point that leads to cancer, that is, the original DNA damage (or gene mutation) that occurs, but this alone is often not enough to turn the cell malignant. The cell is likely to be able to correct the problem using DNA repair enzymes (see 'G$_0$ and DNA repair', Chapter 2, p. 30) or even die rather than perpetuate the problem. Cell death in these circumstances is called **apoptosis**, and this ensures survival of only those cells with normal, intact, and viable DNA. We produce many cells each day that have genetic mutations, but they rarely go on to become malignant cells because the problem is corrected or the cell dies. In cases like this, initiation has failed due to the lack of *promotion*.

Promotion is the second effect of the carcinogen. Here, the original damage is sustained by repeating the damage frequently over time with repeated exposure to the carcinogen. This continues until the cell can no longer cope with the onslaught and the DNA mutation is allowed to persist, causing a permanent change in that cell. The option for cell death, apoptosis, also becomes obsolete, making the pre-cancerous cell immortal. The cell now stands a good chance of becoming malignant. Promotion takes time to achieve, often years, and this is why repeated exposure to the carcinogen is needed throughout that time span to sustain the damage and, therefore, cause the cancer. Just one or a few exposures to the carcinogen may not be enough to sustain promotion and thus will not cause cancer. This is one reason that smoking is such a disastrous habit to acquire. Smokers are deliberately exposing themselves to the same carcinogens every day, repeatedly, usually for years, ensuring both initiation and promotion of malignancy in their lungs and other cells. They are doing exactly what is needed to cause cancer.

Many carcinogenic factors in the human environment have the potential to initiate and promote the onset of malignancy in a cell. Such factors can be classified into:

1. Living organisms, usually **viruses** (see 'The virion', Chapter 4, p. 59), which can infect tissues and cells and leave their own genetic 'fingerprints' behind, affecting the way the cell performs its genetic function.
2. **Chemicals** of many types that can provoke genetic changes by direct damage to the DNA, thus becoming agents of carcinogenesis.
3. **Radiation** of various forms, which can disrupt the DNA and thus seriously disturb gene function.

Chemical agents

Chemicals that could potentially cause us harm are everywhere about us, that is, they are in our food; in the air we breathe; in the cosmetics and cleansing agents we use; in the soil and food-growing agents we use, for example, such as pesticides; in our drugs and medicines; in our building materials; and so on. Most chemicals are totally harmless, and many are even essential for our existence, such as in oxygen and food. But carcinogens promote cancer formation in living cells (**carcinogenesis**). Some are **free radicals**, that is, highly reactive chemicals that can damage cells and the DNA.

The carcinogenesis of each of these chemicals is dependent on the duration of exposure, the number and frequency of exposures, the concentration of the chemical, and the individual genetic composition of the person having that exposure. Long and repeated exposures of a carcinogenic chemical greatly increase the risk of developing **neoplastic disease** (= new growths).

The following list is of chemicals that are all carcinogenic to some degree, some more so than others. They are best avoided when possible, or at least to avoid prolonged exposure. Taking protective measures where necessary is always recommended.

List of carcinogenic chemicals

- **Aflatoxins** are released by fungal infections of such crops as corn, peanuts, and tree nuts. The fungal toxin is linked to liver cancer.
- **Arsenic** is found in water, soil, and the air. The organic form is less toxic than the inorganic form. Excessive intake of arsenic has been linked to skin, kidney, bladder, liver, digestive tract, and blood cancers.
- **Asbestos** is a fibrous rock mineral previously used for fire prevention in buildings. It can cause mesotheliomas, that is, benign or malignant neoplasms of the membranes lining the chest and abdomen. This occurs after extensive exposure to asbestos dust, which is inhaled when it is disturbed. Mesotheliomas are becoming rarer due to strict protocols for managing asbestos. **Erionite** is a similar fibrous rock mineral as asbestos with links to lung cancer and mesotheliomas.
- **Benzene** is a product of crude oil. This is released from both burnt and unburnt fuels and is one of the top ten carcinogenic agents. About 78% comes from petrol exhaust, another 9% from diesel exhaust, and another 7% from the evaporation of fuel from vehicles. Air pollution levels in heavy traffic areas rise to peak values between 8:00 a.m. and midday, then again from 4:00 p.m. to 8:00 p.m., that is, corresponding to rush-hour traffic volumes, especially during the winter months. It is also a component of tar in tobacco (see 'Tobacco smoking', p. 48). Benzene is linked to blood cancers.
- **Benzidine** is artificially made from **nitrobenzene**, itself a carcinogen. Benzidine was used extensively in the dye industries prior to the 1970s, but this has reduced significantly since it was found to be linked to bladder and lung cancer.
- **Benzo[α]pyrene** (Figure 3.1a) is the best-known carcinogen found in cigarette smoke.
- **Beryllium** is a highly versatile metal and, as such, is found in a wide range of products. Exposure is mostly through inhalation during the manufacturing process and is linked to lung cancer.
- **Cadmium** is a naturally occurring substance found in very small quantities in the air, water, rocks, and even food. Exposure to significant quantities is seen more in industrial processes using cadmium and cigarette smoking (see 'Tobacco smoking', p. 48). It is linked to lung cancer.

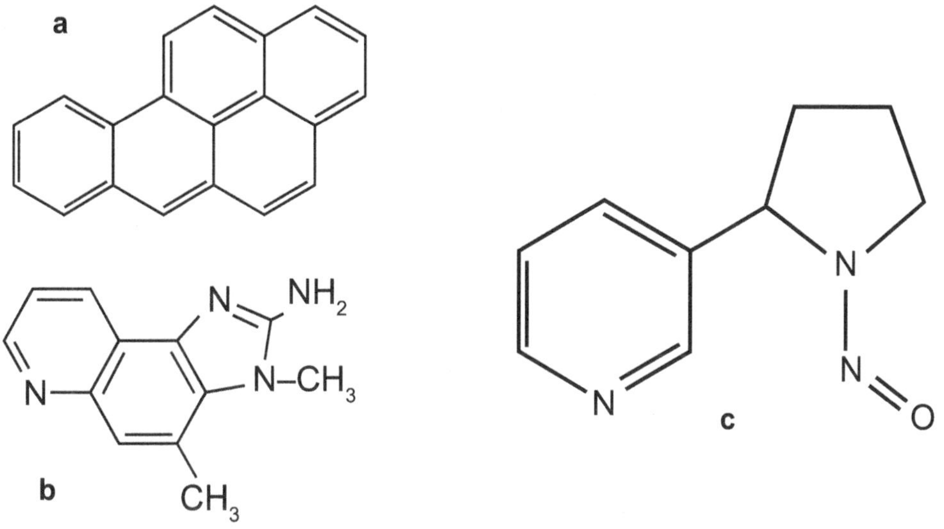

FIGURE 3.1   Chemical structure of three carcinogens: (a) benzo[α]pyrene, (b) 2-amino-3, 4-dimethylimidazo[4,5-f]quinoline (Mel Q), and (c) *N*-nitrosonornicotine.

- **Coal combustion products** include a range of harmful chemicals, some of which are on this list, such as benzene and formaldehyde. Coal combustion products are known to be linked to lung cancer, especially if the smoke from burning coal is inhaled in an enclosed space. Foods treated by being smoked, for example, smoked ham, bacon, and smoked fish, as well as food cooked on an open fire, for example, barbequed (BBQ), will be contaminated with coal combustion carcinogens and, as such, should not be consumed frequently. Incomplete burning of coal produces **soot**, and exposure to soot is known to cause skin, lung, oesophagus, and bladder cancers.
- **Coal tar** is derived from coal and is used extensively, particularly as a road or paving tar. Coal tar contains **polycyclic aromatic hydrocarbons (PAHs)**, a large group of chemical agents that induce cancer. They are mutagenic, that is, they create DNA mutations. Exposure is via inhalation and is linked to skin, lung, bladder, and kidney cancers (see 'Tobacco smoking', p. 48) (Table 3.1).
- **Ethylene oxide** (C_2H_4O) can be in gas form, which is colourless, or in liquid form. It is used in the manufacture of sterilising and fumigating agents. It can be inhaled or ingested and is linked to leukaemia and lymphoid and breast cancers.
- **Formaldehyde** (CH_2O) is a clear, flammable liquid with a strong smell. It is used as a preservative in laboratories for biological specimens or as a fungicide and disinfectant. It can be inhaled as fumes or absorbed through the skin and is linked to myeloid leukaemia and cancers of the upper respiratory tract.
- **Heterocyclic amines (HCAs)** are carcinogenic compounds produced in meats and other foods when fried or roasted at high temperatures. HCAs are mutagenic, that is, promoting gene mutations (see also 'Rosemary', Chapter 18, p. 334).
- **Hexavalent chromium compounds** are a series of compounds based on the metal chromium. They are found in various industries, and industrial exposure to these compounds can cause lung and upper respiratory cancer.

TABLE 3.1 Carcinogenic and toxic agents present in tobacco smoke

Agent	Notes
Acetone	Acetone is a respiratory tract irritant causing headache, tiredness, nausea, and vomiting.
Acrolein	Acrolein is present in tar and is a respiratory irritant involved in a range of diseases, including cancer.
Ammonia	Ammonia changes the way nicotine is delivered to the body so more nicotine will be absorbed, raising the level of addiction.
Arsenic	Arsenic is one of the most dangerous substances in tobacco, causing a range of diseases, including cancer.
Benzene	Benzene is one of the most dangerous substances in tobacco (see 'List of carcinogenic chemicals', p. 42).
Benzo[α]pyrene	A PAH component of tar in tobacco (see 'PAH', p. 47).
Dibenzo[α]anthracene	Another PAH component of tar in tobacco (Figure 3.1a).
Nickel	Nickel is a metal linked to lung cancer.
Cadmium	Cadmium is a poisonous metal, dangerous when inhaled. It causes kidney damage and increased risk of cancers.
Carbon monoxide	Carbon monoxide is a poisonous gas that binds to haemoglobin and prevents oxygen from binding, therefore reducing oxygen levels in the blood.
Radioactive polonium	Polonium is a breakdown product of radium with its own radioactive half-life of 138 days. Most sources of radioactivity are linked to cancer.
Hydrazine	Hydrazine is a toxic compound and possible carcinogen.
Hydrogen cyanide	Hydrogen cyanide is present in tar.
Ethyl carbamate (urethane)	Urethane is used in the plastics industry and is a known carcinogen.
Formaldehyde	Formaldehyde is one of the most dangerous substances in tobacco. It is a component of the tar in tobacco, and it is a carcinogen.
Lead	Lead is a toxic metal linked to nervous system damage and poor development.
Mercury	Mercury is a neurotoxic metal that causes nervous system damage.
Nicotine	Nicotine is the reason for tobacco addiction.
Nicotine-derived N-nitrosamine, 4-(methylnitrosamino)-1-(3-pyridyl)-1-butanone (NNK)	NNK is a by-product of burning nicotine and is linked to adenocarcinoma.
Nitrogen oxides (or oxides of nitrogen)	Nitric oxide (NO) and nitrogen dioxide (NO_2), collectively known at NO_x (or NOX), both respiratory irritants now linked to cancer.
Nitrosamines	Nitrosamines are in food, drugs, and tobacco. Consuming quantities above acceptable levels increases the risk of cancers of the lung, brain, liver, stomach, oesophagus, and bladder.
Nitrosodimethylamine (NDMA)w	NDMA is a carcinogenic and teratogenic, that is, it crosses the placenta and harms the foetus. It can cause cancer of the liver, stomach, prostate, and bladder.
Tar (contains multiple dangerous compounds)	Tar paralyses the mucociliary escalator and accumulates in the lungs. Its contents are carcinogenic.
Toluene	Toluene is present in tar.

- **Mel Q (2-amino-3,4-dimethylimidazo[4,5-f]quinoline)** (Figure 3.1b) is a carcinogen that can be created in meats due to the cooking process. It raises the cancer risk generally but has links to stomach, colon, and kidney cancers.
- **Nickel compounds** are used in a wide number of work environments where nickel and its compounds are found, for example, mining, welding, and casting. Inhalation of nickel compound vapours is common in industry, and it also occurs in smoking. It is linked to lung and nasal cancers.
- **Nitrite**, added to some processed meats as a curing agent and preservative, has been found to be carcinogenic. Bacon, sausages, and ham usually contain nitrite. Excessive nitrite consumption has been linked to breast and prostate cancers.
- **N-nitrosonornicotine** (Figure 3.1c) is a well-known carcinogen of tobacco and tobacco-related products. It is linked to cancers of the liver, kidney, bladder, lung, brain, stomach, oesophagus, and nasal sinus.
- **Trichloroethylene** (C_2HCl_3) is an industrial liquid solvent that produces a sweet-smelling vapour. It is used widely as a cleaning agent. It can be inhaled or absorbed through the skin and is associated with kidney cancer and, possibly, liver cancer.
- **Vinyl chloride** is a colourless gas used primarily to produce polyvinyl chloride (PVC). It is mostly inhaled by those working in PVC production if they are not fully protected. It is linked to cancers of the liver, lungs, brain, and lymphatic system and leukaemia.

Generally, chemical carcinogens cause cancer by adding molecular groups to the DNA bases, that is, the adenine, thymine, etc. These modified bases are then known as **adducts** (Figure 3.2). Adducts may either hide the true nature of the base, that is, hide its identity from the DNA replication process, or distort the DNA double-helix structure. Either way, replication errors occur, which are the primary initiation of cancer.

Obesity and lack of exercise

In addition to all the other health problems linked to obesity, it is now becoming recognised as a risk factor for at least 13 cancers. These include multiple myeloma and uterine, oesophagus, colon, kidney, gall bladder, pancreatic, liver, breast, ovarian, and thyroid cancer. *Obesity* is defined by many authors as having a body mass index (BMI) of 30 or more (see 'Metabolism and energy', Chapter 18, p. 325–327).

Obese people have a more than average risk (73% higher than those of average weight) of having a benign blood disorder, called **monoclonal gammopathy of undetermined significance (MGUS)**. This condition often precedes multiple myeloma (see 'Multiple myeloma', Chapter 7, p. 138). MGUS is the production of abnormal protein from plasma cells. There are no symptoms initially, but if it is discovered, there becomes a need to monitor the person for the development of multiple myeloma. MGUS is also more often found in those who smoke and those who get less than the required amount of sleep.

The risk linked to obesity is more than doubled for some cancers and increased by up to 80% for other cancers when compared with individuals of average weight. And the risk gets worse as the obesity increases. Also, men who gain weight progressively between the ages 17 and 29 years old have a 13% greater risk of aggressive prostate cancer and a 27% greater risk of fatal prostate cancer later in life.

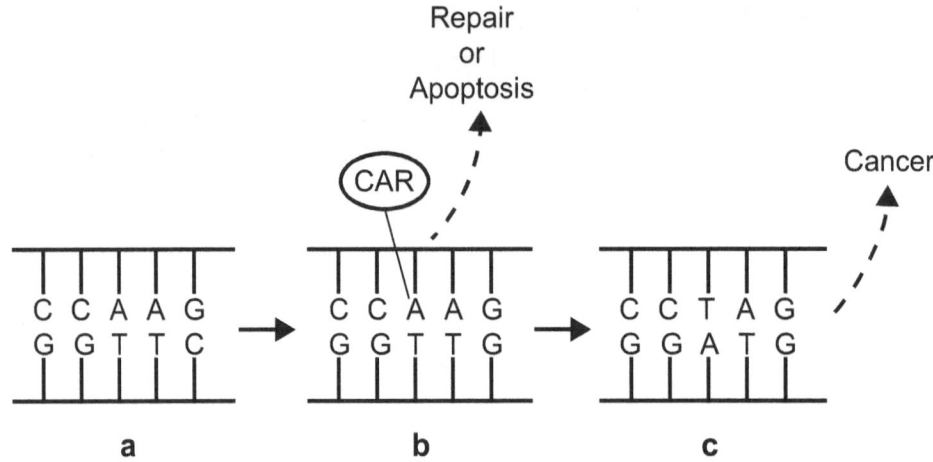

FIGURE 3.2 The mechanism for adduct formation in DNA: (a) A section of normal DNA showing CCAAG sequence. (b) A carcinogen (CAR) forms an attachment with an adenine (A) base. Carcinogens that form adducts are often the end product of cellular metabolism, that is, a metabolite of the original chemical. The link between the carcinogen and the base is an addition reaction, that is, two or more chemicals reacting to form a single molecule. In this case, the damage caused is the swapping of adenine for thymine, forming a CCTAG sequence. This will ultimately cause errors in protein synthesis if it persists. However, at this point, the DNA damage may be either corrected by the cell repair system or the whole cell could be driven to apoptosis (cell death). (c) Any surviving cells may continue towards DNA replication. If so, the cell duplicates the error into many cells, causing significant protein errors, leading to cancer.

The reasons obesity increases the risk of cancer are uncertain, because there are so many factors involved (Figure 3.3). The main causes are likely to be:

1. Changes in hormonal patterns seen in the obese person, especially the increase (↑) in growth factors
2. A persistent state of low-grade inflammation observed in obesity, including an increase (↑) in inflammatory compounds
3. A reduction (↓) in the immune response, including the immune system's reduced ability to fight cancer cells when they arise

(Wallis 2019)

Vigorous intermittent lifestyle physical activity (VILPA)

Linked with obesity, a lack of exercise is also seen to be a high-risk factor for developing cancer. More than three times as many cancers are now linked to lack of exercise than previously thought. VILPA significantly reduces the risk of cancers in addition to reducing the risk of other health problems, such as cardiovascular disease. VILPA means doing a total of about 5 minutes of vigorous activity each day, divided into short periods of 1 minute each, which raises the heart and respiratory rates. Even 3.5 minutes per day can reduce cancer risk by 18%, and 4.5 minutes per day reduces the risk by 32%. These vigorous activities can be part of the daily routine, such

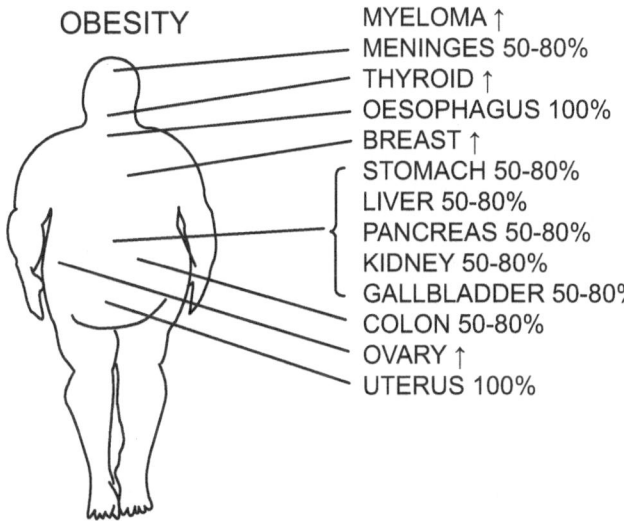

CANCERS AND
INCREASE RISK

REASONS

OBESITY

MYELOMA ↑
MENINGES 50-80%
THYROID ↑
OESOPHAGUS 100%
BREAST ↑
STOMACH 50-80%
LIVER 50-80%
PANCREAS 50-80%
KIDNEY 50-80%
GALLBLADDER 50-80%
COLON 50-80%
OVARY ↑
UTERUS 100%

• Hormone changes
  ↑ Growth factors
  ↑ insulin
• ↑ Substances that promote
  inflammation
• ↓ Immunity
• Changes to microbiome
• Changes to metabolism
• Changes to gene
  expression

FIGURE 3.3   The risk factors for cancer becoming greater with increasing obesity, and the reasons for this. Arrow up = increase; arrow down = decrease.

as housework (vacuum and moving furniture), gardening (mowing the lawn), and shopping (carrying heaving shopping bags).

Air pollution and particulates

Pollutants in the atmosphere are responsible more for respiratory diseases, such as asthma and bronchitis, or for heart disease, rather than cancer, but there are pollutants that can provoke malignant changes in the lungs or elsewhere. Air pollution is considered mostly to be a problem derived from vehicular exhaust and industry, but in cities where aircraft fly over, the jet engines also cause very large amounts of pollution. An example is London, where jets dump 2 million tons of carbon dioxide, 13 thousand tons of nitrogen, and 159 tons of particulates every year.

Particulates are tiny particles of matter than can react with other gases to form obnoxious compounds and can penetrate deeply into the lungs when inhaled. Particulates come in two main sizes, for example, PM10s are particulates 10 μm (micrometres, or one thousandth of a millimetre) or smaller, and PM2.5s are one-quarter of the size of PM10s. Obviously, the smaller the particle, the deeper it can get into the lung and, therefore, the more cellular damage it can do. Examples of PM10s are pollen; smoke from wildfires and waste burning; and dust from multiple sources, such as landfill sites, construction sites, agriculture, and industry. Examples of PM2.5s are emissions from burning wood, oil, petrol, and diesel; very fine dust; and soot.

Many particulates are **polycyclic aromatic hydrocarbons (PAH)** or **nitrated polycyclic aromatic hydrocarbons (nitro-PAH)** (see 'List of carcinogen chemicals', p. 42, and Table 3.1), which are known **mutagenic** agents, that is, they cause gene mutations.

Diesel exhaust is the source of two powerful cancer-causing particulates, **1,8-dinitropyrene** and **3-nitrobenzanthrone**, the latter of the two being a nitro-PAH produced in much larger quantities when the diesel engine is working under a heavy load (Pearce 1997). Both these substances cause mutations in genes that can lead to malignancy. Also, 1,8-dinitropyrene is linked to squamous cell carcinoma, fibrosarcoma, histiocytoma, and chromosomal abnormalities, while 3-nitrobenzanthrone is a potent mutagenic agent linked to squamous cell carcinoma following inhalation from diesel fumes.

Food ingredients

Highly processed foods are now being investigated for their link with cancer. So far, the general conclusion is that the greater the degree of processing, and the greater the quantity of processed food consumed, the higher the rate of cancers. Processed foods contain ingredients which are not used in the home cooking of fresh foods, ingredients such as emulsifiers, artificial sweeteners, and preservatives. Processed meats contain nitrite, which is linked to breast and prostate cancers (see 'List of carcinogenic chemicals', p. 42), and emulsifiers are suspected to be linked to cancers generally but to breast cancers specifically (Stallard 2023).

Tobacco smoking

About 30% of all deaths per year are caused by smoking-related diseases, compared with 2% of deaths caused by air pollution. Smoking is the biggest preventable cause of cancer and other diseases. Everyone has a choice to either smoke or not, and to choose not to smoke is one of the most important single lifestyle choice anyone can make towards a better, healthier life.

The lining of the respiratory tract is mucous membrane that has **cilia**, the delicate, hair-like structures that normally protect the lungs from inhaled particles. Cilia have a wafting motion that sweeps the mucus upwards from the depths of the lung towards the throat. The sticky nature of mucus results in dangerous chemicals, such particulates, sticking to it, and therefore, they get carried out of the lungs to the throat, where they are safely swallowed. This is the '**mucociliary escalator**'. Cigarette smoke contains **tar** that causes lung irritation and, ultimately, lung cancer. Tar is deposited in the lungs and paralyses the cilia. When the cilia are paralysed by smoking, mucus, and anything stuck to the mucus, drains to the depths of the lungs, where it accumulates. Coughing becomes the only way to clear it, that is, the smoker's typical chronic cough, although this is nowhere near as efficient as the mucociliary escalator.

Tobacco contains a deadly cocktail of over 7,000 toxic and carcinogenic substances, the most important of which are shown in Table 3.1 and Figure 3.4. After many decades of research, tobacco smoking has been shown to cause cancer of the mouth, tongue, throat, larynx, trachea, bronchus, oesophagus, breast, lungs, stomach, colon, rectum, bladder, cervix, pancreas, liver, kidney, and blood (acute leukaemia). And it is not just about cancer that is the problem; tobacco smoking also causes a range of non-cancerous diseases, such as heart disease, stroke, bronchitis, emphysema, asthma, and vascular diseases. Smoking also causes faster cognitive decline, leading to dementia. Smoking has now been found to shrink brain volume, and the volume lost from smoking is not replaced, even if the smoker stops the habit. The natural brain volume loss caused by aging is made worse by smoking.

Smoking kills about 8 million people per year worldwide. Lung cancer is the second most common cancer, reaching epidemic proportions, with about 2.2 million new cases of lung cancer in 2020. Smoking causes the presence of activated receptors on the surface of lung cells that bind various growth hormones, including **gastrin-releasing peptide (GRP)**. These receptors

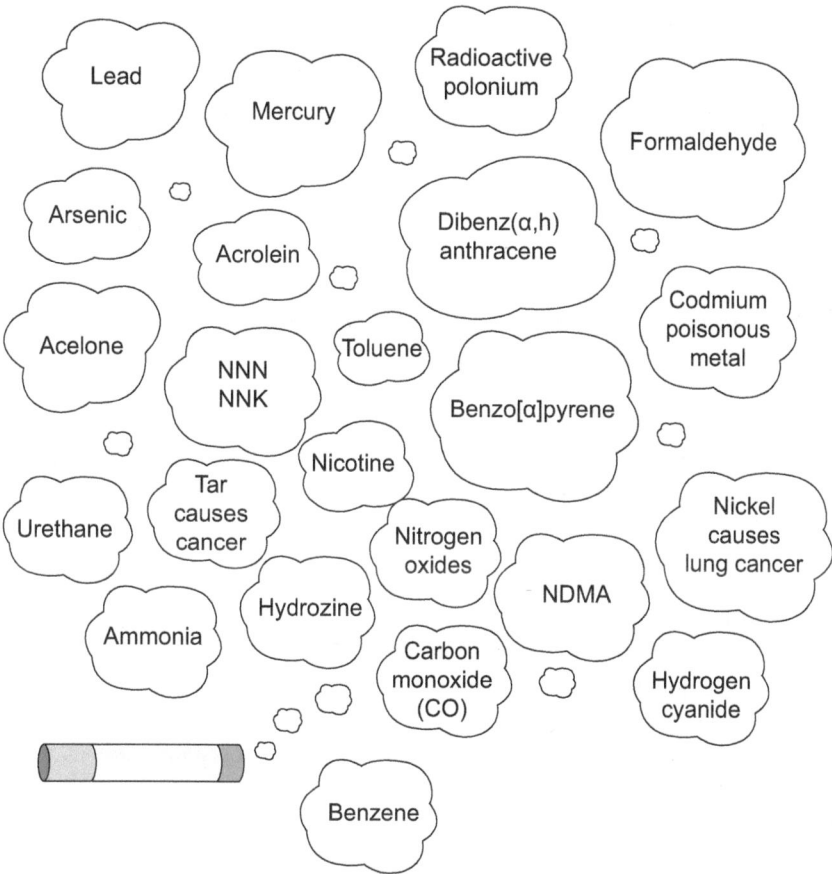

FIGURE 3.4   Some of the 7,000 toxic substances that the smoker is inhaling.

are normally active during lung development in foetal life and are not expected to be active after that. Long-term smoking reactivates these receptors, and this may increase the risk of lung cancer. It appears that once reactivated, these receptors remain active years after giving up the habit, indicating permanent changes in the lung.

Smoking in women is increasing, and thus there is a corresponding rise in lung cancer in women. Mortality rates for women with lung cancer as the cause of death rose dramatically across the world between 1960 and 1980. They increased by 100% in Japan, Norway, Poland, Sweden, and the UK, and by more than 200% in Australia, Denmark, and New Zealand. The increase was more than 300% in the USA and Canada. By 2020, 770,828 female smokers were diagnosed with lung cancer worldwide, and 607,465 had died. Women who smoke also suffer other effects as well. They have a greater number of irregular and painful periods, vaginal dryness, fatigue, lower oestrogen levels, earlier menopause, and worse menopausal symptoms compared to those of non-smoking women.

Passive smoking also increases the risk of lung cancer in non-smokers by 26%, that is, about 600 cases every year in the UK. Passive smokers absorb chemicals called **nitrosamines**, particularly *N*-**nitrosonornicotine** (**NNN**) and **4-(methylnitrosamino)-1-(3-pyridyl)-1-butanone**

(**NNK**) (Table 3.1). These are the by-products of burning nicotine, and therefore, they are only found in tobacco. They cause lung cancer (**adenocarcinoma**) (see 'Non-small-cell lung cancers (NSCLC)', Chapter 9, p. 187), which is common in passive smokers. Mothers who smoke near their babies put the infants' lives at risk. Approximately 80 cot deaths per year in the UK are caused by the infants' passive smoking from their parents' cigarettes.

Smoking is now known to be the biggest avoidable cause of disease and early death in humans. The problem of stopping the population from smoking, especially the younger generations, should be tackled alongside the quest for a cancer cure.

There is also a link between smoking and epigenetic changes, in particular, methylation of CpG islands (see 'Epigenetics: DNA methylation', Chapter 2, p. 36). The epigenetics of two genes are most often involved in two ethnic groups, the *CYTH1* gene (see 'Chromosome 17', Addendum, p. 357) in African American smokers, and the *MYO1G* gene (see 'Chromosome 7', Addendum, p. 349) in Latino smokers. The epigenetic errors affecting these genes increase the risk of cancer progression. The amount of nicotine that smokers inhale can now be accurately measured using **total nicotine equivalents** (**TNE**s) in a urine sample. There is also a high risk that children of parents who smoke will take up the habit. This is not only through children living in a smoking household and learning to smoke from their parents but also 50% of the increased risk is through genetic inheritance (see also 'Epigenetics', Chapter 2, p. 36).

The situation with vaping is currently different because it is a relatively new habit, and it tends to be more popular in younger people. Therefore, there has not been the decades of long-term research into vaping that tobacco smoking has had. At present it appears that vaping is not safe, partly because some of the chemicals in vaping oil are the same as in cigarettes, such as formaldehyde and acrolein (Table 3.1). At best, these cause bronchial and lung irritation, and in the long term, they can cause lung damage. Smoking tobacco and e-cigarettes is now known to cause the same epigenetic changes (see 'Epigenetics', 'DNA methylation', Chapter 2, p. 36) in cheek cells that are seen in lung cancers. Since lung cancer develops in a longer time frame, it is likely that this, and maybe other cancers, will eventually be linked to vaping.

A British study (Kingman 2004) that was conducted over 50 years, beginning in 1951, shows quite clearly the following:

1. That half of all smokers will die from their habit.
2. That smoking *shortens your life expectancy by ten years*.
3. That stopping smoking at any age improves health and life expectancy.
4. That smoking is now recognised as the *top health hazard in the world*.

Some smokers, when they are told that they have cancer, will stop smoking, but others will not. Those who do not stop smoking after a cancer diagnosis tend to suffer worse pain, worse fatigue, and worse emotional problems than those that do stop the habit. However, among those that do stop smoking, most start smoking again after a while. Very few remain non-smokers for life. Such is the power of addiction.

The bottom line is that the human lung is not expected to accept anything other than air, and forcing it to accept other substances can, and will, cause harm. Surely, the case for *not* smoking, and *not* vaping, is now overwhelming.

Environmental factors: radiation

Radiation comes in four main forms, *alpha*, *beta*, *neutron*, and *electromagnetic*, for example, gamma.

Alpha (α) radiation

Alpha particles are two neutrons and two protons combined (Figure 3.5). Such 'large' particles (by atomic standards) are weak and relatively slow and are incapable of penetrating the skin. Therefore, alpha particle radiation is only considered to be dangerous to people if it is consumed in our diet. An example of alpha particle radiation is the radioactive material used in smoke alarms.

Beta (β) radiation

These are high-energy electrons (Figure 3.5) which are much smaller than alpha particles and are very much faster-moving. They are therefore harder to stop than alpha. Unlike alpha particles, electrons technically have no mass and are therefore capable of deep penetration of human tissues. This makes them more dangerous to health when people are exposed to them.

Electrons, the outer components of atoms, can gain or lose energy. The more energy electrons gain, the faster and more excited they become, moving rapidly into positions further away from the nucleus of the atom. Eventually, the electron gains enough energy to fly off the atom and become a free entity. It is these free electrons, travelling at great speeds, that are beta radiation. With high speeds and high energy, coupled with no mass, the electrons have considerable penetration and ability to cause damage.

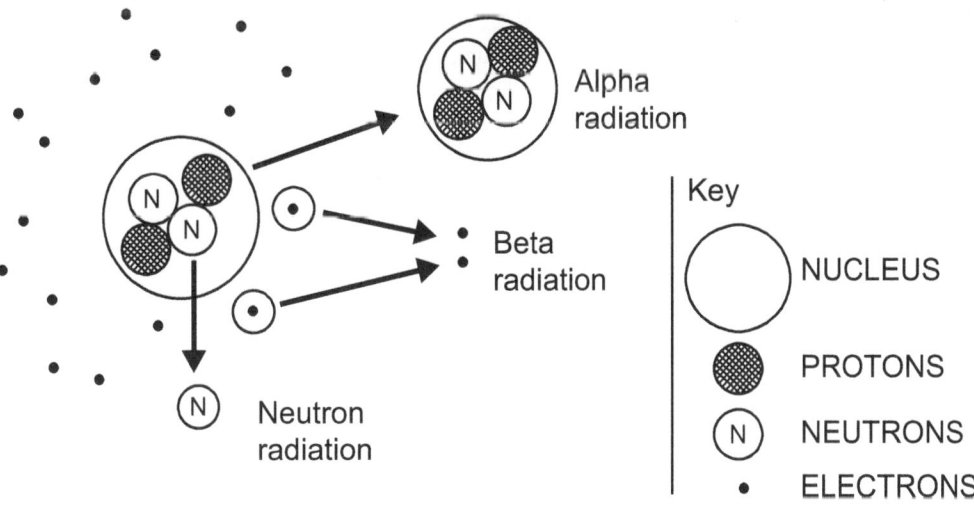

FIGURE 3.5   Different forms of radiation: alpha (two protons and two neutrons), beta (electrons), and neutron radiation (neutron particles).

Neutron radiation

This is a stream of high-energy **neutrons** (Figure 3.5), that is, particles from the nucleus of an atom that have no charge, neither positive nor negative. To obtain such particles, the nucleus must be split, and this is called **fission**, or 'splitting the atom', an event that happens in nuclear reactors or nuclear explosions. This makes exposure for most people remote. Neutron radiation is more penetrating that alpha or beta radiation, but less penetrating than gamma radiation. However, because the neutron particle has a large mass (in atomic terms), it is considerably damaging.

Electromagnetic radiation

This is part of the **electromagnetic spectrum**, which is a way of classifying a particular group of energies that occur in a waveform rather than particles. Many forms of these energies exist, as shown by the spectrum, including *light*, *X-rays*, and *radio waves*. Being a wave means that it has a pattern of peaks and troughs (or ups and downs), in the same way that ripples on a pond have high points (the peaks of water) and low points (the troughs of water). And like pond ripples, electromagnetic waves move outward from the source, but at much greater speeds than pond ripples. The distance measured from the top of one peak to the top of the next peak is the **wavelength** (Figure 3.6).

Obviously, the shorter the wavelength, the more waves will be able to pack into a metre. This is the **frequency**. The shorter the wavelength, the greater the frequency, that is, each peak arrives at its destination more frequently if the wavelength is short. Conversely, the longer the wavelength, the lower the frequency, that is, each peak arrives far less frequently if the wavelength is long. It is the difference in the wavelengths, and thus in the frequency, that distinguishes one waveform from the next. In this spectrum, different forms of waves are presented according to:

1. Their *wavelengths*, measured in **metres (m)**, or subdivisions of a metre, such as **centimetres (cm)** (Figures 3.6 and 3.7)
2. Their *frequency*, measured in **hertz (Hz)**, or variables of this, for example, **megahertz (MHz)**

High frequency is at one end of the spectrum, low frequency at the other (Figure 3.7). Long-wavelength (low-frequency) waves include radio waves, followed by microwaves. The frequency increases considerably as we pass through infrared and visible light. Very-high-frequency waves include ultraviolet light, X-rays, and gamma rays. Along with increasing frequency, we

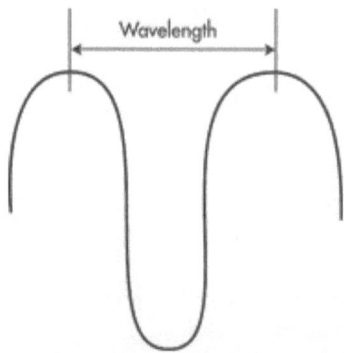

FIGURE 3.6 The measurement of a wavelength. This is the distance from one peak to the next.

Wavelength [in metres]

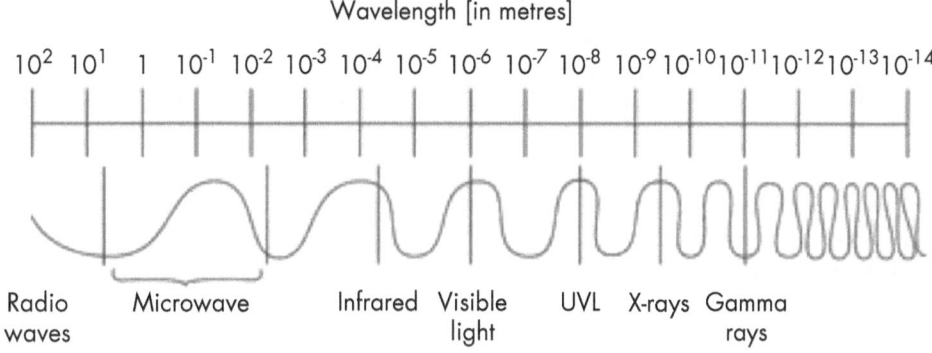

FIGURE 3.7   The electromagnetic spectrum.

also see an increase in the levels of energy. The high frequency of ultraviolet light, and even the higher frequencies of X-rays and gamma rays, means that these waves have high energies compared with radio waves, and this means greater penetration of tissues and potential tissue damage.

The terms **ionising radiation** and **non-ionising radiation** are used to indicate energy levels. Ionising radiation is high-energy, enough to remove electrons from atoms, creating **ions**, or charged particles, whilst non-ionising is lower-energy, that is, insufficient energy to affect electrons. Ionising radiation is more damaging to DNA than non-ionising radiation.

Gamma radiation (or **gamma rays**) has an extremely high frequency (10^{-10} cm, or 10^{-12} m), that is, a wavelength of only 1/10,000,000,000 cm long (one ten thousand millionth of a centimetre from one peak to the next), and therefore, it has extremely high energy, which is what makes it dangerous to cells and tissues. It has the high level of energy required to dislodge electrons from atoms, making it a source of *ionising radiation*, which is what happens inside the cells when exposed to a gamma radiation source. Such ionising radiation causes damage to DNA and therefore increases the cell's risk of turning malignant. Gamma radiation is found coming from some rocks and soil, from radon gas, and as cosmic radiation from the sun and outer space. All these are natural background sources of radiation to which we are all subjected (see 'Background radiation', p. 54). Man-made sources of gamma radiation include X-rays and nuclear contamination from atomic energy plants or nuclear weapons. Fortunately, we can avoid X-rays, unless they are necessary, and nuclear fallout is extremely rare, that is, it accounts for less than 1% of all the typical human lifetime exposure to gamma rays.

X-rays have a wavelength that is longer than that of gamma rays, that is, between 10^{-9} and 10^{-10} meters (Figure 3.7). This is still very short, and therefore, it is a high-energy ionising radiation. Excessive exposure to X-rays is dangerous and should be kept to a minimum. X-ray dosage is measured in **RAD**s, that is, **radiation absorbed dose**, or in **SI** (**International System of Units**) units, it is the **gray (Gy)**, a measure of the energy absorbed per unit mass of body tissue (see also 'Artificial sources of radiation', p. 57).

Electromagnetic radiation with a wavelength between 10^{-2} m (or 1cm) and 10 m is called **microwave** radiation (Figure 3.7). Microwaves are produced inside a **magnetron** (see Figure 17.3, Chapter 17, p. 312), and this can be another potential source of radiation. Microwave ovens (wavelength of about $10^{-2} \times 20$ m, or 20 cm) and mobile phones (wavelengths from 22 cm up to about 3 m or more) both use microwaves. These wavelength values fall into the non-ionising category for radiation, which means that they are less damaging to cellular structures but are still a potential health hazard and should be used with caution. Microwaves heat water by increasing the energy of the water molecules, and this is the basis by which the microwave oven works to heat food. It is also the reason mobile phones have received a great deal of interest in terms of their health hazard potential. The brain contains water, and extensive use of the mobile phone close to the head may raise the temperature of this water. Whilst mobile phone manufacturers and distributors support their product as safe for human use, the reports of brain tumours associated with extensive mobile phone use cannot be ignored. Claims that radiation levels used in mobile phones are well below radiation guidelines should be treated with caution, because it very much depends on the length of exposure, and ultimately, the only really safe level of radiation is zero. *Anything* above this carries some degree of risk, no matter how small, and should not be considered as totally safe.

Some people spend long periods talking on their mobile phone, and clearly, this excessive exposure to microwave radiation can only be bad for the brain cells adjacent to the transmitter. Some people claim to have suffered memory losses, dizziness, fatigue, and headaches, and even fits, when they use their mobile phone for long periods. This shows that the radiation is having some adverse effect on the brain, and it is a warning sign that further brain exposure to mobile phone radiation could lead to more serious consequences, such as malignancy. Limiting the use of the mobile phone to an absolute minimum is clearly a sensible precaution, and some people do keep mobile phones for emergencies only. One group of people who should *never* use mobile phones, other than in extreme emergencies, are children. The growing and developing brain is more prone to potential radiation effects than the adult, mature brain. And adverse effects on the developing brain may be permanent, so again, a sensible precaution would be not to issue children with mobile phones as routine. Given that children do not need the phone at school and that most calls that are made, by adults and children alike, are not necessary, that is, they are made solely because the phone is conveniently there, it makes sense to avoid this form of radiation. However, with the continuing growth of sales in the mobile phone industry, most people are prepared to take the risk, and therefore, there may be an increased in problems such as brain tumours.

Some people can be seen both smoking and talking on the mobile phone at the same time. This is courting the twin carcinogenic hazards of cigarette tar and mobile phone radiation at the same time. This is throwing all caution to the wind and shows that these individuals appear to have no regard for their future health.

Background radiation

Radiation is an environmental factor from which we cannot completely escape, but we do have some power to reduce exposure to a minimum. We are constantly subject to what is termed **background radiation** (Figure 3.8), that is, natural radiation sources which, between them. provide a constant level of radiation to which we are all exposed. The main sources of background radiation are (1) the *rocks* beneath us, (2) sunlight (i.e. *ultraviolet light* from sunshine), and (3) *cosmic radiation.*

Radiation from rocks

The *soil* and *rocks* are both a source of generally low levels of gamma radiation; the amount depends entirely on the nature of the rocks beneath you. Granite, and other forms of igneous (fire-formed) rocks, may yield a slightly higher proportion of radiation than sedimentary rocks, such as clay, which would usually yield none. Some rocks may test for various levels of

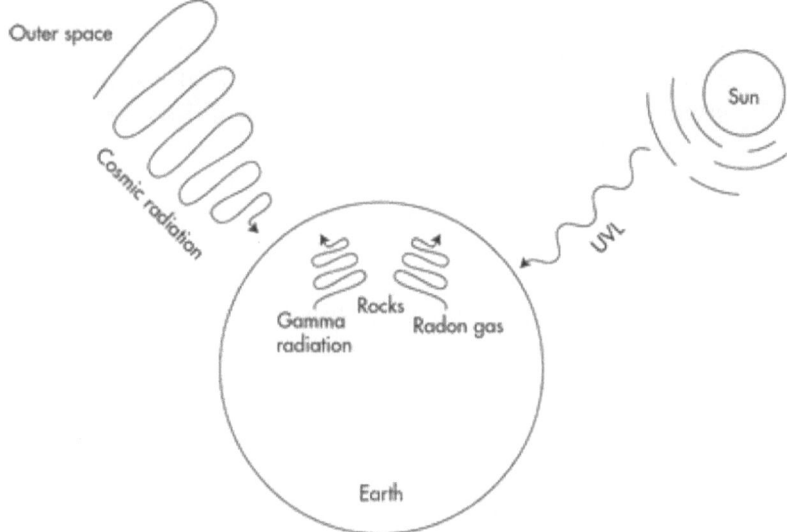

FIGURE 3.8   Sources of natural (background) radiation. *UVL* = ultraviolet light.

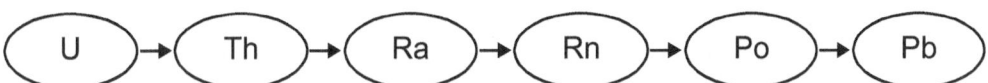

FIGURE 3.9   A simplified chain of products from uranium decay. Uranium (U) is found in certain rocks. Over time, it decays and changes first to thorium (Th), then to radium (Ra). Thorium and radium further decay to radon (Rn), a gas that leaks from the Earth into the atmosphere. Radon can be inhaled into the lungs in an enclosed space. Further decay of radon leads to polonium (Po), which is found in tobacco and can attach to dust, water vapour, or air particles and, as such, can also be inhaled. Decay of polonium results, ultimately, to the formation of lead (Pb).

radiation if they have been contaminated with radioactive elements during the time they were deposited. This applies also to the fossils within those rocks. In some cases, radioactive dinosaur bones have been found and may be present in some fossil collections. Soil is derived from the underlying rocks, with organic matter mixed in, and is also a potential source of radiation, particularly if the soil is derived from subterranean igneous rocks.

Thorium is a naturally occurring radioactive metal found in rocks and soils and groundwater, in areas where it had been naturally deposited. It is part of the process of uranium decay (Figure 3.9). It has been mined and used in various industries, although its use is declining with safer alternatives. Although thorium could be in any rocks anywhere, the risk is low, that is, it becomes part of background radiation. Any exposure would be by inhalation, by ingestion, or through the skin. Thorium is linked to liver, lung, pancreas, and bone cancers.

Radon gas is a radioactive product of the decay process of **uranium** (Figure 3.9). Radioactive decay releases sub-atomic particles, that is, α (**alpha**) and β (**beta**) (Figure 3.5), as part of the process. Radon gas comes from the soil, and thus ultimately from the uranium in rocks, particularly concentrating in volcanic rocks (e.g. granite) or limestones and sandstones. When liberated into the open air, radon gas disperses with no harmful effects. In fact, radon gas itself causes no health risk to humans from the outside of the body. However, in enclosed spaces, such as in a house, it is potentially more harmful as it is then breathed in. Radon itself decays to form radioactive 'daughters', which release alpha particles (Figure 3.9). These are not harmful from outside the body, but if the radon daughters are inhaled directly into the lungs, it increases the risk of lung cancers. The UK national average of radon activity in houses is 20 Bq (becquerels) per cubic metre, causing a lifetime risk of lung cancer of 1 in 300 people. Action is needed if the level in a house rises to 200 Bq per cubic metre, the equivalent to a lifetime lung cancer risk of 1 person in 30. One of the radioactive daughters of radon gas is a solid particle called **polonium** (Figures 3.4 and 3.9, Table 3.1), which attaches itself to dust, water, tobacco, or smoke particles in the air, and this facilitates its inhalation into the lungs.

Cosmic radiation

Cosmic radiation comes from space (Figure 3.10), mostly from stars, including our own star, the sun. It also includes more distant stars that explode at the end of their lifespan, quasars, pulsars, and radiation from black holes. This term includes several different radiation elements contributing to an overall effect. These elements include atomic particle matter made up from approximately 2% electrons, 85% protons, 12% helium nuclei, and 1% heavier nuclei. In addition, there are photons, that is, packages of electromagnetic light energy, particularly ultraviolet light, which has a shorter wavelength than visible or infrared and, therefore, has more energy. Plus, there are higher-energy particles of various kinds, including microwaves and X-rays. At ground level, cosmic radiation accounts for about 10% of the background radiation, but it increases in intensity with altitude because the atmosphere, which affords some protection, gets thinner at higher altitudes and thus provides less protection. This causes an increased risk of radiation exposure to flight crew of aircraft who are exposed to this increase on a daily basis and those passengers who fly long distances regularly. The occasional flight here or there is not a problem, but regular air travellers are warned that they are exposing themselves to greater radiation levels, sometimes 100 to 300 times more than that encountered at sea level. Therefore, the more you fly, or the higher you fly, the greater the risks. Aircraft are not built to protect the occupants against this important radiation source, for very practical reasons. Lead shielding is the only truly effective protection, and the weight of lead makes this economically impossible. Because this radiation is ionising (see 'Electromagnetic radiation', p. 52), exposure to it causes damage to DNA. This predisposes the cell to increased risk of malignancy, especially those cells that reproduce rapidly, such as blood cells, sperm, and ova. Some studies have shown aircrew to have higher than average numbers of cancers, including cancer of the brain, prostate, skin, breast, colon, and blood (leukaemia) (Kahn 1999). This is also a major problem for astronauts, who are likely to suffer the greatest risks of all, and one that needs addressing before any long manned space flights are attempted.

Ultraviolet light (UVL) radiation

Ultraviolet light (UVL) is a longer wavelength (100–400 nm) but is also part of the more hazardous forms of ionising radiation, and again, exposure to it should be strictly limited (see Figure 13.4, Chapter 13, p. 247). Sunlight is the most important natural source of UVL (Figure 3.8), but man-made sources, such as sunbeds, are also potentially dangerous if used for too long. The big danger is skin cancer, since it is the skin that receives the main dosage (see 'Neoplastic disorders of the skin', Chapter 13, p. 246), but UVL also causes premature ageing of

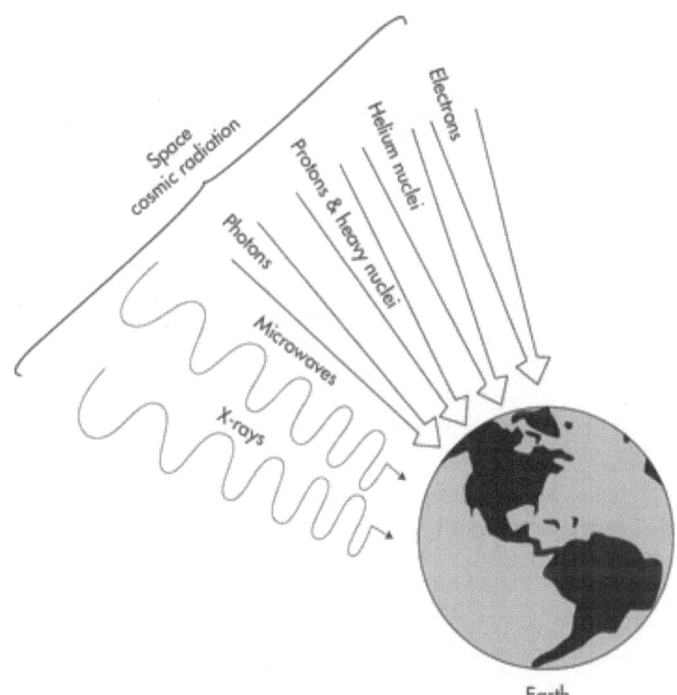

Earth

FIGURE 3.10   Cosmic radiation. This is a collection of atomic particles, photons, microwaves, and X-rays from outside the Earth.

the skin. Protective skin lotions and wearing protective clothing help filter out the harmful UVL when exposure is inevitable, but deliberate sunbathing or use of the sunbed should be avoided or limited. Exposure to the sun should be restricted to those parts of the day when sunshine is less intense. **Visible** and **infrared lights** are forms of non-ionising radiation, having not enough energy to release electrons from atoms (Figure 3.6).

Artificial sources of radiation

Artificial sources of radiation are very important to consider because exposure to these sources could, at least in theory, be reduced to a minimum or eliminated entirely. What humans produce, humans should be able to avoid. In practical terms, this is not always possible, and so artificial sources of radiation must be part of the equation when calculating risks. The use of X-rays in medicine has proven extremely valuable in the diagnostics of many disorders, both in the standard X-ray form seen in hospitals associated with departments such as accident and emergency and as the newer forms of X-ray equipment, such as **computerised axial tomography** (**CAT** or **CT**) scans (Coutts 2002). Whatever their form, medical X-rays should be used only when essential, and then with great caution (Blows 2002). X-rays are measured using a unit called the **rad** (**radiation absorbed dose**), whilst the **standard international** (**SI**) equivalent of this is the **gray** (**Gy**), the unit for measuring the X-ray energy absorbed per unit mass of body tissue. This is the energy that causes tissue damage, 1 Gy being 1 J (joule) of absorbed energy per kilogram of body tissue. One standard chest X-ray delivers about as much energy to the tissues as does background radiation over ten days or so (see 'Radiotherapy', Chapter 17, p. 310).

All electrical equipment produces electromagnetic radiation to some extent, particularly televisions and visual display units (VDUs), and sitting in front of these for too long, or too close, is not good for the health.

Stress in cancer

Stress does not cause cancer, but it may be a contributing factor in promoting cancer progression where tumours already exist that have originated from other causes. In lung cancer, and maybe for other cancers also, stress has been found to cause:

- A weaker immune system, for example, fewer T cells.
- More fibronectin (see 'Tissue invasion', Chapter 6, p. 123).
- Altered hormonal levels, that is, stress raises the blood cortisol level, a glucocorticoid hormone.
- Increased neutrophils, which form **neutrophil extracellular traps** (**NET**s). This helps the cancer spread. The raised cortisol level promotes the formation of NETs (see 'Neutrophils', Chapter 6, p. 121).

Key points

Carcinogenesis

- *Carcinogens* are anything that both initiates and promotes changes in the DNA, leading to cancer.
- *Mutagens* promote mutations in DNA; *mitogens* promote mitosis, leading to excessive cell growth.
- Viruses, chemicals of many types, and radiation can be carcinogenic.
- Cigarette smoke contains tar that causes lung irritation and lung cancer.
- Cigarettes contain a deadly cocktail of over 7,000 toxic substances.
- Chemical carcinogens damage DNA by attaching adducts.
- Obesity increases the risk of multiple cancers.

Radiation

- Radiation comes in four main forms, alpha (α) (two neutrons and two protons combined), beta (β) (high-energy electrons), electromagnetic (energy in waveform), and neutron (high-energy neutrons).
- Ionising radiation has enough energy to causes electrons to be ejected from atoms, creating ions. Non-ionising radiation does not eject electrons.
- The *wavelength* is the measure from the peak of one wave to the peak of the next.
- X-rays have a longer wavelength than gamma rays but are still high-energy ionising radiation.
- The electromagnetic spectrum has radio waves at the low-energy end, and gamma rays at the high-energy end, with visible light close to the centre.
- X-ray dosage is measured in units called the rad (radiation absorbed dose).
- The standard international (SI) equivalent is the gray (Gy), the unit for measuring the X-ray energy absorbed per unit mass of body tissue.
- Background radiation is found everywhere and comes from rocks, the sun, and cosmic radiation. It is generally low-energy and harmless.

4

THE CAUSES OF CANCER 3

Viruses and hormones

Introduction

Having looked at genes (Chapters 1 and 2) and carcinogenic chemicals and radiation (Chapter 3), here we look at viruses and hormones that have the potential to initiate and promote cancer development. Viruses are responsible for the least number of human cancers, about 10%. The difference, however, is that they are transmitted from one person to another, so it becomes possible to catch the virus and risk developing the cancer. On the other hand, they are potentially preventable.

Whether or not viruses are 'alive' in the true sense of the word is a matter of debate. Unlike human cells, they have no organelles. Therefore, they can only reproduce through the mechanisms provided by the cells that they have invaded. Outside the body, in the environment, viruses are inert and are awaiting the opportunity to infect more cells. New viruses derived from intracellular replication gain access to the blood and lymph and travel around the body to invade other cells. They also collect in body secretions for the chance to infect other bodies through coughing and sneezing, kissing, and sexual intercourse. A few viruses change the very nature of the cell they invade, that is, they change it to become malignant.

The virion

A **virion** is a completely intact virus, just as it would exist in the environment. In this state, virions consist of a lipid outer envelope surrounding a protein nucleocapsid containing nucleic acid. This is either **deoxyribonucleic acid (DNA)** or **ribonucleic acid (RNA)**, but never both together

DOI: 10.4324/9781003389125-4

(Figure 4.1). This makes a useful means of classifying virions, that is, into DNA viruses and RNA viruses. There are many variations on this basic structure, producing a range of different virions.

The RNA virions have very little effect on human cancers, although they are involved to a greater extent in animal tumours. The exceptions are the **human immunodeficiency virus (HIV)** and the **human T cell lymphotropic virus (HTLV)** (see following list). Contrary to this, DNA virions are more often involved in the cause of human cancers (known as **oncoviruses**). The following are the best-known oncoviruses:

DNA viruses

- *Epstein–Barr virus* (**EBV**), also called **human herpes virus 4 (HHV4)** (Figure 4.2a), is a DNA vi.rus that causes various lymphomas, including **Burkitt lymphoma**, a tumour of the lower jaw (see Table 7.7, Chapter 7, p. 145), and nasopharyngeal cancer (Pecorino 2021). EBV produces a protein called **EBNA1 (Epstein–Barr nuclear antigen 1)** which binds to human chromosome 11 during infection and breaks chromosome 11 in half. This creates an unstable genome which can lead to cancers (Frappier 2023).
- *Human papillomavirus* (*HPV*) (Figure 4.2b), a DNA virus that causes most cases of cervical cancer and some cases of oropharyngeal cancers. It is spread by sexual contact, and the risk increases with each additional sexual partner. Subsets of the virus are known, with HPV16 and HPV18 accounting for 70% of cervical cancers.
- *Hepatitis B virus* (*HBV*) (Figure 4.2c) and *hepatitis C virus* (*HCV*) are both causes of **hepatocarcinoma**, a liver cancer (see 'Hepatocellular carcinoma (HCC)', Chapter 8, p. 174) (Murray et al. 2020). In addition, HCV can cause non-Hodgkin lymphoma.
- *Human herpes virus 8* (*HHV8*, a DNA virus) (Figure 4.2d) causes **Kaposi's sarcoma**, a rare skin vascular neoplasm that can spread to become a lymphoma (see 'Vascular tumours', Chapter 13, p. 250). It functions in situations where the immune system is reduced, as in **acquired human deficiency syndrome (AIDS)** (see 'Human immunodeficiency virus, HIV', p. 61).

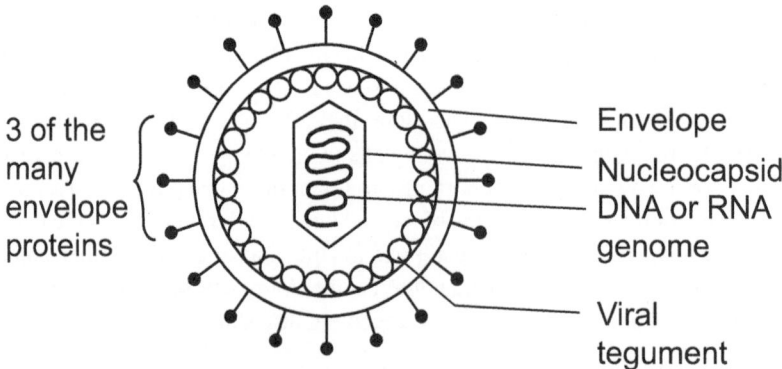

3 of the many envelope proteins

Envelope

Nucleocapsid

DNA or RNA genome

Viral tegument

FIGURE 4.1 The basic structure of a virion. This consists of an internal protein nucleocapsid containing either DNA or RNA. The core is surrounded by a lipid envelope with an inner layer of tegument. On the surface are various proteins which have a range of functions, including some acting as receptors for binding substances and others necessary to gain entry to a host cell.

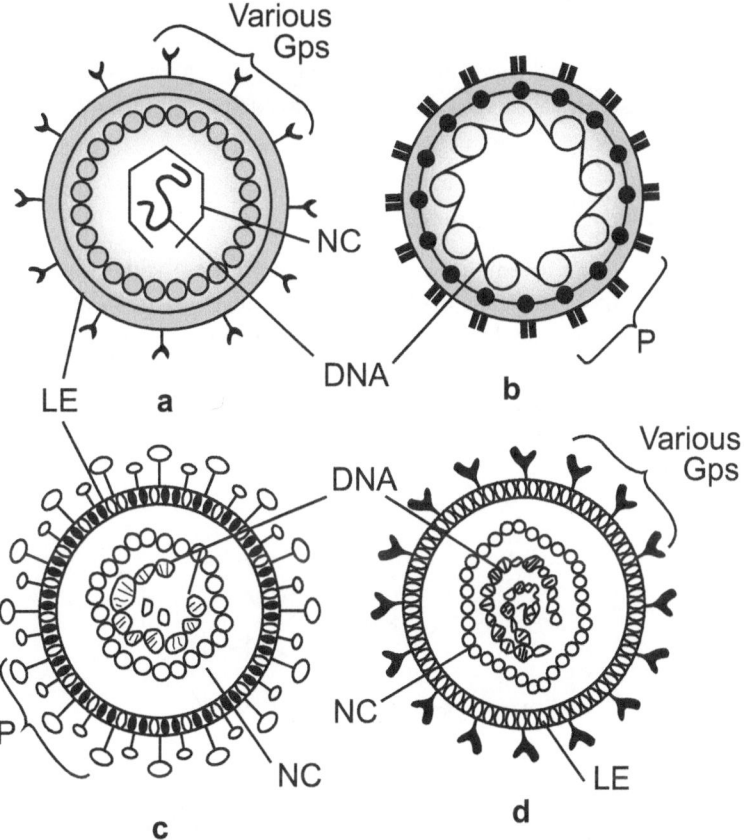

FIGURE 4.2   Four DNA cancer-causing virions: (a) EB virus; (b) human papillomavirus (HPV); (c) hepatitis B virus (HBV), (d) human herpes virus (HHV8). All four are DNA viruses. *GPs* = glycoproteins; *LE* = lipid envelope; *NC* = nucleocapsid; *P* = proteins.

RNA viruses

- *Human T cell lymphotropic virus type 1* (*HTLV-1*) is the only RNA retrovirus known to cause cancer in humans. It can cause **adult T cell leukaemia** (**ATL**) in about 2% to 5% of infected patients and is linked to lymphoma.
- *Human immunodeficiency virus* (*HIV*), an RNA retrovirus that does not cause cancer itself but weakens the immune system, and this increases the risk of malignancies caused by other viruses. It causes **acquired immunodeficiency syndrome** (**AIDS**), which increases the risk of **Kaposi's sarcoma** (see 'Human herpes virus 8 (HHV8)', p. 250, and 'Vascular tumours', Chapter 13, p. 250), **non-Hodgkin lymphoma** (see 'Non-Hodgkin lymphoma', Chapter 7, p. 144), and **Epstein–Barr virus–related lymphoma** (see 'Epstein–Barr virus', 'Human herpes virus 4, HHV4', p. 60).

Note 1: This list identifies different human herpes virus (HHV) by a numbering system (e.g. HHV2, HHV4, etc.), and the numbers not shown are those types that are not involved in human cancers.

Note 2: Retroviruses are so called because they have RNA cores that are used by the virus to create a DNA copy, a process that is a reversal of the normal process of generating an RNA copy from DNA (*retro* = backward). It must first copy its RNA into DNA using the enzyme **reverse transcriptase**. Once the viral DNA copy is available, it follows the mechanism seen in DNA viruses.

The mechanism by which a virus causes cancer

Viruses cause cancer by first invading a cell, a hijacking process which usually requires the virion to fuse with the outer membrane on the host cell surface (Figure 4.3). The cell will then engulf the virus into the cytoplasm by a process called **endocytosis**, that is, the invagination of the virus into a vacuole with the cytoplasm. The virion will de-coat, that is, strip off the outer protein coat, a process carried out by the cell's own lysosomal enzymes. This exposes the nucleic acid core, which can now be accessed for replication.

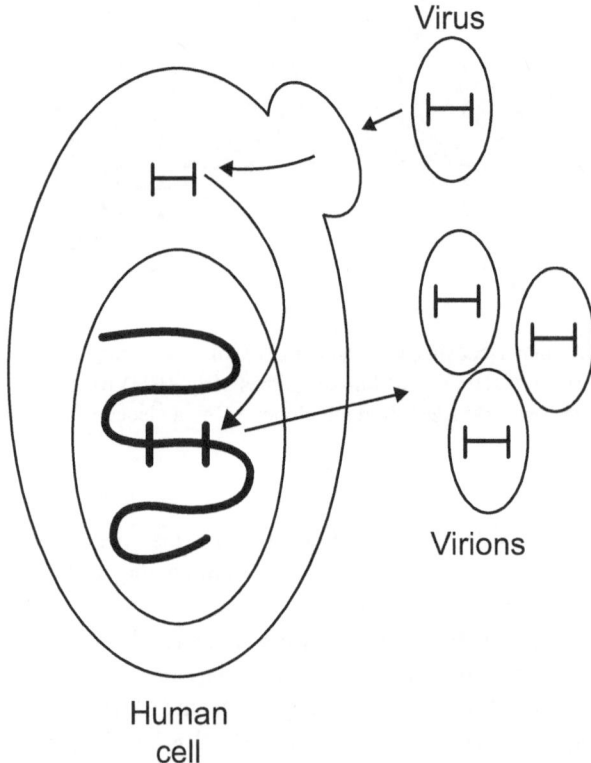

FIGURE 4.3 The creation of a viral provirus. The virion infects the cell and releases the viral genetic material. Only DNA can be inserted into DNA, so if the viral genetic material is RNA, a DNA copy is made first. The viral DNA is incorporated into the host DNA within the nucleus of the cell. Here it is called a provirus. Activation of this provirus causes production of new virions, and these leave the cell, taking copies of the viral genetic material with them.

Some RNA viruses can produce messenger RNA, which can then be directly used to produce viral proteins by the ribosomes, thus bypassing the nucleus. Retroviruses can also make a DNA copy of the viral RNA genome for incorporation into the host genome, creating a **provirus**. DNA viruses can simply copy the viral genome to produce a provirus. The provirus is a stretch of viral DNA placed within the host's normal DNA.

V-onc, provirus and viral replication

Proviruses can remain dormant for various time spans, sometimes for many years, or begin the process of viral replication immediately. The mechanism involved in activating a provirus is not fully understood. Eventually, the provirus will start the process of viral protein replication. This is the same as for the host cell proteins (see 'Genes and protein synthesis', Chapter 2, p. 25). The difference is that the ribosomes are producing viral proteins, which can then be assembled into new virions. These will burst free from the host cell and maybe infect other cells. The eruption of the virions is likely to kill the host cell.

This is how viral infections, such as the common cold, spread throughout the body. But to cause cancer requires additional processing only seen in the specific virions listed earlier. These particular virions may take on board a copy of a gene from the host cell that controls growth,

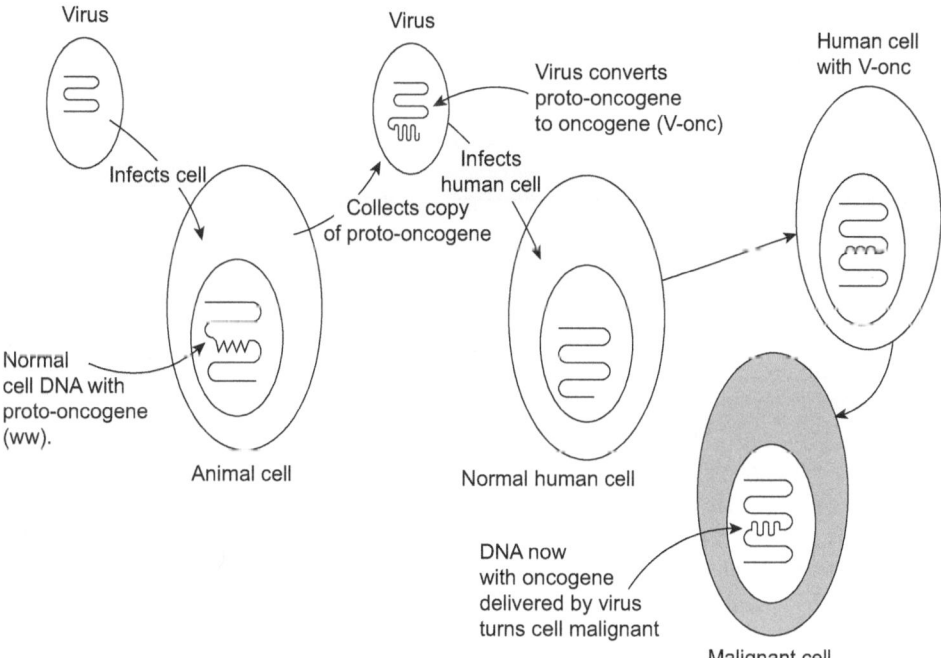

FIGURE 4.4 A virus causes cancer by first infecting an animal cell. The new virions produced pick up one of the animal proto-oncogenes and incorporate it into the viral genetic material. The virus then converts the proto-oncogene to an oncogene (mutation) and then infects a human cell. The oncogene is implanted into the human DNA, and it triggers malignancy in that cell.

that is, a gene called a **proto-oncogene** (see 'Genes and tumour development', Chapter 2, p. 25). These genes control growth in the cell, but the copy taken by the virion can be altered (or mutated) to create an **oncogene**. In a virus, this is known as a **v-onc**, or viral oncogene.

For the virus to use the cell for its own purpose of replication, the virus must ensure three things:

1. The cell will proceed through its own cell cycle, which involves it moving into S phase, and not get held up in the G_1 phase (see Figure 1.6, Chapter 1, p. 7).
2. The virus must prevent the cell from going into apoptosis so it will not die.
3. The virus will induce inflammatory processes and increase growth pathways.

The virion is not only responsible for this change but can also be spread by the virus through cross-infection to other people and lodge in the new host cell. The provirus will then introduce a potentially cancer-causing oncogene (the v-onc) into the new host. Examples of this process have also been recorded, where a virion has introduced oncogenes into human cells which were originally animal proto-oncogenes as a result of cross-infection from non-humans to humans

Viral therapy for cancers

Since virions are excellent carriers of genes and excellent at transplanting those genes into cells, especially modified virions could be used to deliver treatment to kill malignant cells. These are referred to as **oncolytic viruses (OVs)**. There are various approaches to this form of treatment; for example, some viruses kill the malignant cells directly, whilst others recruit the immune system to kill the cells, or do both (Roberts 2022). Oncolytic viruses take advantage of the differences between cancer cells and normal cells, so they attack and kill only cancer cells. Viruses replicate within cells, and on erupting from the cell, the cell dies (see 'Provirus and viral replication', p. 63).

They may be natural viruses or genetically engineered:

- An example of a natural human virus is the *reovirus* that attacks cancer cells having defective *Ras* cell signalling pathways. The *Ras* family of genes includes *NRAS* (chromosome 1), *HRAS* (chromosome 11), and *KRAS* (chromosomes 12) (see Addendum, p. 342, 352, and 353, respectively). Mutations of the *Ras* gene family render cancer cells more susceptible to *reovirus* infection, and such mutations are found in 20% to 30% of cancers generally, and up to 90% of pancreatic, lung, and colon cancers.
- An example of a genetically modified virus is the *adenovirus* called **Onyx-015**. The unmodified virus only replicates in human cells because it has a gene that inactivates the protein p53 (see 'Gene TP53, chromosome 17', Addendum, p. 356). Modification of the virus removes this gene so it is unable to replicate in normal cells. Cancer cells of many kinds actively disable *TP53*, and therefore, the only cells Onyx-015 can replicate in are cancer cells.

Once oncolytic viruses have replicated within cancer cells, they erupt from the cells. The newly released viruses then infect other cancer cells, and the process is repeated (Figure 4.5). But a secondary effect is just as important. The burst cancer cells release their contents into the surrounding environment. The contents include viral proteins and tumour antigens. This release causes a large response from immune cells in the environment, notably T cells and macrophages (Figure 7.2, Chapter 7, p. 131), which are then primed to attack and kill other cancer cells that

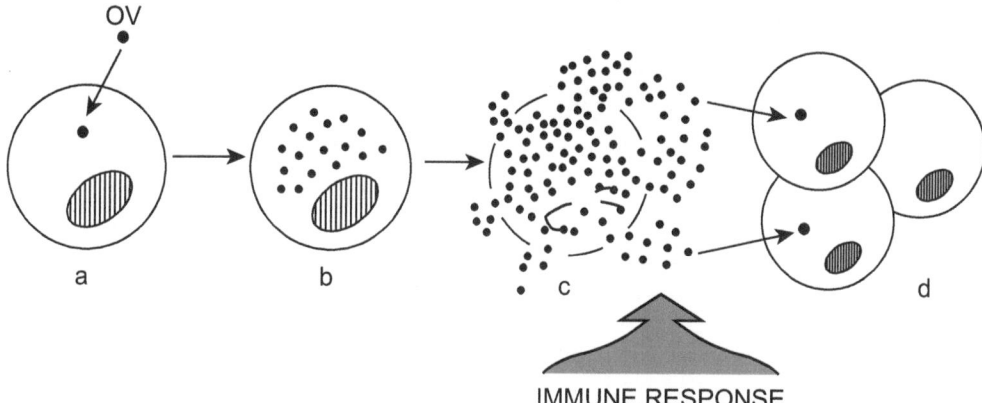

FIGURE 4.5 Oncolytic virus (OV) action: (a) The OV is introduced into the tumour and infects the cancer cell. (b) The OV replicates within the cancer cell. (c) The cancer cell erupts and dies, releasing thousands of new OVs. The release of many OVs triggers an immune response. (d) Other cancer cells get infected by the newly replicated OVs, and the process repeats.

also have these antigens. This creates a huge boost to the local and systemic immune system (Figure 4.5).

The problem is that T cell activity diminishes with time for various reasons, and the immune response may then decline. This is sometimes referred to as *T cell exhaustion*. To maintain the good work started by the viruses, a hormone called **leptin** was found to support T cell activity. Leptin is normally associated with the regulation of food intake and body weight. However, T cells also need leptin to function normally. Cancer cells appear to have low leptin levels, and T cells have high levels of the leptin receptors that bind leptin. Providing additional leptin increases T cell activity. This is achieved by adding the leptin gene to the oncolytic virus. This forces the cancer cell to produce leptin. Increased leptin levels inside the cancer cell provide the leptin needed by the T cell.

It is hoped that trials like this will develop products available for clinical treatment within a few years. Such oncolytic virus treatment is likely to be very effective when used in combination with other existing therapies. Also, viral vaccines have been in use for many years now, and vaccine technology is at an advanced stage. Therefore, it is hoped that oncolytic viruses can be available as vaccines for individuals that are at risk of certain cancers, such as melanoma (see 'Viral vector vaccines', Chapter 5, p. 108).

Hormones

Growth is partly triggered and modified by biochemical agents called **hormones** (Table 4.1).

Hormones are produced by glands of the **endocrine system**. The name *endocrine* means that the glandular product goes directly into the blood. Hormones are of two types:

1. Proteins, derived from amino acids
2. Steroids, derived either from fatty acids or cholesterol

TABLE 4.1 The hormones related to growth in humans

	Glandular origins	*Function related to growth*
Protein hormones		
Growth hormone	Anterior pituitary	Promotes growth and anabolism in normal cells
Thyroid hormones (T$_3$ and T$_4$)	Thyroid gland	Promotes metabolism essential for normal growth
Insulin	Pancreatic islet (beta cells)	Promotes glucose uptake by cells (energy source for growth), and promotes protein synthesis
Parathyroid hormone	Parathyroid gland	Regulates bone growth (together with calcitonin) by controlling calcium levels in blood
Calcitonin (or calcitriol)	Thyroid gland	Regulates blood calcium levels (with parathyroid hormone), controlling bone growth
Steroidal hormones		
Cortisol	Adrenal cortex	Regulates metabolism, including energy uptake required for growth;
Female oestrogen and male testosterone	Female ovary and male testes; small quantities from the adrenal cortex.	promotes bone and muscle growth and reproductive development

Hormones travel in the blood to all parts of the body from the gland where they were produced but only affect the cells and organs that have receptors that can bind that hormone, that is, the **target organs** (Figure 4.6). They regulate cellular activity, including cellular reproduction and development, by activating genes that encode for further protein production. This is cellular signalling, and it involves hormone synthesis and secretion, transportation in the blood, recognition of specific receptors and binding to those receptors, relay of the signal through the cytoplasm to the nucleus, and transcription of genes. Finally, the hormones must be broken up and removed in order to prevent their overactivity.

Protein hormones

As with all proteins, these hormones are synthesised from amino acids. They are encoded by genes within the specific glandular cells, and they pass through the regular protein synthesis process (see Figure 2.1, Chapter 2, p. 26). After they have reached their target cells, they bind to cell surface receptors. This triggers the internal cellular process of signalling the genes to begin their activity related to growth (Figure 4.7).

Steroidal hormones

Steroids are produced by specific glandular cells using cholesterol as the substrate[1] (Figure 4.8).

Steroidal hormones are lipid-based and tend to be smaller than protein hormones, so they can pass through the outer membrane of the cell, a phospholipid layer, and bind to receptors inside the cytoplasm, or even inside the nucleus. Protein hormones are too large to cross the membrane and must bind to cell surface receptors (Figure 4.9).

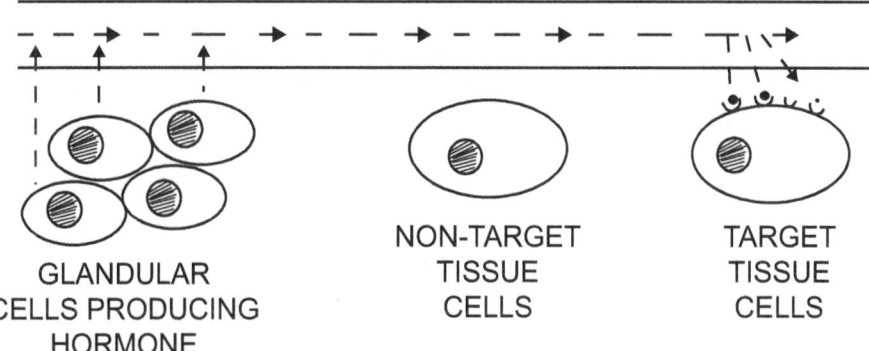

FIGURE 4.6   Hormones from gland to cells. Glandular cells secrete hormone into the blood, which carries it around the body. Those tissue cells without receptors for binding the hormone are not the target of the hormone and thus remain unaffected. Target tissue cells, that is, those cells with receptors, bind the hormone, and this causes activity of these tissues, for example, gene transcription and protein synthesis.

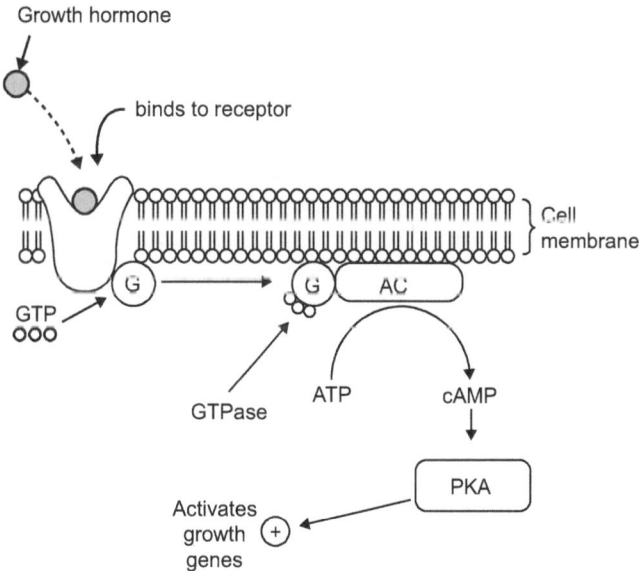

FIGURE 4.7   The effect of growth hormone. On binding to the receptor, growth hormone activates a G protein by binding guanosine triphosphate (GTP). This combined G protein with GTP then activates adenylyl cyclase (AC). Both the G protein and AC are membrane-bound. To get the message to the nucleus, AC must produce cyclic adenosine monophosphate (cAMP) from adenosine triphosphate (ATP). cAMP conveys the message to phosphokinase A (PKA), which activates growth genes.

Source: Simplified from Figure 2.2, Chapter 2, p. 28.

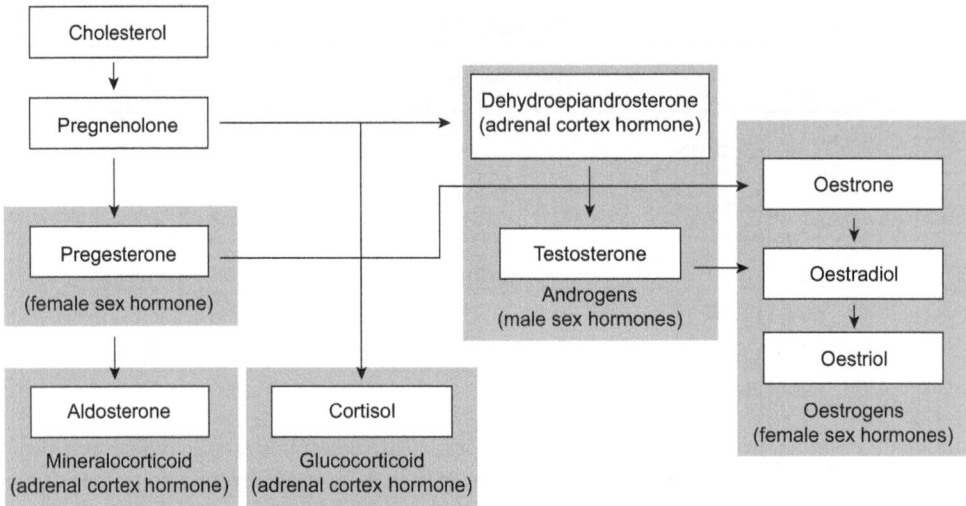

FIGURE 4.8 Synthesis of steroidal hormones. These hormones come from cholesterol in the adrenal cortex (mineralocorticoids and glucocorticoids), and in the ovaries and testes (oestrogens [♀] and androgens [♂]). The arrows in the diagram show the conversion of one product to the next, a process that requires enzymes. Aldosterone conserves sodium from the renal tubule, and cortisol has wide-ranging functions, including an anti-inflammatory and anti-stress role, and helps maintain blood pressure. The sex hormones (androgens and oestrogens) also have wide-ranging effects on bone and muscle growth and development, and they are essential for the development of the genitalia and maintenance of the functions of the ovaries and testes.

Source: After Blows (2022).

Once the steroid hormone has locked onto a receptor, the two components together form a 'hormone–receptor complex'. This complex then binds to the 'gene promoter' DNA sequence of the target gene. Gene promoters are short portions of DNA adjacent to a gene. If the promoter is activated, for example, when a hormone–receptor complex binds, this starts the replication of that gene, leading to protein synthesis (Figure 4.10).

Pituitary gland

The production of hormones is largely controlled by other hormones produced in the pituitary, a small gland at the base of the brain. This is further controlled by the hypothalamus, part of the brain connected to the pituitary by the pituitary stalk (Figure 4.11). Pituitary gland hormones (Table 4.2) are also released directly into the blood and have their own target organs and cells.

The hypothalamus is in ultimate control of two major hormonal systems. Both systems act via the pituitary gland (Figure 4.12). They are:

1. **The hypothalamic-pituitary-adrenal (HPA) axis**, which results in cortisol release from the adrenal cortex (Table 4.1)

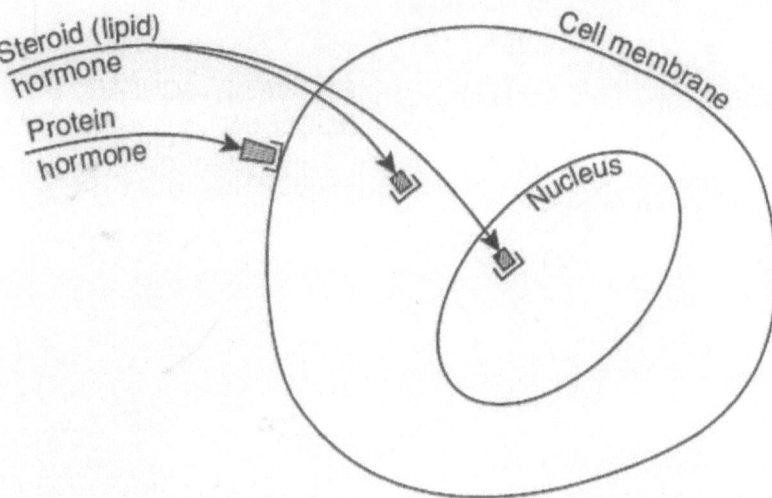

FIGURE 4.9 Hormones and receptors. Protein hormones are too large to enter the cell, so they bind to the surface receptor. Steroid hormones are smaller and are based on lipids, the same as the cell membranes, so they can enter the cell and bind to receptors in the cytoplasm or nucleus.

Source: After Blows (2022).

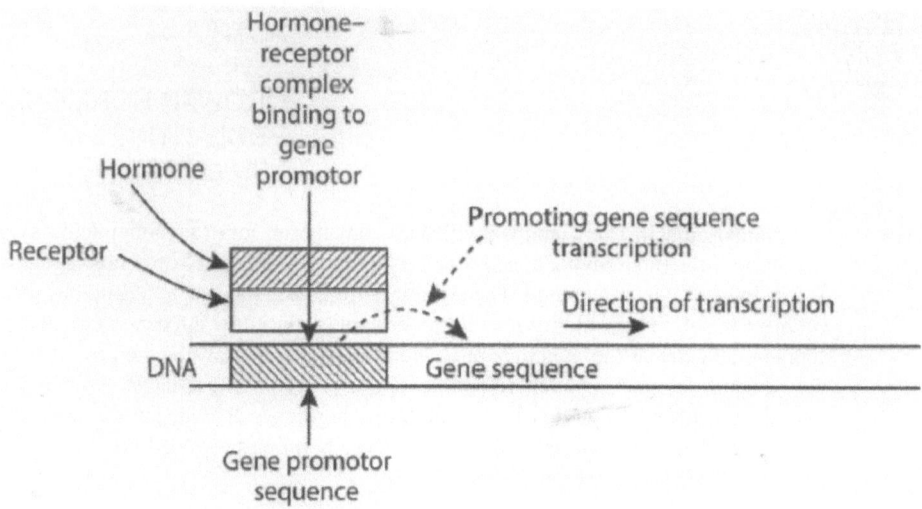

FIGURE 4.10 The steroid hormone–receptor complex. This binds to the gene promoter sequence next to the required gene. The promoter sequence then triggers the start of gene transcription, that is, replication of the gene as the first stage of protein synthesis (see also Figure 2.1, Chapter 2).

Source: After Blows (2022).

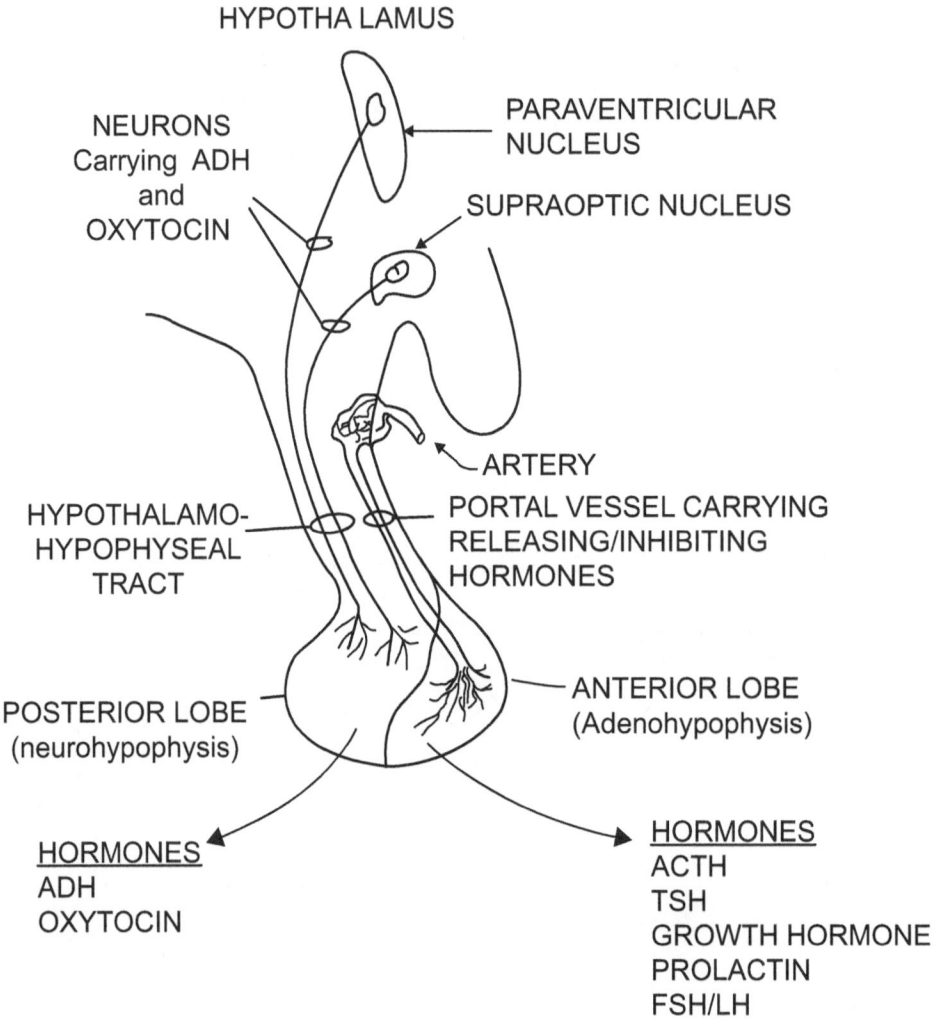

HYPOTHALAMUS

PARAVENTRICULAR NUCLEUS

NEURONS Carrying ADH and OXYTOCIN

SUPRAOPTIC NUCLEUS

ARTERY

PORTAL VESSEL CARRYING RELEASING/INHIBITING HORMONES

HYPOTHALAMO-HYPOPHYSEAL TRACT

ANTERIOR LOBE (Adenohypophysis)

POSTERIOR LOBE (neurohypophysis)

HORMONES
ADH
OXYTOCIN

HORMONES
ACTH
TSH
GROWTH HORMONE
PROLACTIN
FSH/LH

FIGURE 4.11 The pituitary gland. This gland is divided into an anterior lobe (adenohypophysis) and a posterior lobe (neurohypophysis). Each lobe releases different hormones (as shown, and in Table 4.2) into the blood. The hormones from each lobe are controlled by different mechanisms. The posterior lobe hormones are produced by the paraventricular and supraoptic nuclei of the hypothalamus and drain down neurons to the posterior lobe before being released. The anterior lobe hormones are produced in the anterior lobe, but this is controlled by releasing or inhibiting hormones arriving in the blood from the hypothalamus via a portal vein.[2] One of these hormones is gonadotropin-releasing hormone (GnRH) (see 'Hormonal therapy', p. 71).

Source: Modified from Blows (2022).

2. **The hypothalamic-pituitary-thyroid (HPT) axis,** which results in the release of thyroid hormones T_3 (triiodothyronine) and T_4 (tetraiodothyronine) (Table 4.1)

The pituitary gland and hypothalamus together control the hormonal balance by **negative feedback systems**.[3] They measure the amount of hormone in the blood and control the amount

TABLE 4.2 The pituitary hormones, the lobes they come from, their target organs and functions

Hormone	Pituitary lobe	Target organ	Function
Antidiuretic hormone (ADH)	Posterior	Kidney	Conserves water from the renal tubules
Oxytocin	Posterior	Uterus	Promotes labour during delivery
Adrenocorticotrophic hormone (ACTH)	Anterior	Adrenal cortex	Stimulates cortisol production
Thyroid-stimulating hormone (TSH)	Anterior	Thyroid gland	Promotes metabolism essential for growth
Growth hormone	Anterior	All growing tissues	Promotes growth, especially during childhood
Prolactin	Anterior	Female breasts	Promotes breast milk
Follicle-stimulating hormone (FSH)	Anterior	Ovaries and testes	Promotes development of the ova and the sperm
Luteinising hormone (LH)	Anterior	Ovaries and testes	Promotes ovulation and testosterone production

released sufficiently to stabilise the normal blood levels. They do this by adjusting the level of pituitary hormones released. In this manner, the blood level of any hormone should not be too high or too low. If abnormally high or low levels are discovered by blood tests, the problem may be over- or underproduction of the gland that produces that hormone or a problem with the pituitary gland (see 'Pituitary tumours', Chapter 14, p. 71).

Hormonal treatment of cancers

The sex hormones are the **oestrogens** (female) and **androgens** (male). These are discussed in the relevant chapters (see 'Introduction: the oestrogens', Chapters 11, p. 206, and 'Introduction: The androgens', Chapter 12, p. 229). **Oestradiol** is the most potent of the oestrogens, and the most potent androgen is **testosterone**. These hormones promote normal cellular and tissue growth and development. The same will happen with cancer cells that respond to these hormones because they have the relevant receptors, that is, they often increase the rate of tumour development. Hormones can sometimes act as carcinogens, that is, they can contribute towards the causation and promotion of certain tumours. These are notably breast cancers, but also endometrial and ovarian tumours in women, prostate and testes tumours in men, and thyroid tumours in both sexes. Oestrogen can initiate and promote breast cancer progression. Prolonged exposure to oestrogen, such as in hormonal replacement therapy (HRT) and through oral contraceptives, increases the risk of breast cancer (Pecorino 2021).

Tumour cells with oestrogen receptors are said to be **ER+**, that is, **oestrogen receptor positive**, and they may also be **progesterone receptors** positive (**PgR+**) as well. Male cancer cells may be **testosterone receptor positive** (**TR+**), particularly those cancers associated with the reproductive tract.

Hormonal therapy is the use of drugs to reduce the effects of hormones (notably oestradiol) that would otherwise promote breast cancer growth. Anti-oestrogens (Table 4.3) work by binding to the oestrogen receptors (ER) in breast cells that are ER positive (ER+) (see 'Breast cancer', Chapter 11, p. 208), and this prevents the oestrogens from binding and therefore eliminates the growth these hormones would promote. The difficulty is that in breast cancers, not all

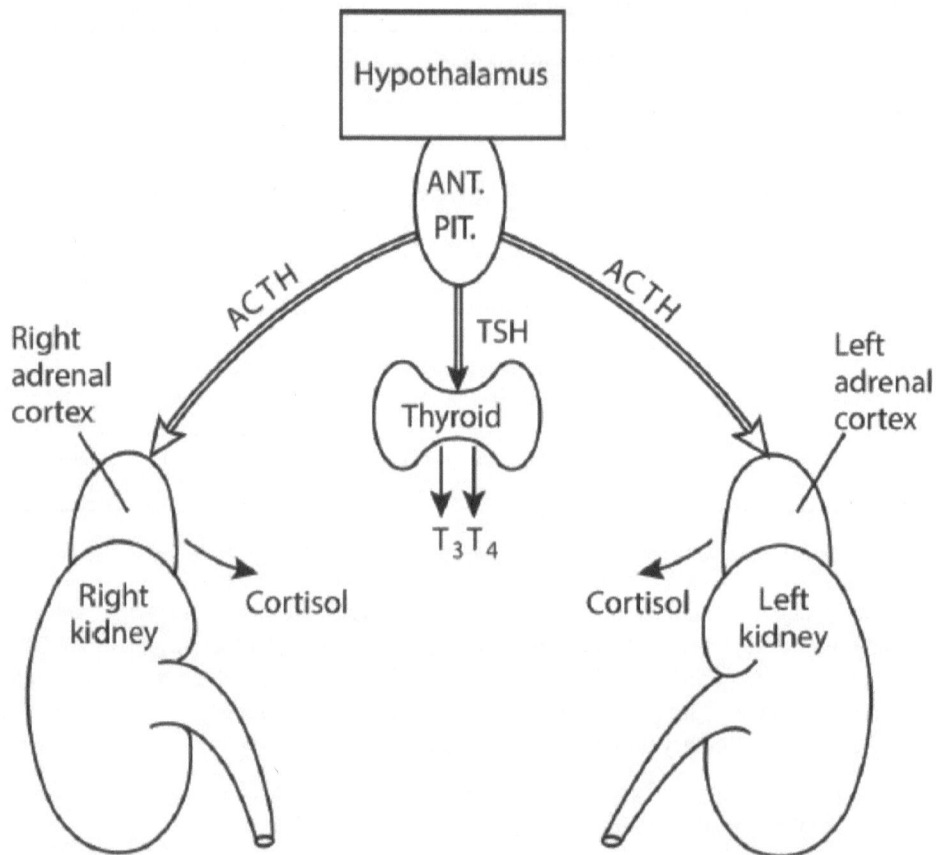

FIGURE 4.12   The HPA and HPT axes. The hypothalamic-pituitary-adrenal (HPA) axis is where ACTH releases cortisol from the adrenal gland on top of the kidney, and the hypothalamic-pituitary-thyroid (HPT) axis is where TSH releases thyroid hormone (T_3 and T_4) from the thyroid gland that is positioned below the larynx.

Source: After Blows (2022).

malignant cells are ER+. Many cells may be oestrogen receptor negative (ER−, that is, without ER) and therefore would not respond to this type of treatment. Some tumours are a mix of ER+ with ER− cells, and since only ER+ cells respond to anti-oestrogen treatment, the tumour may regress but not respond completely. Another approach is the use of drugs that reduce the amount of oestrogen produced, that is, the aromatase inhibitors. Given that not all breast cancers will respond to hormonal therapy, it is considered as an adjunct (or additional) therapy alongside other treatments.

The drugs used in hormonal therapy are (Table 4.3):

- **Anti-oestrogens**, used in ER+ breast cancer, are **tamoxifen**, **fulvestrant**, and **toremifene**. They block oestrogen receptors to prevent oestrogen from binding. They may be used in prophylaxis to prevent further malignant growth in the breast after the tumour, and any spread of the disease, has been eradicated.

- **Aromatase inhibitors** are drugs that block the function of **aromatase**, an enzyme that converts the androgens to oestrogens (Figure 4.13). This significantly reduces the amount of oestrogen produced. These drugs are **anastrozole**, **exemestane**, and **letrozole**. Anastrozole not only treats breast cancer but can also now be given as a preventative measure, that is, prophylaxis, in women at high risk of the disease. This means those women with a family history of carrying the BRCA1 or BRCA2 gene mutations (see 'The genetics of breast cancer', Chapter 11, p. 216). In this preventative role, anastrozole works better than tamoxifen, with fewer side effects.
- **Progesterone therapy** is used to relieve symptoms in women with advanced breast disease involving metastatic spread that is not responding to other treatments. Progesterone cannot be given directly by mouth but is given orally as a precursor, called a **progestogen** (the drug is **megestrol acetate**).

TABLE 4.3 Drugs used in hormonal therapy

Drug	Mode of action	Cancer treated
Abiraterone acetate	Anti-androgen	Prostate cancer
Apalutamide	Anti-androgen	Prostate cancer
Bicalutamide	Anti-androgen	Prostate cancer
Darolutamide	Anti-androgen	Prostate cancer
Enzalutamide	Anti-androgen	Prostate cancer
Flutamide	Anti-androgen	Prostate cancer
Fulvestrant	Anti-oestrogen	ER+ breast cancer
Tamoxifen	Anti-oestrogen	ER+ breast cancer
Toremifene	Anti-oestrogen	ER+ breast cancer
Anastrozole	Aromatase inhibitor	ER+ breast cancer
Exemestane	Aromatase inhibitor	ER+ breast cancer
Letrozole	Aromatase inhibitor	ER+ breast cancer
Diethylstilbestrol	Synthetic oestrogen	Breast cancer (post-menopausal); prostate cancer
Degarelix	Anti-gonadotropin-releasing hormone	Prostate cancer
Relugolix	Anti-gonadotropin-releasing hormone	Prostate cancer
Lanreotide	Somatostatin analogue	Neuroendocrine tumours
Octreotide	Somatostatin analogue	Neuroendocrine tumours
Megestrol acetate	Synthetic progestogen	Breast cancer

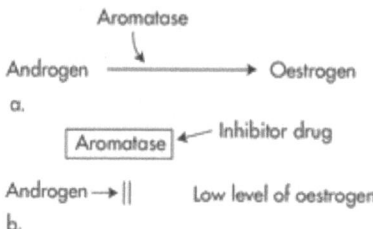

FIGURE 4.13   Aromatase inhibitors: (a) The enzyme aromatase converts androgens to oestrogen. (b) Aromatase inhibitor drugs block the enzyme and therefore reduce the oestrogen levels (see also Figure 11.7, Chapter 11, p. 220).

- **Anti-androgen** drugs (Table 4.3) are used to treat prostate cancer. Similar to oestrogen, androgens promote cell growth in males, notably the reproductive system, including the prostate. By blocking androgen receptors, the growth effect of androgens is reduced.
- **Anti-gonadotropin-releasing hormone (anti-GnRH)** drugs, that is, **degarelix** and **relugolix**, block the release of the gonadotropins **follicle-stimulating hormone (FSH)** and **luteinising hormone (LH)** from the **anterior pituitary** (Figure 4.11). In males, LH normally promotes testosterone production from the testes (Table 4.2). GnRH comes from the hypothalamus, and by blocking GnRH, the release of LH is reduced. Less LH reduces testosterone production from the testes. Many forms of prostate cancer thrive on testosterone as a growth factor, and by reducing testosterone in circulation, these drugs prevent testosterone stimulation of cancer growth.
- **Somatostatin analogue** drugs (Table 4.3) enhance the action of the natural **somatostatin**, which is produced by the hypothalamus, the stomach, the pancreas, and the bowel.

Some of the normal somatostatin functions are:

1. *Inhibiting* other hormones, that is, it reduces insulin and digestive hormone production.
2. *Controlling* stomach and bowel emptying.
3. *Blocking* growth hormone release from the pituitary gland (Table 4.2).
4. *Preventing* the fast reproduction of cells.

The somatostatin analogue drugs lanreotide and octreotide enhance these activities, and by increasing functions 3 and 4 on this list, they help slow down tumour growth. They are especially useful in controlling the symptoms of **carcinoid syndrome** (see 'Carcinoid syndrome', p. 74).

Carcinoid syndrome[4]

Some neuroendocrine tumours (NETs) are responsible for the production of large quantities of hormones and other proteins, more than what is normally required. This particularly applies to **serotonin**. This substance is normally involved in a wide range of physiological processes, such as multiple brain activities, for example, sleep, memory, pain, and learning, and numerous body activities, for example, biological rhythms, feeding, temperature regulation, movement, sexual activity, and social behaviour. Excessive amounts of serotonin and hormones, found in the blood from NETs, cause the following symptoms:

- Unpredictable skin flushing of the neck, face, and chest (occurs in 80% of people with carcinoid syndrome)
- Diarrhoea, often three times or more per day (occurs in 70% of people with carcinoid syndrome)
- Abdominal pain, palpitations, oedema of the lower limbs, and wheezing
- **Telangiectasis**, which are red marks on the skin due to bleeding from damaged skin capillaries

Cancers of the endocrine system

Pituitary gland tumours

Pituitary neuroendocrine tumours (PitNET) are mostly slow-growing benign adenomas. They are grouped into two types: those that produce hormones causing hormonal excess, that is, *secreting adenomas* (Table 4.2), and those that do not produce hormones, that is, *non-secreting adenomas*. Together they account for around 17% of brain tumours.

Symptoms of secreting adenomas are dependent on which hormone, if any, is produced in excess:

- **Prolactinomas** produce too much prolactin. They are the most common type of secreting pituitary tumours. In women, they cause excess milk production and menstruation failure, infertility, and reduced libido. In men, they can cause erectile problems.
- **Somatotroph adenomas** produce excess growth hormone. This can cause a condition called **acromegaly**, with overgrowth of feet, hand, and lower jaw in adults and excessive growth spurts in children.
- **Corticotroph adenomas** produce excess ACTH, which overstimulates the adrenal gland to produce too much cortisol. This results in the symptoms of **Cushing syndrome**, that is, weight gain, raised blood pressure, and a red rounded face.
- **Thyrotroph adenomas** produce too much TSH, which causes the thyroid gland to produce excess thyroid hormones, T3 and T4. The result is **hyperthyroidism**, the symptoms of which are weight loss, tremor, palpitations, and sweating.

Non-secreting adenomas are usually larger than secreting tumours, and they put increasing pressure on surrounding tissues, not least on the normal part of the pituitary gland, and disturbing its functions. Pressure can also occur on other tissues, causing headache, especially on the optic nerve, causing vision loss.

Thyroid gland tumours

Thyroid gland tumours occur in various forms, depending on which of the two main types of cells it originates from. The cell types are *follicular cells* and *parafollicular (C') cells*, which produce the hormone calcitonin (Table 4.1). These tumours include:

- **Papillary thyroid cancer**, the commonest form, is derived from follicular cells. It is more common in women in their 30s and 40s. It is slow-growing, and if metastases do occur, they are likely to spread to the neck lymph nodes.
- **Follicular thyroid cancer** is also derived from follicular cells. It most common in women aged 40 to 60 years. Metastases can occur in the lungs or the bones.
- **Oncocytic cell (Hürthle cell) thyroid cancer**, also called **oxyphil cell cancer**, is a rare tumour derived from oxyphilic cells, which have some similarities to follicular cells. They can be benign, called **oncocytic adenomas**, or malignant, which can spread to other parts of the body. They are most often found in women older than 40 years.
- **Medullary thyroid cancer** is a rare cancer derived from parafollicular ('C') cells. Most cases (about 75%) are sporadic, meaning, they are not inherited. The remaining 25% are due to an inherited familial gene mutation, the *RET* proto-oncogene (see 'Chromosome 10', Addendum, p. 351). The mutation causes the 'C' cells to grow, producing excess calcitonin. This inherited gene is part of the **multiple endocrine neoplasia type 2 (MEN2)** syndrome (see 'Multiple endocrine neoplasms (MEN1 and MEN2)', p. 76), which includes diseases of the parathyroid and adrenal glands. Medullary thyroid cancer can spread to other parts of the body, such as the liver or the lungs.

- **Anaplastic thyroid cancer** (**ATC**) is a rare but highly aggressive tumour that has a poor prognosis. Diagnosis is often made after the spread of metastases. It occurs in about 1–2% of thyroid tumours, mostly seen in women over 60 years old. The cells are strongly undifferentiated and look very abnormal. Treatment options are limited, and the tumour is often resistant to therapy.

Adrenal gland tumours

There are several different adrenal gland tumours which are either benign or malignant. They include:

- **Adrenal adenomas**, which are benign tumours that usually do not have any symptoms.
- **Phaeochromocytomas** are rare tumours forming in the medulla of the gland. Most are benign, but some can become malignant, with metastases spreading to other parts of the body. They often produce too much adrenaline and noradrenaline, the natural hormones from the adrenal medulla. An excess of these hormones can cause symptoms such as sweating, tachycardia (fast heart rate), raised blood pressure, headaches, and anxiety.
- **Adrenal cortical cancer** (**ACC**) is a rare, aggressive cancer of the adrenal cortex that can spread to the lungs, the bones, or the liver. It can sometimes cause excess production of the hormones cortisol and aldosterone, or the sex hormones, that is, oestrogens and androgens (Figure 4.8). This can cause symptoms such as raised blood pressure, diabetes, weight gain, and excess hair growth. ACC can also grow quite large and cause a painful lump in the abdomen.

Multiple endocrine neoplasms (MEN1 and MEN2)

These are rare, inherited gene disorders encompassing cancers of several specific glands. There are two recognised types:

1. **MEN1** (Wermer syndrome) is seen as multiple cancers of the glands. There are more than 20 tumour types that may be involved, but notably tumours of the parathyroid. Also seen are tumours of the pituitary gland, and a tumour affecting the stomach, duodenum, and pancreas, known as a gastroenteropancreatic tumour. They are mostly benign, but some can become malignant.
2. **MEN2** (Sipple syndrome) is dominated by a medullary thyroid tumour (see 'Thyroid gland tumours', 'Medullary thyroid cancer', p. 75) in all cases. This is derived from the thyroid 'C' cells, which do not produce thyroid hormone. In addition, MEN2 includes either an adrenal tumour, called a phaeochromocytoma (see 'Phaeochromocytoma', p. 76), or a hyperparathyroidism, that is, overactive parathyroid glands due, usually, to a tumour or hyperplasia. The tumour may cause excessive release of **parathormone**, a hormone that regulates calcium. Hyperparathyroidism causes brittle bones and calcium deposits in multiple organs.

Key points

Viruses

- Viruses cause the least number of human cancers.
- They spread by way of the respiratory contact (coughing, etc.) or through sexual contact.

- Viruses consist of a protein outer shell with either DNA or RNA core.
- They reproduce inside human cells.
- Some viruses can collect a proto-oncogene from one human cell and mutate it to become a v-oncogene, which then infects another cell and causes malignancy.

Hormones

- Hormones fall into two groups, the protein and steroid (lipid-based) hormones.
- They bind to receptors on target organs or cells.
- The two groups function differently to activate genes related to growth.
- Some hormones are normally involved in activating growth genes, and these can also increase growth in tumours.

Hormonal therapy

- Oestradiol is the most potent of the female hormones, and the most potent male hormone is testosterone.
- These hormones increase the rate of tumour development if the cancer cells have receptors that bind the hormone, that is, are ER+.
- The classes of hormonal therapy drugs are anti-oestrogens, anti-androgens, aromatase inhibitors, anti-gonadotropin-releasing hormones, and somatostatin analogues.
- Synthetic oestrogen and progesterone can be used is specific circumstances.
- Carcinoid syndrome occurs when neuroendocrine tumours (NETs) produce too much hormones and serotonin.

Endocrine cancers

- Endocrine tumours, such as those of the pituitary, thyroid, or adrenal glands, can be benign or malignant.
- Some can produce excess hormones, which is what often causes the symptoms.

Notes

1 *Substrate* is the original substance from which the hormone is derived; in this case, it is cholesterol.
2 A portal vein has capillaries at both ends. Only two exist in the body, that is, the large hepatic portal vein from the gut to the liver (Chapter 8), and the tiny hypothalamo-hypophyseal portal vein within the pituitary stalk, as shown in Figure 4.8.
3 The reason this is *negative* feedback is that the hypothalamus and pituitary will do what they can to reverse what is happening in the blood; that is, if blood hormone levels rise, the hypothalamus/pituitary will try to lower it, and vice versa. This is part of **homeostasis**, the mechanisms adopted by the body to stabilise the internal environment.
4 A *syndrome* is a collection of signs and symptoms that correlate with each other and are usually seen in a specific disorder.

5

IMMUNOLOGY AND IMMUNOTHERAPY

- An introduction to the immune system
- The chemical defences
- Immunotherapy
- Cancer vaccines
- Key points

An introduction to the immune system

To protect the body against potential harm, the immune system is composed of tissue barriers, multiple cells of different types and functions, and a battery of chemical agents.

Immunity can be divided into two main types:

1. **Innate**, or **non-specific immunity**
2. **Adaptive**, also called **acquired** or **specific immunity**

The difference between these two forms is fundamental to our understanding of how our defences work (Figure 5.1).

Innate (non-specific) immunity

This is a system which defends the body against *entry* of unwanted agents. As such, it does not require the agents themselves to be recognised by the system; it just needs to know that these agents are not part of the individual, that is, they are **non-self** and are considered *foreign* to the body. The system then keeps them out of the body, as best as it can, under quite difficult circumstances. There are four categories of non-specific immunity: (1) physical barriers, (2) chemical barriers, (3) cellular barriers, and (4) species differentiation.

1. **Physical barriers** are structures like the skin and mucous membranes. They are therefore mostly on the outside of the body and form an impenetrable layer. **Skin** has an outer

DOI: 10.4324/9781003389125-5

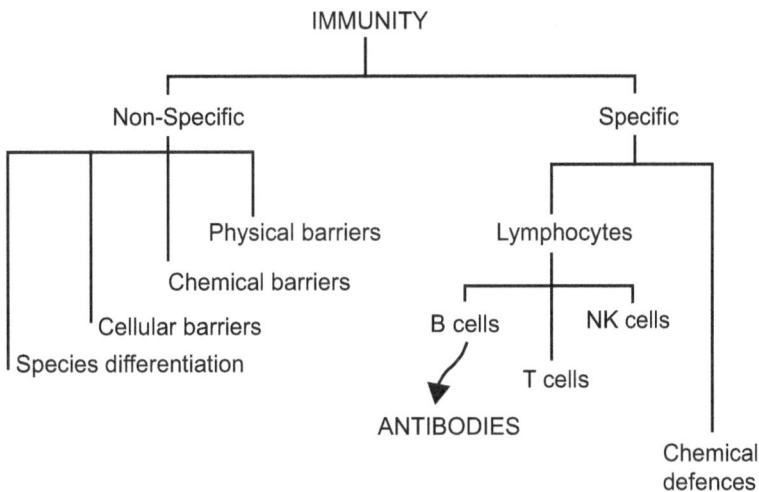

FIGURE 5.1 A classification of the immune system. It is divided into adaptive (specific) and innate (non-specific), and the different components of each part.

layer that consists of **keratinised stratified epithelium** (see 'Structure and function of skin', Chapter 13, p. 241). The very outer layer of this is dead tissue, and as such, it is almost impossible for most organisms to get through this layer. This is despite many organisms living on the surface as **commensals,** that is, organisms that live on the body but cause it no harm. Very few organisms are capable of penetrating intact skin. However, if that outer dead layer of the skin is broken, the defence barrier is lost and the surface commensals would gain entry to deeper layers, where they may possibly become **pathogenic,** that is, a disease-causing organism, and begin the process of setting up an infection. Skin covers about 98% of the body surface, and the gaps caused by various natural openings, for example, the mouth, nose, and others, are similarly protected by mucous membrane.

Unlike the outer layers of skin, mucous membrane is living tissue and is therefore more suitable for lining surfaces inside the body that are daily subjected to outside environmental agents. The best examples of these are the lining of the digestive tract, which is subject to environmental agents in food and drink, and the lining of the respiratory tract, which is subject to environmental agents in the air. Mucous membrane produces the sticky substance **mucus,** which traps these foreign agents and takes steps to eliminate them back to the environment. The lungs are particularly difficult to keep clean from unwanted polluting agents in the air. The mucous membrane of the respiratory tract traps the inhaled agents on the sticky mucus. The cells of the membrane have tiny hair-like structures called **cilia** which sweep repeatedly backwards and forwards, giving a brush-like action, sweeping the mucus, and its trapped agents, upwards towards the throat and out of the lungs. It is known as the **mucociliary escalator,** and it delivers the contaminated mucus to a point in the throat where it can be swallowed. In the stomach, the unwanted agents can be destroyed by the acid conditions there. Smoking paralyses this mucociliary action, and the mucus, laden with harmful agents, drains by gravity further down into the lungs, where it can accumulate and cause harm.

2. **Chemical barriers** include **hydrochloric acid** in the stomach, which has a very low **pH**, that is, a strong acid, and therefore, any unwanted environmental agents that are swallowed, as may be found in food or drink, will be destroyed by the acid before entering the body.[1]

3. **Cellular barriers** are cells that destroy any unwanted foreign agents that get into the body. **Phagocytes** are cells that engulf and destroy the foreign agent. This involves the phagocytes surrounding the foreign agent and taking it into their cytoplasm encased in a membrane. Inside the cytoplasm of the phagocyte are other membrane-bound organelles, called **lysosomes** (see Table 1.1, Chapter 1, p. 5), that contain digestive enzymes. Merging the membrane-bound foreign agent with the lysosomes destroys the foreign agent. **Macrophages** are a major phagocytic cell in both the blood and body tissues. Blood cells called **neutrophils** also have phagocytic activity. Other blood cells are part of the innate immunity, that is, **eosinophils**, which attack invading parasites and are involved in allergies, and **basophils**, which attack bacterial and viral antigens and are involved with allergies and the blood clotting mechanism (see Figure 7.2, Chapter 7, p. 131). **NK (natural killer) cells** are cytotoxic lymphocytes that attack and destroy human cells that are either malignant or virally infected (see 'Natural killer (NK) cells', p. 91). **Mast cells** are present in connective tissue, and they release heparin, which stops blood clotting, and histamine and cytokines, which cause inflammation (Figures 5.4 and 5.12).

4. **Species differentiation** means that certain diseases are suffered by a particular species and not by others. For example, dogs do not catch measles; it's a human disease. The question is why? To catch a disease, it is necessary first for the organisms to **colonise** the body. But this is not enough, as they can be removed, for example, by handwashing with soap, which is an excellent way of removing colonised organisms on the hands.[2] To overcome the possible removal, the organisms must be able to stick to the cells and tissues that they colonise, a process called **adhesion**. If they can stick to the tissues, they stand a chance of invading the body and causing disease. In species differentiation, a particular species is immune from the disease simply because the organisms have no means of sticking to the cells of that species, that is, they are unable to demonstrate adhesion in that species. Sometimes the organism can create certain gene mutations, which increase their sticking ability, and this allows them to adhere to a wider number of species. This is when they have *crossed the species barrier*.

The term *foreign agent* indicates something from the environment that is not part of the body, but not all foreign agents are harmful. Food, for example, is a foreign agent that is both valuable and essential to the body. A better term is **antigen**, which is also a foreign substance, often a protein, but one that causes a reaction from the immune system. In fact, the term **immune response** means the reaction between the body's immune system and an antigen. This immune response, or reaction, is designed to eliminate the antigen from the body as it is seen by the immune system as potentially harmful and must be removed. Antigens are mostly proteins, such as bacteria, viruses, and pollen, but sometimes they are other substances, such as dust particles. It is the nature of the immune response to antigens that is the role of specific immunity.

Adaptive (acquired or specific) immunity

Some cells of the blood plasma and the lymphatic system, called **lymphocytes** (one of our types of **leucocytes**, or **white blood cells**, **WBC**) (see 'Blood cell formation', Chapter 7, p. 130), are genetically triggered to respond to a particular antigen and not to any others. One lymphocyte, for example, may be triggered to respond to the flu virus but will not respond to anything else. There are two types of lymphocytes, B cells and T cells.

B cell lymphocytes

B cell lymphocytes are formed in the bone marrow, where they stay until fully mature. B cell lymphocytes are activated by contact with the antigen to which they are specific. Often, one B cell will be activated in this way, but many more will be needed, and these will be obtained by multiple divisions of the original activated cell. This produces a colony of many thousands of cells, all active against the same specific antigen. B cell lymphocytes, when activated, convert into **plasma cells**, which then start to release proteins called **antibodies** (Figure 5.2).

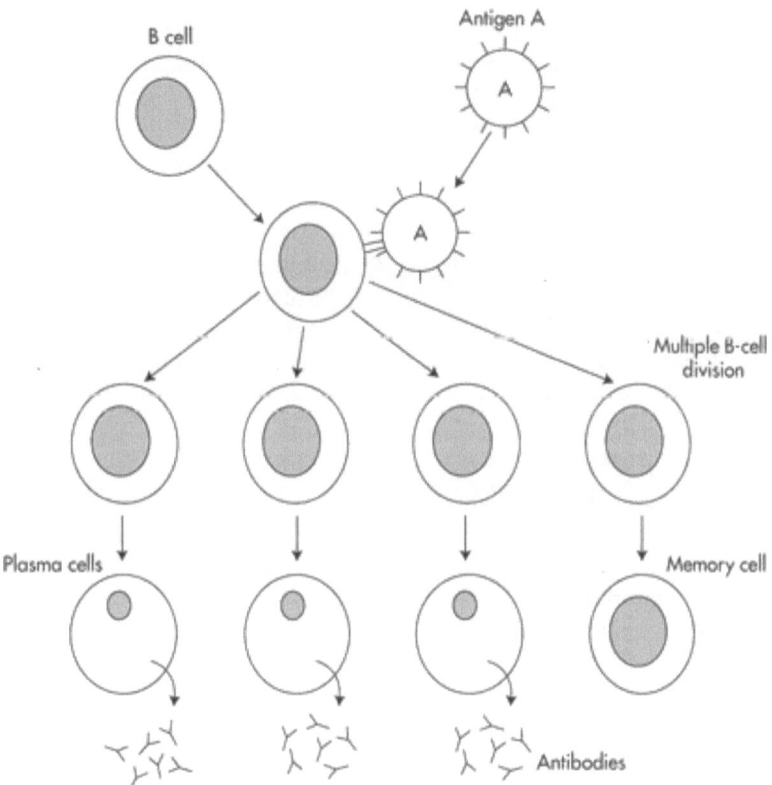

FIGURE 5.2   B cell activation. The B cell shown is specific for antigen A. On meeting with antigen A, the B cell goes through multiplication. The daughter cells mostly become plasma cells that produce antibodies. These antibodies are also specific for antigen A. Some activated B cells will become memory cells.

These antibodies carry the same specificity as the parent B cell, that is, they will bind to the same antigen. This type of immune reaction, that is, using antibodies, is known as **humoral immunity**. By binding to the antigens, antibodies provide a wide range of valuable functions, all of which are important in the fight against the antigens. However, in the case of living antigens, for example, bacteria, they do not actually kill the antigens. This task is left to cells that are dedicated to the role of killing antigens.

Antibodies carry out a range of functions against their specific antigens.

They can:

1. Render many antigens harmless, especially viruses and some **protozoans**, that is, single-cell animals that can sometimes enter the body as an antigen.
2. Neutralise some toxins, for example, **tetanus toxin**, a dangerous poison that causes the disease **tetanus**. This toxin is released by the bacterial organism *Clostridium*.
3. Prevent adhesion of some organisms, and thus, prevent tissue invasion.
4. Immobilise certain antigens, especially bacteria that use tail-like structures called **flagella** to move.
5. Activate the complement system (see 'The complement system', p. 91).
6. Form complexes with antigens, and these complexes become the targets for phagocytosis.

Being proteins, antibodies are also known by the nature of the protein they are made from, namely, **immunoglobulins (Ig)**, which means *globular proteins of the immune system*. There are five main classes (or types) of immunoglobulins: IgA, IgD, IgE, IgG, and IgM.

Immunoglobulin A (IgA) (Figure 5.3) makes up 15–20% of the total blood plasma immunoglobulins. They are important for the protection of surfaces against antigen invasion. IgA is found in various secretions that bathe surfaces, such as lachrymal fluid bathing the surface of the eye, mucus covering the surface of the digestive and respiratory systems, saliva protecting the mouth, breast milk where it protects the surface of the infant's digestive tract, sweat protecting the skin surface, and bile.

Immunoglobulin D (IgD) (Figure 5.3) occurs as a trace quantity within the total blood plasma immunoglobulins. It is found on the surface of many B cell lymphocytes and may have a role in the activation of these B cells.

Immunoglobulin E (IgE) (Figure 5.3) occurs as a trace quantity of the total blood plasma immunoglobulins, but the level is often raised in individuals who suffer from allergies. IgE is different in having the ability to bind not only to antigens but also to **mast cells** at the same time (Figure 5.4). Mast cells are found in many tissue types, and they contain a cocktail of chemicals which induce **inflammation** when released, particularly a chemical called **histamine**. It seems strange that we have stored chemicals that cause inflammation. Inflammation causes pain and discomfort. Histamine, and other similar chemicals, induces inflammation because it is through inflammation that the immune system works properly. By binding to mast cells, IgE can cause the release of the inflammatory chemicals at that moment when the antigen also binds to the IgE (Figure 5.4). In this way, the inflammation coincides with the presence of an unwanted antigen. Increased amounts of IgE lead to an inappropriate amount of mast cell activation and inflammation, as seen in allergic disorders such as hay fever, contact dermatitis, and asthma.

Immunoglobulin G (IgG) (Figure 5.3) accounts for 70–75% of the total blood plasma immunoglobulins. It is the second antibody to respond to infections getting into the body but is the most important of the antibodies in the fight against infection. It is mostly found in blood plasma

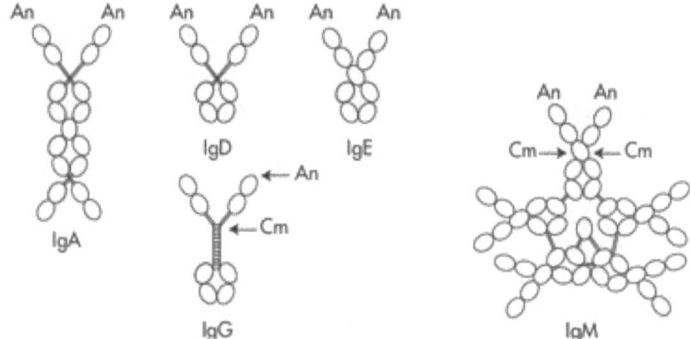

FIGURE 5.3 The five classes of immunoglobulins (antibodies). The antigen-binding sites (An) occur at the ends of the molecule, and the complement binding sites (Cm) are at the hinge area.

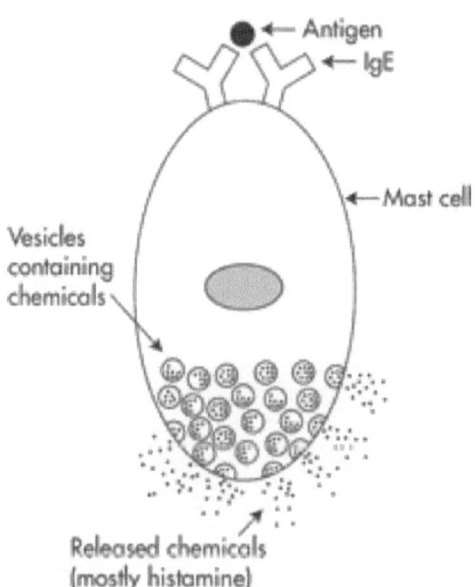

FIGURE 5.4 Chemical release from a mast cell. Two IgE molecules are cross-linked by a binding antigen on the surface of a mast cell. This causes the release of chemicals, particularly histamine, from the mast cell.

and tissue fluids. It crosses the placenta and provides immunity for the unborn child during pregnancy and remains in the child's blood, providing up to nine months' immunity following birth.

Immunoglobulin M (IgM) (Figure 5.3) accounts for 10% of the total blood plasma immunoglobulins. It is the first antibody to respond to an infection, but being a large molecule, it is confined to the blood. It therefore is unable to fight the infection in tissue fluid, which then becomes the role of IgG. The initial surge in IgM at the start of an infection usually gives way to IgG when levels of this secondary antibody are raised enough. IgM is, however, the best antibody for activating **complement** (see 'The complement system', p. 91), a process known as **complement fixation**.

Antibodies are 'Y'-shaped proteins with an antigen-binding site at the end of the two 'arm-like' extensions and a site at the junction of these extensions for activating complement (Figure 5.5).

IgE has a mast cell binding site at the end of the other extension of the molecule. IgA consists of two molecules joined (Figure 5.3), and IgM consists of five molecules joined (Figure 5.3), a structure known as a **pentamer**.

There are two types of B cells, that is, B1 and B2. B2 cells are produced and mature in the bone marrow, and on activation, they will manufacture IgG, IgA, and IgE. B1 are also produced in the bone marrow but mature outside of the bone marrow, and when activated, they produce mostly IgM.

The use of antibodies by the body falls into two classes:

1. **Active immunity** is the term used when the body produces its own antibodies in response to an invading antigen.
2. **Passive immunity** is the term used when the body uses antibodies from an outside source, that is, they are not produced by the body that uses them.

Natural immunity occurs when the cause of the antibody production is purely natural, that is, caused by nature. **Artificial immunity** is when antibody production is caused by human

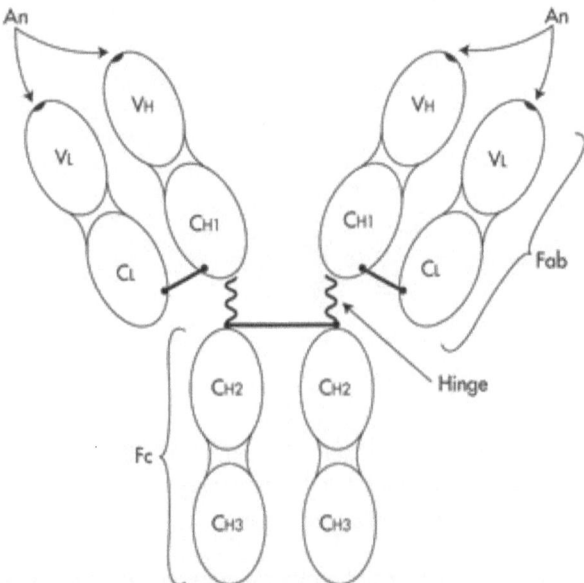

FIGURE 5.5   The simplified structure of an antibody. The protein domains are V (variable) and C (constant). The chains are L (light) and H (heavy). The heavy chain has four domains; one is variable, and three are constant. The light chain has two domains, one variable and one constant. The *Fab* segment is the antigen-binding fragment, while the *Fc* segment is the crystallisable fragment. The antigen-binding site (*An*) is at the end of the Fab segment. A hinge region in the middle allows movement of the two Fab arms. The molecule is held together by bonds, shown as cross-bridges. (See Figure 7.4, p. 139, for abnormal variations that occur in multiple myeloma.)

TABLE 5.1 The mechanisms of active/passive and natural/artificial immunity

	Active immunity	*Passive immunity*
Natural	Catch the disease and recover	Breastfeeding (IgA) and through the placenta (IgG)
Artificial	Vaccination	Injection of antibodies

intervention. Table 5.1 shows the combination of active or passive with natural or artificial immunity.

Table 5.1 shows that *passive natural immunity* involves IgA and IgG both protecting the baby before and after birth. IgA in breast milk is an important factor in choosing breastfeeding, at least for the first few months. Vaccination has become a major mechanism for *active artificial immunity* against infections, and anti-cancer vaccines have become an important way of fighting and preventing cancers. Similarly, the injection of specific anti-cancer antibodies (an *artificial passive immunity*) is a promising prospect.

B cell surface molecules

B cells produce antibodies, and they can use antibodies as part of their cell surface receptors and markers. B cell antigen receptors (BCR) are IgM and IgD, plus **CD79A** (alpha chain) and **CD79B** (beta chain) (see 'CD (cluster of differentiation) system', p. 90), forming a combination receptor which is important for antigen binding and B cell activation. Other co-receptors that modulate B cell activation are **CD19**, **CD20**, and **CD21**. CD21 binds a **complement protein** called **C3d**, which also binds to the antigen and enhances B cell activation.

The adhesion molecule **CD54**, also called **ICAM-1**, that is, **intracellular adhesion molecule-1**, facilitates 'B cell to T cell' binding, as well as 'T cell to T cell' and 'T cell to antigen-presenting cell' (APC) binding, which is necessary for cooperation between the two lymphocyte systems with the APC (see 'T cell activation', p. 87).

T cell lymphocytes

T cell lymphocytes learn specificity in the **thymus gland** (*T* = thymus). The thymus gland is located just above the heart (Figure 5.6).

During childhood, immature T cell lymphocytes migrate from the bone marrow, where they are produced and develop, to the thymus gland. Here they take on a specificity, that is, learning to respond only to one antigen (Figure 5.7). They then spend their existence in the blood, the tissues, or the lymph nodes, waiting to contact that antigen. When they meet with this specific antigen, they will react in a manner that is designed to destroy that antigen. The thymus gland is like a finishing school for T cell lymphocytes, where they will learn their most important lesson, that is, which antigen they should destroy. Those that fail this process and do not acquire a specificity will pay the ultimate price and be destroyed. The gland is most active during human childhood, after which most lymphocytes are enriched with a specificity to one of a range of harmful antigens the body is likely to encounter. After puberty, the thymus gland gradually reduces in size and function but never entirely disappears.

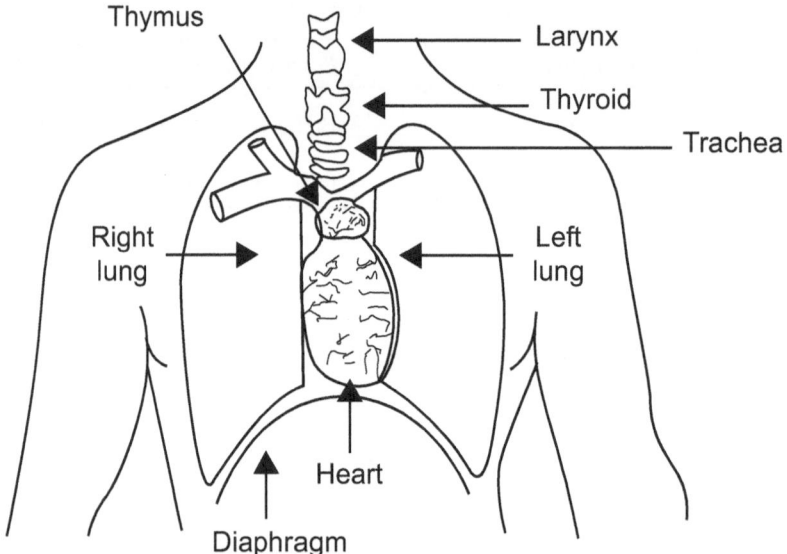

FIGURE 5.6 Location of the thymus gland. The thymus gland is in the chest immediately above the heart.

Source: Redrawn from Martini et al. (2023).

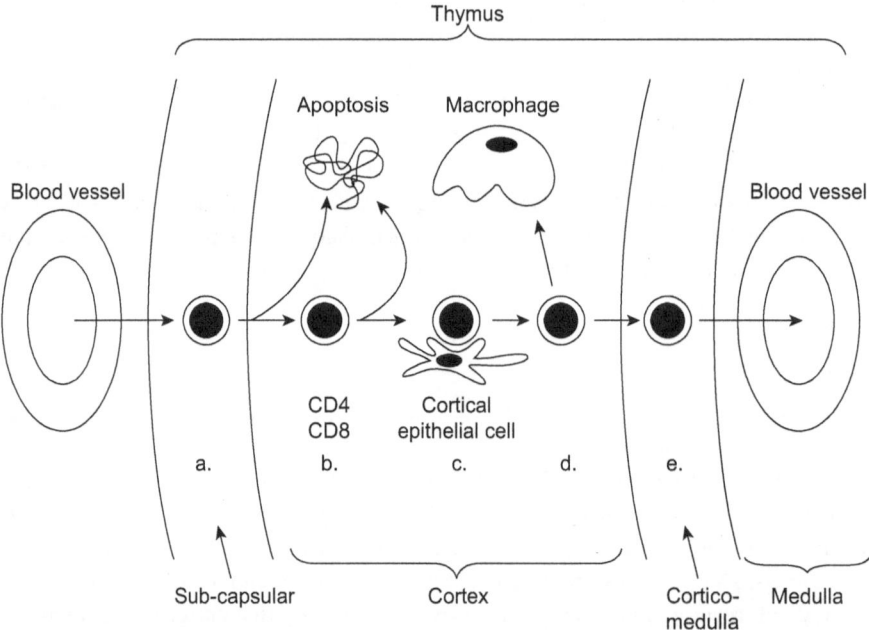

FIGURE 5.7 T cell lymphocyte maturation through the thymus: (a) The immature T cell enters the gland from the blood into the sub-capsular region. (b) In the cortex, it gains its CD4 or CD8 status. If there are problems at this stage, the cell will go to apoptosis (cell death). (c) The T cell gains its specificity and learns to not respond to 'self' (the body's own cells). Failure to learn this causes it to go be phagocytosed by macrophages. (d) Final adjustments to the T cell receptor (TCR) are made before entry into the medullary blood supply as a mature T cell.

T cell activation

The specific immunity related to T cell activation is known as **cell-mediated immunity**. T cells do not activate so easily as B cells, even when coming face to face with the antigen to which they are specific. Follow this scenario in combination with Figure 5.8:

1. If the T cell meets up with the same antigen to which it is specific, nothing happens.
2. It becomes necessary, first, for the antigen to be engulfed by a particular phagocyte called an **antigen-presenting cell (APC)**, also known as a **dendritic cell (DC)**.
   These cells can migrate between lymphoid and non-lymphoid tissues.
3. The APC destroys the antigen and expresses, that is, exposes, some of the antigen proteins onto its surface.
4. When the APC shows these exposed antigen proteins to the same T cell, nothing happens.
5. What the APC must do is produce some of its own proteins to expose on its surface *in combination* with the antigen proteins. These 'home-grown' proteins are one of the classes of proteins known as **major histocompatibility complex (MHC)**.

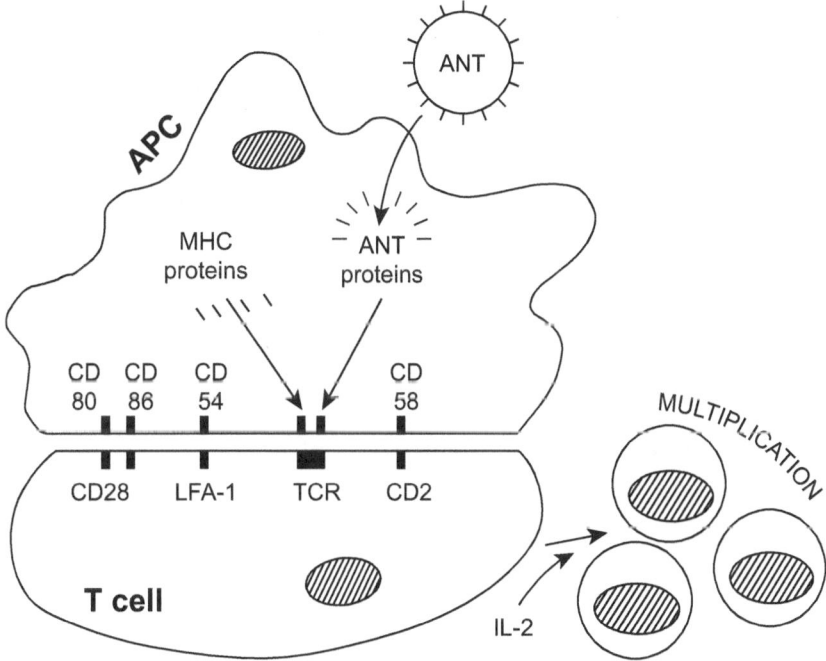

FIGURE 5.8   Activation of a T cell. The antigen (*Ant*) is engulfed and broken up by an antigen-presenting cell (*APC*). Antigen proteins (*Ant*) will be expressed on the APC surface in combination with major histocompatibility complex (MHC) proteins produced by the APC. The T cell binds to the APC using the binding molecules LFA-1 (binds to CD54), CD2 (binds to CD58), TCR (binds to the MHC/antigen protein complex), and CD28 (binds to CD80 and CD86). Production of Il-2 is important as a stimulation for the process. After activation, the T cell will multiply to form larger numbers which will include memory cells. *CD* = cluster of differentiation (see text, p. 90); *TCR* = T cell antigen receptor; *IL* = interleukin; *LFA* = lymphocyte function antigen; *MHC* = major histocompatibility complex.

There are three classes of MHC proteins: class I, class II, and class III (Figure 5.9).

Class I and II proteins are specifically for exposing onto the surface of a cell, and in the correct combinations, they act as cell markers, to identify 'self', that is, those cells that belong to the body, from 'non-self', that is, foreign cells. This is similar to name badges worn by individuals to identify those who belong to that particular institution from those who do not.

6. Once produced, the correct combination of MHC class proteins with the antigen proteins is exposed to the T cell, which is then activated and multiplies into larger numbers. The cytokine **interleukin 2 (Il-2)** (see 'Cytokines and chemokines', p. 94) is produced to aid the process.

T cell surface molecules

Proteins on the cell surface act as **markers**, as **adhesion molecules** (see 'Species differentiation', p. 80), as **antigen-binding sites**, and as **activation molecules**.

Adhesion molecules allow two cells to interlock together, a vital process for several reasons, including cell activation and the killing of antigens. Antigen-binding sites allow lymphocytes to recognise and bind only their specific antigens and activation molecules to facilitate the switching on of inactive cells, that is, inactive cells are said to be in the *resting state*.

There are two major types of activated T cells developed in the thymus gland: the **T helper** (T_H) and **T cytotoxic** (T_C) cells.

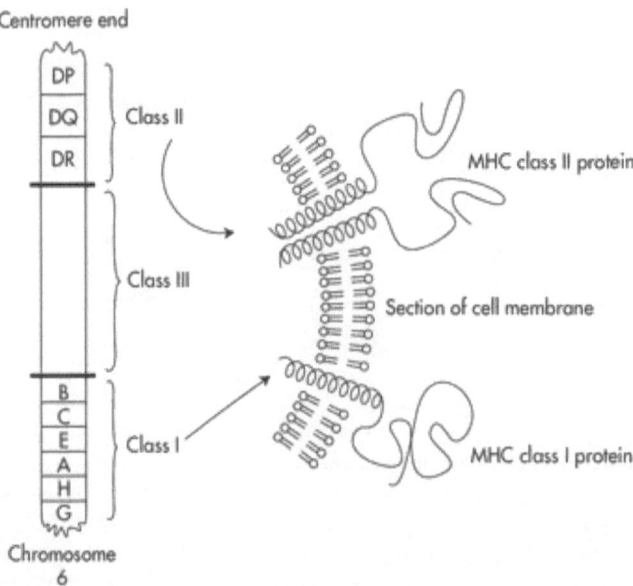

FIGURE 5.9 Part of chromosome 6. Genes code for the MHC proteins class I, II, and III. Classes I and II are cell-surface transmembranous receptor proteins. Class III genes code for complement proteins (see 'The complement system', p. 91).

The **T$_H$ cells** fall into two main types:

- **T$_H$1s**, which produce chemicals called **cytokines** (see 'Cytokines and chemokines', p. 94), which are important for killing intracellular organisms, that is, those inside the cell, and for the generation of T$_C$ cells.
- **T$_H$2s**, which also produce cytokines that are important for B cell multiplication. T$_H$ cells do not directly kill antigens, but they provide a much greater opportunity for the T$_C$ cell to kill the antigens.

The **T$_C$ cell** actually kills the antigen. They do this by developing close contact with the antigen, followed by a lethal disruption of the antigen membranes, and the antigen then dies. T$_C$ cells produce proteins called **perforins**, that is, pore-forming proteins, which are stored in granules within the cytoplasm. On close contact with the antigen, the perforins are released from the granules into a confined space formed between the two cells. The perforins become incorporated into the membrane of the antigen, forming holes, which lead to the disruption of the membrane. The activated T$_C$ cell also produces **granzymes**, that is, proteolytic[3] enzymes, which disrupt the structural cytoskeleton[4] and cause degradation of the target cell chromosomes. This leads to the death of the antigen. This close contact is essential because release of the perforins and granzymes from a distance would not be effective (Figure 5.10). Close contact is achieved largely through the role of the T$_H$ cells, which therefore increase the kill rate of the T$_C$ cells enormously.

In addition, there are two other types of T cells. The **Tregs cells** (**regulatory T cells**, previously **T suppressor cells**) reduce the immune response and restore the immune system to a normal state after the response is no longer required (see 'The tumour and its microenvironment: regulatory T cells', Chapter 6, p. 120).

The **T$_D$ cell** (**T delayed hypersensitivity cell**) launches a prolonged defence against persistent antigens when an acute response has failed. Activation of delayed hypersensitivity T cells can trigger a complex interplay of immune cells and cytokines that could result in tissue damage.

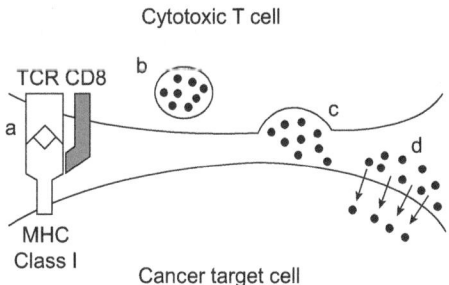

FIGURE 5.10   The cytotoxic T cell killing a cancer cell: (a) The T cell binds to the cancer cell using the MHC class I–TCR/CD8 receptors. (b, c) It releases perforins and granzymes (shown as black dots) from the storage site within vesicles in the T cell. (d) The perforins create holes in the cancer cell membrane, and granzymes break down cancer proteins, causing the cancer cell to die.

CD (cluster of differentiation) system

This is an important protocol for the identification of more than 400 cell surface molecules. These are receptors that occur on various leukocytes, including T cells, at different stages of their development in the thymus gland (Figure 5.7). The list of CD surface molecules is considerable, but here are a few important examples:

- **CD2**, a cell-signalling component and adhesion molecule that binds **CD58** (Figure 5.8) (see 'T cell acute lymphoblastic leukaemia', Chapter 7, p. 135, and 'T cell lymphoma', Chapter 7, p. 145).
- **CD3**, a cell-signalling component, part of the TCR (T cell receptor) complex that binds antigen.
- **CD4**, a co-receptor for MHC class II proteins along with TCR found on T helper and other immune cells.
- **CD8**, a co-receptor for MHC class I proteins, along with TCR, found on T-cytotoxic and other immune cells.
- **CD19**, a B cell surface antigen (B4) found in most B cell malignancies and is a target for CAR T and CAR NK cells (see 'Adaptive cell therapy (ACT)', p. 99) and MAB (see 'Monoclonal antibodies (MABs)', p. 102) cancer treatments.
- **CD20** is a B cell transmembranous protein that acts as a calcium channel. It may be involved in B cell lymphomas and chronic B cell lymphocytic leukaemia. It is the target for several drug treatments.
- **CD22**, a transmembranous B cell protein receptor present in most B cell malignancies and is therefore the target of several MAB cancer treatments (see 'Monoclonal antibodies (MABs)', p. 102).
- **CD28**, a receptor for stimulating T cell activation when binding with **CD80** and **CD86** (Figure 5.8).
- **CD44** is a transmembranous glycoprotein receptor–binding hyaluronic acid and metalloproteinases (MMPs) and involved in cell adhesion, cell migration, and cell signalling (see 'CD44', Chapter 6, p. 118).
- **CD54**, a receptor that binds to the integrin[5] LFA-1 during T_C cell activation (Figure 5.8).
- **CD154**, a receptor for stimulating APC and T cell activation when binding with **CD40** and MHC proteins.
- **CD95**, the **Fas apoptosis pathway receptor**, which leads to programmed cell death (apoptosis) if activated by binding to the Fas ligand (FasL) (see 'FAS, chromosome 10', Addendum, p. 352).

Memory cells

Both B cell and T cell lymphocytes produce **memory cells** when they are activated by antigen exposure. Memory cells created after a first exposure to the antigen persist in the circulation and lymphatic system and provide a rapid and stronger defence should the same antigen return and a second exposure occur. Memory T cells rapidly convert to T_C cytotoxic cells and attack the antigen, while memory B cells quickly convert to plasma cells and secrete antibodies when faced with a second or subsequent exposure to their specific antigen. In this way, memory cells provide rapid removal of antigens when they return after the first exposure. This is why we catch diseases many times, but whilst the first exposure causes symptoms, it also creates the memory cells. After that, the memory cells eliminate all subsequent exposures to the antigen before any symptoms arise.

Monocyte/Macrophage cells

These cells are derived from the myeloid cell line in the bone marrow (see 'Blood cell formation' and Figure 7.2, Chapter 7, p. 131). They exist as monocytes at first in circulation but convert to macrophages when they pass out of the blood and into tissues. Macrophages are phagocytic cells, that is, they engulf foreign antigens, such as bacteria and viruses, and break down their proteins. Some macrophages become **antigen-presenting cells** (**APC**s) (Figure 5.8, p. 87).

Natural killer (NK) cells

NK cells are another form of lymphocyte also called a **large granular lymphocyte** (**LGL**), and these are important for our innate (non-specific) immune defences against cancer cells and viral-infected cells. As the name suggests, they are bigger than the average lymphocyte and contain many dark granules. Like other white cells, NK cells are derived from the bone marrow and occupy most body tissues. They form 5–15% of the total lymphocytes in blood plasma. They kill viral-infected and tumour cells, and they do this by the same mechanism as that used by T cells when they kill antigens. The NK cells' granules contain enzymes called **perforins** and **granzymes**. These are liberated when in close contact with the antigen membrane. Perforin acts similar to the lytic complex of the complement system (see 'The complement system', p. 91) in making a hole in the membrane through which granzymes can then enter. Granzymes are proteolytic (protein-digesting) enzymes which cause the antigen cell to die. NK cells exposed to the cytokine **interleukin 2** (**Il-2**) become **lymphokine-activated killer** (**LAK**) cells. These cells have been used in clinical trials to kill malignant cells (see 'CAR–natural killer (CAR NK)', p. 101).

The approximate percentages of the different lymphocytes in circulation are T helper cells 55%, T cytotoxic cells 25%, B cells 10%, and NK cells 10%.

The chemical defences

The complement system

The binding of antibodies to the antigen allows the activation of a chemical chain reaction called the **complement system** (Figure 5.11). This consists of a series of nine proteins that must be activated in a particular sequence in order to function. In the absence of such activation, they remain dormant in the blood plasma. The complement system is activated either via the **classical pathway** or the **alternative pathway**. Complement proteins are identified by the letter 'C', so the nine proteins are labelled C1, C2, C3, and so on to C9. Some are split in the process into two components 'a' and 'b'; notably, C3 becomes C3a and C3b, and C5 becomes C5a and C5b. Some of these protein combinations are enzymes called **convertases** which continue the process by converting specific proteins. Convertases are shown in boxes in Figure 5.11. There are four main products of complement activation: chemotaxins, opsonins, anaphylatoxins, and the lytic complex (Figure 5.11).

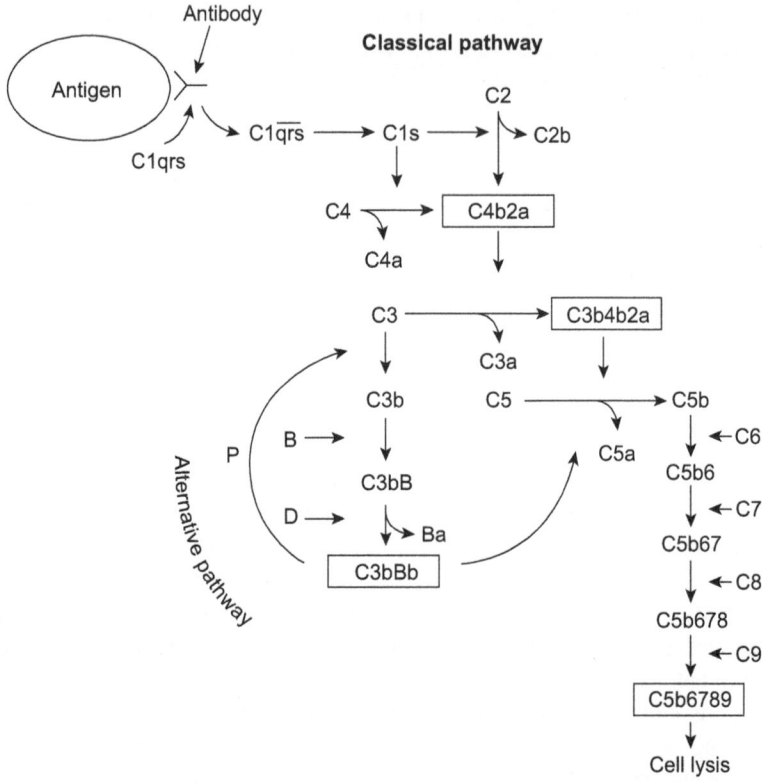

FIGURE 5.11   The complement (C) system. Each protein is numbered (C1, C2, etc.), and combinations in boxes are enzymes called convertases. C proteins can be split by convertases into two portions, a and b. C1qrs is first activated by the binding of an antibody to an antigen. The activated C1s component splits off and converts C2 and C4 to their respective a and b parts. C4b combines with 2a to form C3 convertase that splits C3 into C3a and C3b. The cascade follows either the classical or alternative pathways, both of which split C5 to C5a and C5b. Combining C5b with C6, C7, C8, and C9 forms the lytic complex (C5b6789) that can lyse (break down) antigen cell membranes. B, D, and P are additional factors needed for the alternative pathway, and c3bBb is an alternative C3 convertase.

Chemotaxins (C3a, C5a)

These are chemicals which attract white cells of most kinds to the scene of the antigen. The advantage of this is the concentration of body defensive cells at the site where they are needed most.

Opsonins (C3b)

These are chemicals that label antigens for phagocytosis by coating the surface. Macrophages need to know what cells to destroy by phagocytosis at the scene, so they are labelled by a coating of opsonins. This often means that macrophages will engulf and destroy a complex of antigens with antibodies attached, known as the **immune complex**.

Anaphylatoxins (C3a, C5a)

These are chemicals that cause inflammation to occur. C3a and C5a have a dual role, as chemotaxins and anaphylatoxins. How C3a and C5a cause inflammation is shown in Figure 5.12. **Inflammation** is vital for the function of the immune response, even though it may produce unpleasant symptoms for us. This is because inflammation results in dilation of blood vessels, called **vasodilation**, which brings more blood, and therefore more white cells, to the scene of the antigen. It also causes greater permeability of the capillary wall, allowing white cells like macrophages to pass from the blood into the tissues. Inflammation increases the efficiency of the immune system considerably.

Lytic complex (C3b, C5b, C6, C7, C8, C9)

This is a chemical complex called **MAC (membrane attack complex)** that can kill the antigen by breaking down the antigen membranes.

The acute-phase proteins

These are a collection of liver-produced proteins which are normally in low quantities but increase rapidly following the introduction of an antigen in the body. Their purpose is to activate the complement system, to increase **opsonisation** (see 'Opsonins (C3b)', p. 92), and to limit the tissue damage. They are also important in tissue repair. A major protein in this group is **C-reactive protein (CRP)**, which directly activates the complement system, via the **alternative pathway** (Figure 5.11), and acts as an **opsonin** (see 'Opsonins (C3b)', p. 92). The main activity of acute-phase proteins is against bacterial infections, so they do not play a big role in the body's fight against cancer.

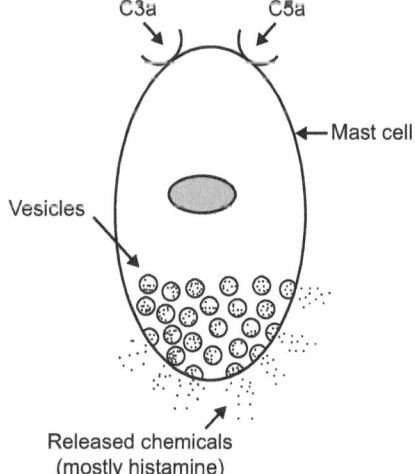

FIGURE 5.12 C3a and C5a release of chemicals from a mast cell. The complement components C3a and C5a are anaphylatoxins, that is, they can cause inflammation by degranulation of mast cells, similar to IgE binding to mast cells (Figure 5.4).

Cytokines and chemokines

Cytokines are soluble chemicals of small molecular size produced when required by a wide variety of cells in response to stimulation of some kind. They are usually related to the immune system and tend to have a local effect in mediating cell-to-cell communication within the same tissue. There are some exceptions that work systemically. As cell-signalling agents, they bind to either themselves (**autocrine activity**) or to other cells nearby (**paracrine activity**). As such, they induce many cellular responses, including growth (protein synthesis), cell differentiation, chemotaxis (see 'Chemotaxins (C3a, C5a)', p. 92), and cellular activation. Some are causes of inflammation, and these are the **pro-inflammatory cytokines** (e.g. Il-2, TNFα, IFNγ), while others reduce inflammation, the **anti-inflammatory cytokines** (e.g. Il-4, Il-10, Il-13). Some cytokines activate cellular growth and are therefore significant in the treatment of cancers. **Growth factors** are substances that cross the line between hormones and cytokines. They are naturally produced substances which are specifically required for cellular growth and tissue healing (Table 5.2).

Interleukins (Il)

These are cell-signalling chemicals between lymphocytes and coordinate immune cell activity. They bind to specific receptors on T_C cells and NK cells and lymphokine-activated killer (LAK) cells. They work in combination with other cytokines in a cascade effect. There are several kinds, called **Il-1**, **Il-2**, **Il-3**, and so on. When these are produced by lymphocytes, they are often referred to as **lymphokines**, or **monokines** if produced by monocytes. Some of these interleukins are growth factors in the sense that they induce proliferation in numbers of specific cells (Table 5.3).

TABLE 5.2 Cytokines and growth factors related to growth in humans

	Origin	*Function*
Cytokines		
Interleukin 2 (Il-2)	T cells	Promotes growth and activates T cells and NK cells
Interleukin 8 (Il-8)	Monocytes	Promotes blood vessel growth
Interleukin 6 (Il-6)	Fibroblasts, lymphocytes, and macrophages	Activates T cell lymphocytes and causes fever
Tumour necrosis factor alpha (TNF-α)	Macrophages, B cells, activated T cells, neutrophils, and mast cells	Slows tumour growth, causes fever and inflammation, and is involved in immune functions
Growth factors		
Fibroblast growth factor (FGF)	Variety of cells	A family of factors stimulating growth in many tissues
Transforming growth factor β (TGF-β)	Platelets, T cells, endothelium, and macrophages	Promotes protein synthesis and thus growth in connective tissues
Epidermal growth factor (EGF)	Duodenal glands	Promotes stem cell growth and epithelial growth
Insulin-like growth factor	Liver cells	Promotes bone and soft tissue growth
Platelet-derived growth factor (PDGF)	Platelets, smooth muscle cells, and macrophages	Promotes growth in fibroblasts, smooth muscle, and monocytes

TABLE 5.3 The major interleukins

Interleukin	Notes and function
Il-1α and Il-1β	Derived from macrophages and many other cells, they cause fever, activate lymphocytes, induce acute-phase protein production, activate vascular endothelium, cause cells to produce Il-6, and mobilise neutrophils.
Il-2	Derived from activated T_H and NK cells, it increases proliferation and efficiency of T cells, B cells, and NK cells and increases the formation of immunoglobulins.
Il-3	Causes increased proliferation of bone marrow cells (to increase WBC production).
Il-4	Derived from activated T cells, it activates B cells, increases T cell proliferation, and increases IgG and IgE immunoglobulin proliferation.
Il-5	Growth of eosinophils, B cell activation, and increases IgA response.
Il-6	Derived from fibroblasts, B cells and T cells, macrophages, and bone marrow cells, it activates T cell lymphocytes, causes fever, and increases acute-phase protein production.
Il-8	Chemotaxis of neutrophils.
Il-10	Activates B cells, reduces macrophage activity, and induces activity of T_H1 cells.
Il-12	Activates NK cells and induces activity of T_H1 cells.

Interferons (IFNs)

These are a group of **glycoproteins** (proteins with sugars attached), of which there are two types: **type I**, comprising **IFNα** and **IFNβ**, both binding to the same receptors, and **type II**, comprising **IFNγ**, which binds to its own receptor. Interferons are pro-inflammatory cytokines which are antiviral in nature, which means they are secreted by many cells when they are virally infected.

IFNα is coded for by more than 20 genes on chromosome 9. It is antiviral, reduces growth in both normal and malignant cells, increases NK cell activity, and influences cell differentiation.

IFNβ is coded for by one gene on chromosome 9. It is very similar to IFNα in that it is also antiviral, reduces growth of both normal and malignant cells, and increases NK cell activity. The paracrine effect of IFNα and IFNβ on surrounded cells causes a reduction in protein synthesis, which helps shut down virus replication in those cells (see 'Provirus and viral replication', Chapter 4, p. 63). They are both also active in regulating inflammation.

IFNγ is coded for by one gene on chromosome 12. It has a similar antiviral role but also has a part to play in the activation of immune cells, such as macrophages, and the development of specific immunity. It also causes a reduction of growth in both normal and malignant cells.

Tumour necrosis factors (TNF)

TNF (also called TNFα, or **cachexin**), binds to two cell surface receptors, TNFR1 and TNFR2. Binding to these receptors results in activation of any one of three pathways all leading to gene transcription. One pathway is involved in cell survival, cell proliferation, inflammation. A second pathway is involved in cell differentiation and proliferation, and a third pathways results in the production of pro-apoptosis factors, resulting in cell death (see 'Cachexia', Chapter 18, p. 328).

Leukotrienes, thromboxanes, prostaglandins, and prostacyclin

These are chemical groups derived from the **phospholipids** that make up part of the cell membrane (Figure 5.13). The lipid components of cell membranes act as a reserve to produce these substances. The enzyme **phospholipase A$_2$** converts the phospholipids from the membrane to **arachidonic acid**. It is then acted on by the enzyme **cyclo-oxygenase (COX)** to produce **thromboxanes** and **prostaglandins (PGs)**, which are classed as **PGA** to **PGI**. PGI$_2$ is also known as **prostacyclin**. Alternatively, arachidonic acid can be converted to **leukotrienes** if acted on by the enzyme **lipoxygenase**. Thromboxanes, prostaglandins, and leukotrienes are inflammatory mediators, that is, causing inflammation, which is essential for the efficient function of the immune system (Conlon et al. 2019). Thromboxane is an important mediator in the process of blood clotting, that is, it promotes blood clotting, and in normal circulation, this must be constantly opposed by the production of prostacyclin.

Prostacyclin is also produced from arachidonic acid in endothelial cells lining blood vessels. Here, prostacyclin helps prevent platelet aggregation, and therefore prevent blood clotting, during normal circulation of blood (see 'Blood cell types: platelets', Chapter 7, p. 132), and prostacyclin can cause vasodilation (Germann and Stanfield 2016).

In addition, there are other chemical agents related to cellular growth, and these are listed in Table 4.1 (Chapter 4, p. 66).

Cytokine release syndrome, or '**cytokine storm**', is a set of symptoms caused by a large release of cytokines into the bloodstream as a result of some therapies, notably CAR T therapy (see 'Adaptive cell therapy (ACT)', p. 99). The symptoms are fever, nausea, vomiting, low blood pressure, confusion, shortness of breath, cough, headache, tiredness, skin rashes, and muscle pain. It can become very serious and even life-threatening.

Chemokines

These are more than 40 small molecules which are chemo-attractants, that is, they are involved in *chemotaxis* (see 'Chemotaxins (C3a, C5a)', p. 92) and immunoregulation of various

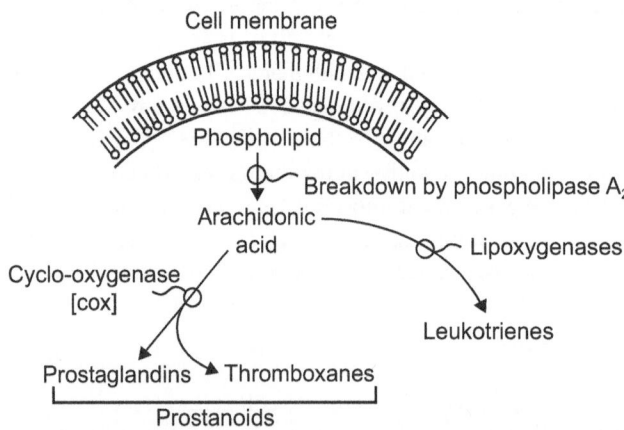

FIGURE 5.13 The production of prostanoids and leukotrienes. Cell membrane phospholipids can be used to form arachidonic acids, and then the subsequent production of prostanoids and leukotrienes from arachidonic acid.

leucocytes, including lymphocytes, monocytes, NK cells, neutrophils, and memory cells. They are produced by a wide variety of cells, such as platelets, T cells, and macrophages.

The different types of chemokines include:

- CXC chemokines, for example, CXCL1 to CXCL17
- CC chemokines, for example, CCL1 to CCL28 (see 'Brain secondary tumours', Chapter 14, p. 265)
- CX3C chemokine, called CX3CL1
- XC chemokines, called XCL1 and XCL2

Immunotherapy

Immunotherapy is the process of increasing the immune system's anti-cancer activity in killing tumour cells. It involves using monoclonal antibodies, modified immune cells, cytokines, and the prospect of anti-cancer vaccines for the future. Surveillance by the immune cells and their products, for example, antibodies, is normally directed against foreign agents, often from the environment invading the body, such as viruses and bacteria, that is, **antigens**. Virally infected cells will attract the attention of the immune surveillance, but only a small number of tumours are caused by viruses.

Malignant cells produce surface antigens that are specific to cancer, and they provoke an immune response. These are mostly proteins known as **tumour-associated antigens**, which occur on tumour cell surfaces (Table 5.4). Some of these antigens, and even some DNA from tumour cells, circulate in the blood or lymph and get excreted in the urine. Such circulating tumour cell products are called **biomarkers**, that is, if present in the blood or urine, they indicate the presence of a specific tumour (Table 5.4) (see also NHS Galleri Trial[6]).

The immune response to tumour antigens is initially strong, and many tumour cells are destroyed and eliminated from the body. This initial phase is known as the *elimination phase*.

TABLE 5.4 Some of the known tumour antigens, or biomarkers, used in diagnosis

Tumour antigen	Found in association with
Prostate-specific antigen (PSA)	Prostate cancer
Melanoma antigen expression (MAGE)	Melanomas
Renal antigen expression (RAGE)	Melanomas, kidney tumours
Carcinoembryonic antigen (CEA)	Colon cancers
Common acute lymphoblastic leukaemia antigen (CALLA)	Leukaemia
Mucin	Breast and ovary cancers
Alpha-fetoprotein (AFP)	Ovarian and testicular cancers
Cancer antigen 125 (CA125)	Ovarian cancers
Cancer antigen 15-3 (CA15-3)	Some breast cancers
Carbohydrate antigen 19-9 (CA19-9)	Pancreatic cancer
Human chorionic gonadotropin (hCG or beta-hCG)*	A wide range of cancers
Human epidermal growth factor receptor 2 (HER2)	Breast cancers

*hCG is also known as a pregnancy test.
Note: A more comprehensive list of biomarkers can be found online at NIH/NCI (2021).
Source: Pecorino (2021).

However, this response declines with time, the time being dependent on the aggressive nature of the tumour. The response passes through the second phase, the *equilibrium phase*, where the number of new and surviving cancer cells is equal to the number killed. The third phase occurs when tumour cells escape from the immune response, the *escape phase*, by suppressing the immunity and even enrolling immune cells to act towards promoting tumour cell survival and proliferation (Figure 5.14). This final phase is the time when metastases are allowed to leave the original tumour and circulate around the body before causing secondary tumours elsewhere (Chapter 6).

Another problem is that the immune system is less efficient against solid tumours, as these are difficult to penetrate, and they are made from a mix of cancer cells with variations in mutations and cell surface markers. So specific immunity may attack some cells, but not others. This is the reason for solid tumour biopsy and analysis, followed by individualised therapy. In development are drugs which target **Fas receptors** (see 'CD95', p. 90, and 'Chromosome 10', Addendum, p. 352), which occur on the surface of cells that line tumour blood vessels. These drugs trigger cell apoptosis (cell death) through these receptors. The death of these cells causes disruption to the blood supply to the tumour.

The purpose of immunotherapy is to restore phase 1 of the immune response as much as possible, and to promote the immune system in its initial role of eliminating the tumour. The strategies currently used in immunotherapy are:

- Oncolytic viruses
- Use of cytokines
- Adaptive cell therapy
- Monoclonal antibodies, including immune checkpoint inhibitors (ICI)
- Gene editing, base editing, and prime editing
- Cancer vaccines

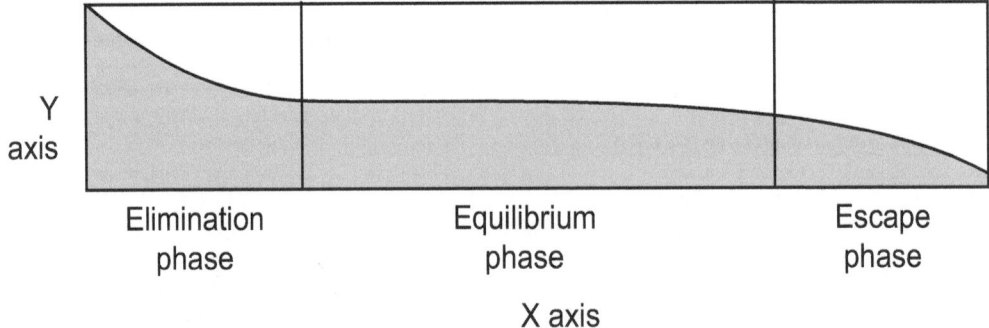

FIGURE 5.14   The three phases of immune response to tumour cells. The *elimination phase* is where the response is initially strong and the tumour cells are dying. This immune response (shaded area) declines over time to the *equilibrium phase*, where the tumour is growing at the same rate as tumour cells are dying. Further decline in the immune response leads to the *escape phase*, where the tumour outgrows the immunity and can develop metastases. The Y axis is the strength of the immune response, and the X axis is time, which varies significantly in each phase between different tumours.

Oncolytic virus therapy (OVT)

These are viruses modified to only infect and kill tumour cells. They kill the tumour cells by the process of lysis, that is, onco*lytic*, which means the breakdown of the tumour cell structure. In addition, the fact that they are viruses, that is, foreign antigens, increases the immune response to the cells, thereby reversing immune suppression. Whilst several are in clinical trials, currently, only one such virus is available for use in human patients, called *talimogene laherparepvec*. It is a modified live herpes virus used to treat unresectable metastatic melanoma. It is given by injection directly into the melanoma lesion. This topic is discussed in Chapter 4 (see 'Viral therapy for cancers', Chapter 4, p. 64).

Use of cytokines

Cytokines (see 'Cytokines and chemokines', p. 94) have been used to improve cancer treatment in any of the following ways:

- Interfering with, and blocking, the way cancer cells grow and replicate
- Stimulating the immune cells to kill cancer cells
- Promoting cancer cells to produce chemicals that attract immune cells to attack them

The pro-inflammatory cytokines interferon-alpha (IFNα) and interleukin 2 (Il-2) (Table 5.3) were used for the treatment of cancers (Conlon et al. 2019). Now, the drug aldesleukin, a synthetic version of interleukin, is used for renal cell carcinoma, but other cytokines, such as the interferons, are not generally used now, as better treatments are available and new targeted cytokine drugs are in development.

Adaptive cell therapy (ACT)

Adaptive T cell therapy involves modifying and proliferating the patient's own immune cells so they are adapted to recognise and kill malignant cells with greater efficiency. They are modified by genetic engineering after removal from the patient, and they are then grown in large numbers and returned to the patient. There are several types of ACT.

Chimeric antigen receptor T cell (CAR T or CART)

This therapy consists of T cells collected from the patient to which are added a gene that codes for a specific receptor, that is, a **chimeric antigen receptor (CAR)**. The gene gets into the T cell via a harmless virus. The T cells are then replaced into the patient's circulation. The receptor has three components (Figure 5.15):

- An extracellular domain that binds to the cancer cell
- A transmembranous domain that passes through the carrier cell membrane, for example, T cell
- An intracellular domain within the carrier cell

This receptor allows the T cell to bind to specific cancer cell antigens, and then it kills the cancer cell. They appear to be very effective against leukaemia. The process sometimes has side effects,

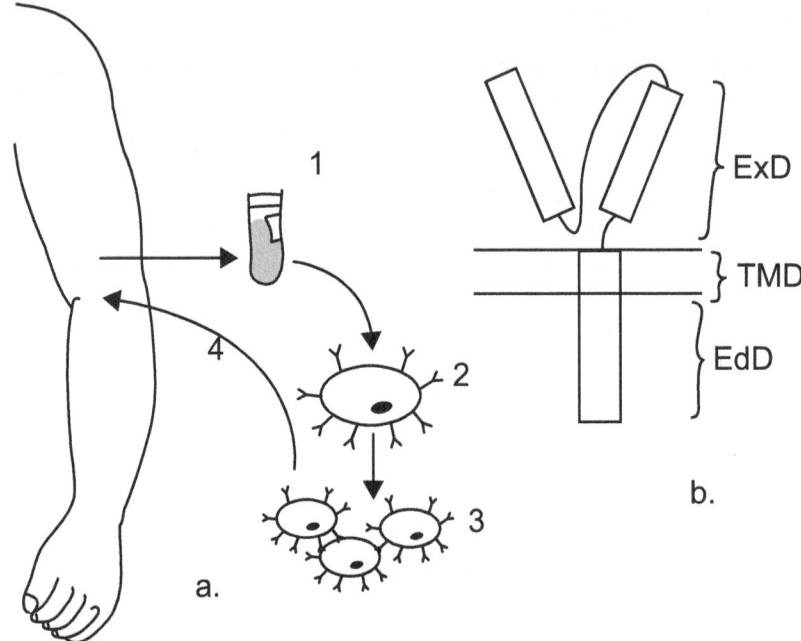

FIGURE 5.15   Chimeric antigen receptor (CAR T) therapy: (a) (1) Blood is taken from the patient. (2) T cells are purified and modified to express the CAR molecule that targets the patient's particular cancer. (3) The CAR T cells are grown in large numbers (called expansion). (4) Millions are then infused back into the patient. The process takes between 21 and 35 days. (b) Structure of a CAR showing EdD (endodomain; inside the cell), ExD (extra-cellular domain; outside the cell), and TMD (transmembranous domain, passing through the cell membrane). Successive generations of CAR show variations in the endodomain.

especially when the T cell attacks and kills healthy cells that carry the same target antigen. This could cause a **cytokine storm** (see 'Cytokine release syndrome', p. 96). To overcome this, certain proteins, called **adapters**, can be used to keep the T cell receptors separate from the target antigen yet still connected with, and active against, the cancer cell. The adapter fits into the T cell receptor and binds to the target antigen on the cancer cell. Should a side effect occur, drugs that are currently in development will be used to deactivate the adapter or make the adapter switch from one tumour antigen to another. Adapters could also be made to act only in specific environments, such as the environment inside tumours (Le Page 2023). Further development of the CAR molecule has produced five generations of CARs with extended intracellular domains. Each generation provides better intracellular signalling, leading to better cellular activation and proliferation.

CAR T cell therapy works best in liquid cancers, for example, blood cancers. Their effectiveness appears to decline over time against solid tumours and may fail completely. Interleukin 10 (Il-10) can be engineered to boost CAR T cell therapy, which then works well on established tumours and helps prevent relapse. CAR T cells can also sustain good activity if they have higher FOXO1 protein, which acts as a master switch for activating 41 other genes. CAR T cells boosted with FOXO1 protein suppress tumour activity over longer periods.

CAR natural killer (CAR NK) cell therapy is another ACT technique using CAR technology. NK cells (see 'Natural killer cells', p. 91) have been equipped with chimeric antigen receptors (CAR NKs). Further genetic modification extends the NK cells' abilities from CAR-dependent to CAR-independent cell-killing activity. NK cells also release cytokines GM-CSF (**Granulocyte-macrophage colony-stimulating factor[7]**), TNF-α, and IL-3, which reduce the effects of cytokine release syndrome (see 'Cytokine release syndrome', p. 96). CAR NK cells that target CD19 on B cells have been used against B cell tumours. NK cells require the cytokine interleukin 15 (Il-15), which is important for NK cells to proliferate and survive. Now, modified CAR NK cells can express this cytokine (CAR19/Il-15) and attack B cell tumours that express CD19. They have shown to be effective, are safe to use, and may be available in the future for 'off-the-shelf' treatments.

CAR macrophages (CAR M) cell therapy allows macrophages to infiltrate the tumour microenvironment (TME) and remain in tumours better than CAR T or CAR NK cells. Macrophages are derived from monocytes and are phagocytic (see 'Monocyte/macrophage cells', p. 91). CAR M therapy has developed with the introduction of CAR M cells derived from **pluripotent stem cells (CAR iMac)** (see 'Cellular differentiation' and Figure 7.1, Chapter 7, p. 129–130) as a possible alternative to CAR T therapy. Several generations of CAR M have been developed, each new type having variations within the intracellular component of the receptor.

Tumour-infiltrating lymphocyte (TIL) therapy

This therapy involves collecting the patient's T cells that have already penetrated the tumour. They are then activated and grown into large numbers before being returned to the patient. They are not only active specifically against the tumour but also, in large numbers, the tumour can be overwhelmed and killed (Figure 5.16).

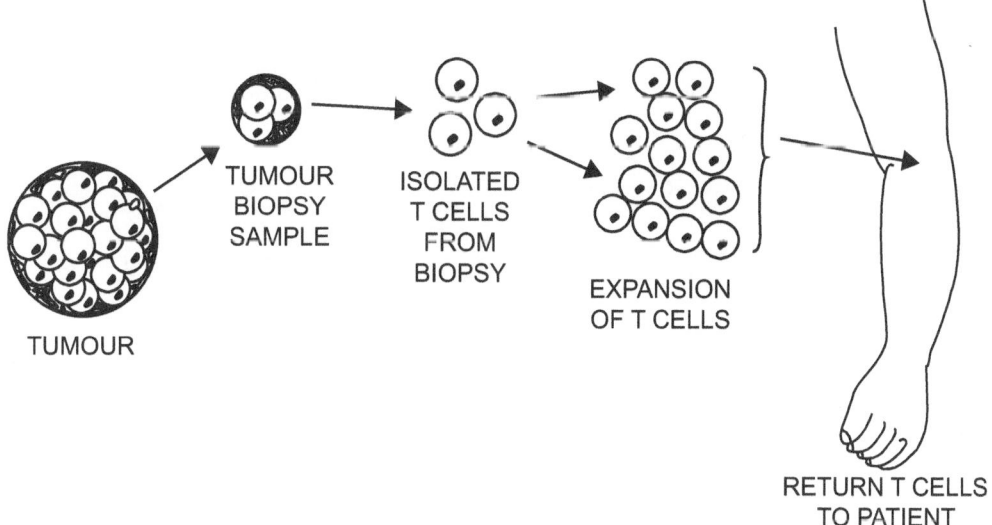

TUMOUR BIOPSY SAMPLE

ISOLATED T CELLS FROM BIOPSY

EXPANSION OF T CELLS

TUMOUR

RETURN T CELLS TO PATIENT

FIGURE 5.16 Tumour-infiltrating lymphocyte (TIL) therapy. A biopsy of the tumour provides T cell lymphocytes, which are already specific to that tumour, to be isolated and grown in large numbers (expansion) before being returned to the patient.

Engineered T cell receptor (ECR)

This therapy involves collecting T cells from the patient that have not yet become specific for the tumour and engineering them with a new receptor that targets the tumour. They are then grown in large numbers and returned to the patient. This form of approach allows T cells to become very specific to the cancer type that the patient has, that is, personalised cancer therapy.

ACT has to overcome two problems: (1) the cost, as they are expensive to produce, and (2) the high risk of 'off target' reactions, that is, adverse reactions away from the tumour, such as **cytokine release syndrome** (see 'Cytokine release syndrome', p. 96). Work is in progress to improve CART and to reduce the costs.

Monoclonal antibodies (MABs)

Monoclonal antibodies have been developed specifically against certain antigens found on tumour cells or immune cells. In each case, the drug name ends with '-mab', which means 'monoclonal antibody' (Table 5.5). They work in the following ways:

- Some block growth factor signals that cause the cancer cells to divide.
- Some stop cancer cells from taking up proteins necessary for cell division.
- Some carry cancer drugs (see, 'Monoclonal antibodies (MABs) known as antibody–drug conjugates (ADCs)', p. 105) or carry radiotherapy, that is, radiolabelled MABs (see 'Radioimmunotherapy', Chapter 17, p. 310), and deliver these to cancer cells.
- Some are *immune checkpoint inhibitors* (*ICIs*) (Table 5.5).

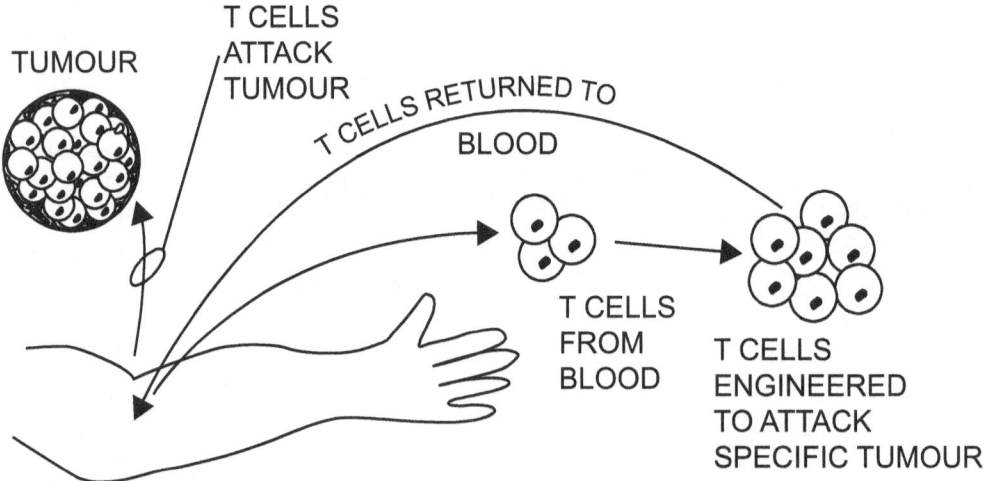

FIGURE 5.17   Engineered T cell receptor (ECR) therapy. T cells collected from the patient's blood are subject to genetic engineering to make them specific for that tumour. They are grown in large numbers before being returned to the patient to attack the tumour.

TABLE 5.5 The 35 monoclonal antibody drugs in the current BNF: a selection including some *ICI*s

Drug name	Mode of action	Cancers treated
Amivantamab	Blocks epidermal growth factor receptor (EGFR) and mesenchymal–epithelial transition (MET), that is, the transition from mesenchymal to epithelial cells. (See 'Bispecific antibodies', p. 107.)	Non-small-cell lung cancer with EGRF receptors
Atezolizumab	PD-L1 inhibitor. PD-L1 suppresses the immune response to the cancer. The inhibitor blocks that suppression.	Lung, breast, bladder, melanoma, and liver
Avelumab	PD-L1 inhibitor. PD-L1 suppresses the immune response to the cancer. The inhibitor blocks that suppression.	Renal cell carcinoma (Chapter 10, p. 199), urothelial carcinoma (Chapter 10, p. 202), Merkel cell carcinoma (Table 13.1, Chapter 13, p. 245)
Bevacizumab	Blocks vascular endothelial growth factor (VEGF).	Many, including colorectal, lung, kidney, breast, cervical, and ovarian
Blinatumomab	Links cancer B cell protein CD19 with CD3/T cell receptor complex on T cells, activating the T cell to kill the B cell.	Precursor B cell ALL (Chapter 7, p. 134)
Cetuximab	Blocks epidermal growth factor receptor (EGFR).	Bowel, head, and neck
Daratumumab	Blocks the cancer surface protein CD38 and triggers the immune system to kill the cell.	Multiple myeloma
Durvalumab	PD-L1 inhibitor (see 'Immune checkpoint inhibitors', p. 104).	Lung and bladder
Ipilimumab	CTLA-4 inhibitor (see 'Immune checkpoint inhibitors', p. 104).	Melanoma
Mogamulizumab	Targets and blocks CCR4 (C-C chemokine receptor 4) on the surface of cancerous T cells, attracting other immune cells to kill them.	T cell lymphoma
Nivolumab	PD-1 inhibitor (see 'Immune checkpoint inhibitors', p. 104).	Many, including lung, kidney, liver, bladder, melanoma, head, neck, and Hodgkin lymphoma
Panitumumab	Blocks epidermal growth factor receptor (EGFR).	Bowel cancer
Pembrolizumab	PD-1 inhibitor (see, 'Immune checkpoint inhibitors', p. 104, and 'New forms of treatment', Chapter 13, p. 251).	Many, including melanoma, lung, head, neck, gastric, and Hodgkin lymphoma
Rituximab	Targets and blocks CD20 protein.	Non-Hodgkin lymphoma and CLL (Chapter 7, p. 144)
Siltuximab	Blocks Il-6 (Table 5.3, p. 95), preventing it from binding to its receptor. Slows the growth of tumours, producing Il-6.	Multicentric Castleman disease (MCD);[8] ovarian cancer and multiple myeloma

*Monoclonal antibodies (MABs) known as immune checkpoint inhibitors (ICIs)
(Table 5.5)*

These MABs block different *checkpoint proteins* which are found on the surface of cancer and immune cells such as T cells (Figure 5.18).

The main checkpoint proteins are:

- **PD-1 (programmed cell death protein 1)**, a T cell surface protein which, when activated, switches the T cell off.
- **PD-L1** and **PD-L2** are cell surface receptor proteins that bind to PD-1 (i.e. PD-1 ligands) and activate it, thus deactivating the T cell.
- **CD137 (or 41BB)**, a tumour necrosis factor (TNF) receptor.
- **CTLA-4 (cytotoxic T-lymphocyte-associated protein 4)**, a T cell surface protein that also acts as an 'off switch' of T cell activity. It is activated by binding to B7 malignant cell surface receptors.
- **LAG-3**, an immune cell surface protein that acts as an 'off switch'.

They act like switches to turn the immune cell activity on or off. This is necessary when the normal function of the T cells is complete and the cell returns to an inactive state. Malignant cells

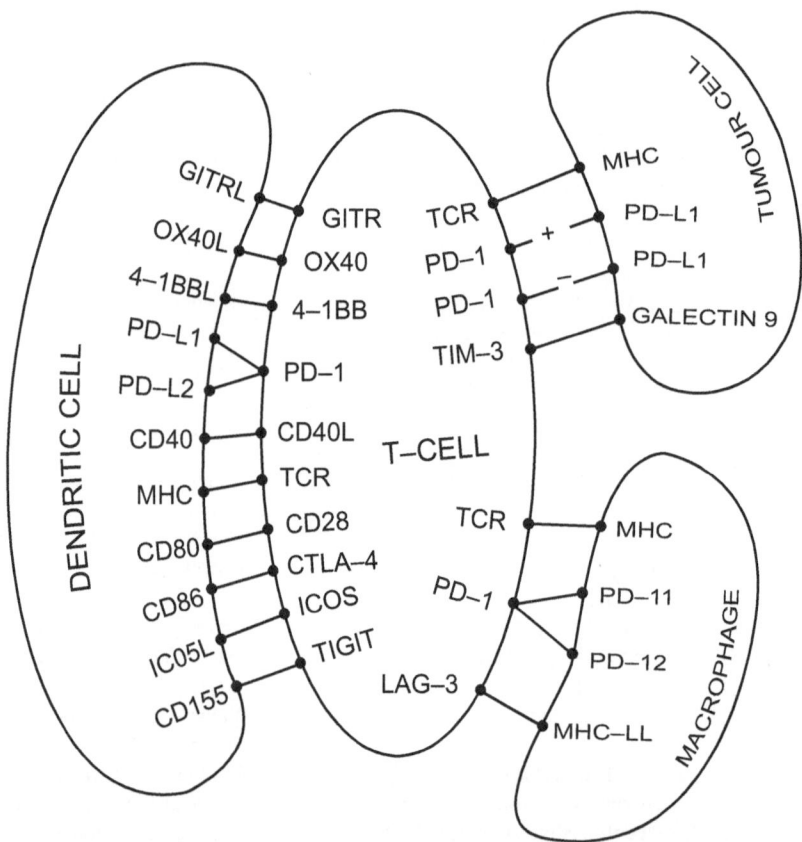

FIGURE 5.18 Checkpoint receptor proteins. The links between T cells, macrophages, dendritic cells, and tumour cells.

develop the ability to use these proteins to switch off the immune cell and therefore downgrade or suppress the immune response, that is, *immune suppression*. ICI drugs block these proteins so the malignant cell cannot switch off the immune cell, which then continues to kill the cancer cell (Figure 5.19). Some malignant cells produce proteins, such as PD-L1, that switch off T cells. These cancer cells are causing the immune suppression. The drugs prevent this and restore normal immune cell activity against the tumour (see also 'Intestinal flora (microbiota or microbiome)', Chapter 8, p. 152).

In addition to ICIs, some small synthetic molecules are being developed to overcome the cost problem linked to synthetic monoclonal antibody use and to reach those parts of the tumour that the much larger antibodies cannot get to. These small molecules block PD-L1 and are currently under development.

Monoclonal antibodies (MABs) known as antibody–drug conjugates (ADCs)

The problem with traditional chemotherapy has been that it attacks not only cancer cells but also normal cells as well, and this causes many of the side effects. The goal has been to try to achieve more targeted therapy, that is, to attack and kill malignant cells whilst not affecting normal cells. This goal is now partly being achieved with the use of a new class of monoclonal antibodies called **antibody–drug conjugates**, or **ADCs** (Table 5.6).

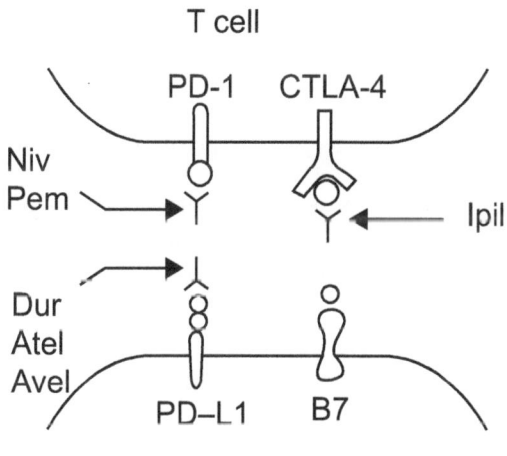

FIGURE 5.19 The function of specific ICIs. Top shows those active on T cell PD-1 and CTLA-4 surface proteins, and the bottom shows those active on PD-L1 malignant cell surface receptors. Without the drugs, PD-1 and PD-L1 would bind, and this connection stops the T cell from killing the malignant cell. Similarly, T cell receptor CTLA-4 would bind to malignant cell B7 receptor, also stopping T cell function. MABs block PD-1, CTLA-4, and PD-L1, blocking these bindings and therefore allowing the T cell to continue to kill the malignant cell. The MABs shown are: *Niv* = nivolumab; *Pem* = pembrolizumab; *Dur* = durvalumab; *Atel* = atezolizumab; *Avel* = avelumab; Ipil = ipilimumab.

TABLE 5.6 Monoclonal drugs that are antibody–drug conjugates (ADCs)

Drug name	Mode of action	Cancers treated
Brentuximab vedotin	A conjugate of a MAB with a drug. The MAB binds to the cancer cell surface protein CD30. The drug monomethyl auristatin E (MMAE) enters the cell and disrupts tubulin, preventing cancer cell replication.	Hodgkin lymphoma. MMAE (monomethyl auristatin E) is toxic and can only be used attached to an antibody (see also polatuzumab).
Inotuzumab ozogamicin	A conjugate of a MAB that targets protein CD22 on malignant B cells with the drug ozogamicin that breaks up DNA beyond repair.	ALL (Chapter 7, p. 134).
Polatuzumab	A conjugate of an antibody with a drug that binds to CD79b protein on lymphoma B cell surfaces. The drug MMAE kills the malignant B cell by blocking tubulin production.	B cell lymphoma. MMAE (monomethyl auristatin E) is toxic and can only be used attached to an antibody (see also brentuximab vedotin).
Trastuzumab deruxtecan	A conjugate of a MAB with the drug deruxtecan. Targets over-expressed HER2 protein (Table 5.4).	Breast and stomach.

An antibody that attaches to a unique cancer cell surface protein is conjugated (joined) to a toxic anti-cancer drug. The antibody attaches to the surface protein on all the cancer cells that express that particular protein. On binding, the drug is released directly into the cancer cell and kills the cell. They would normally spare healthy cells because the healthy cells do not express that particular surface protein. The drugs can be targeted for use in any type of cancer and at any growth stage or spread.

To find out what specific proteins only the cancer cell is producing, a sample from the tumour is collected by biopsy. This sample is examined by 'tumour RNA expression testing'. Laser dissection of the tumour provides a purified sample of cancer cells. RNA from these cancer cells is compared to RNA from healthy examples of the same cell type. This can be done for over 21,000 genes to see which genes are over-expressed. Each ADC targets for one over-expressed cell protein,

Trastuzumab deruxtecan (T-DXd) is the antibody trastuzumab linked to the cytotoxic drug deruxtecan, forming a conjugate. The antibody binds to **human epidermal growth factor receptor 2 (HER2)** in breast cancer (see 'HERs-positive', p. 210, and Table 11.2, Chapter 11, p. 209), and the conjugate then gets taken into the cell. Inside the cytoplasm, the drug component, deruxtecan, detaches from the antibody and kills the cancer cell. On the death of the cell, the cytotoxic drug may be released into the microenvironment. Here it continues to attack and kill other surrounding cancers cells, including those with negative values of HER2, a process known as 'the bystander effect'[9] (Figure 5.20). It becomes important to test tissue from the tumour, taken by biopsy, to see what antigens and receptors are being expressed. That way, the correct antibody–drug conjugate can be used against that tumour. This is individualised tumour management, which is thought, one day, to replace chemotherapy, once antibodies and drugs have been developed against all cancer types.

Occasionally, some ADCs have side effects similar to those of standard chemotherapy (see 'Side effects of cytotoxic therapy', Chapter 16, p. 304). This includes nausea and fatigue. It

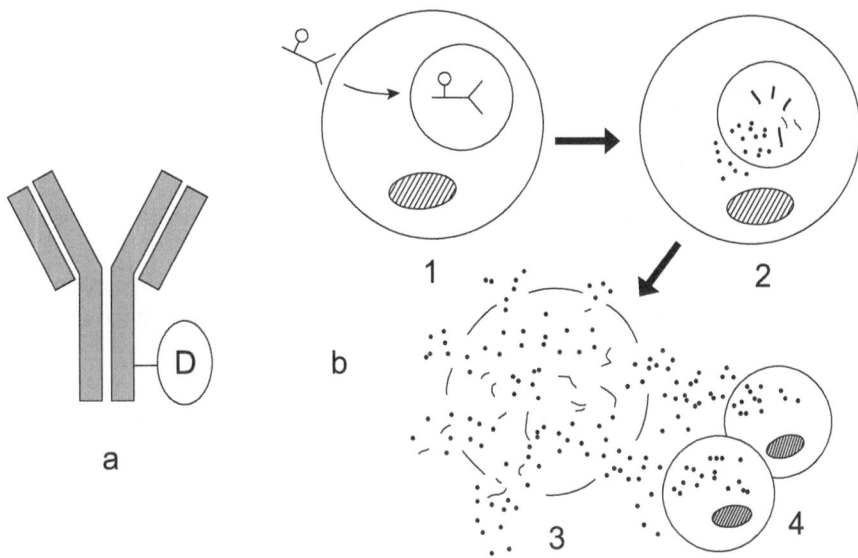

FIGURE 5.20 Antibody–drug conjugates (ADCs): (a) The antibody component of the ADC with the drug (D) attached. (b1) The ADC binds to the cancer cell and enters the cell. (b2) The drug is released. (b3) The drug kills the cell. (b4) The dead cell releases the drug, which continues to attack and kill nearby cells, that is, 'the bystander effect'.

could be due to the bystander effect spreading beyond the tumour and affecting healthy cells or unstable linkage causing the drug to release from the antibody before reaching the target. Better linkages are available now for modern drugs (Madhusoodanan 2024).

Bispecific antibodies

These are antibodies engineered to have two different binding sites, one for the tumour-associated antigens on the cancer cell surface, and the other for the immune cell receptor. This keeps the immune cell linked to the tumour cell. An example is the drug amivantamab (Table 5.5). This drug has three properties, that is, it binds to both EGFR (epidermal growth factor receptor) and MET (mesenchymal–epithelial transition receptor) on the cancer cell and attracts both macrophages and NK cells to the site.

Cancer vaccines

The principle behind all vaccines is the ability to take a small quantity of a specific antigen, usually a protein, which has been rendered harmless and introduce it into the body to stimulate the immune system. This boost to the immune system provides additional cells and antibodies to attack the antigen should it arrive in the body again. Vaccines have been highly successful against foreign organisms, viruses in particular, but also bacteria. In the case of cancer, the antigen introduced in a vaccine is often a unique protein from the surface of the cancer cells that healthy cells do not have, or short pieces of DNA or mRNA that is specific to the cancer.

Vaccines against **human papillomavirus** (**HPV**) and **hepatitis B virus** (**HBV**) (Figure 4.2b and 4.2c, Chapter 4, p. 61) already exist, and therefore, they can reduce the incidence of cancers caused by these virions. Vaccines that protect against infections are **prophylactic**, that is, preventative in nature, and now research is underway to extend this to cancer cells.

Some future cancer vaccines may be aimed at prophylaxis, that is, preventing certain cancers in families that, due to their family history, are at a genetic risk of developing cancer. Some cancer vaccines in current development act as another arm to the treatment regime in people who already have cancer.

Whilst most vaccines tend to be specific, some cancer vaccines in development are an attempt to improve immunity against a wide range of cancers, that is, generic or 'off the shelf' vaccines, by targeting antigens that are produced by many cancer types. One example is a vaccine designed to produce antibodies that bind to proteins encoded by the *MICA* and *MICB* genes in cancer cells. These proteins of the MHC class 1 type (Figure 5.9) alert the immune system to destroy the cancer cell, but the cancer cell can destroy these proteins and survive the immune attack. The vaccine-generated antibodies bind to the MICA and MICB proteins and prevent their destruction.

Other vaccines are using new antigen delivery systems. An example of this is the introduction of an mRNA strand encoding **tyrosinase-related protein-2** (**TRP-2**), a tumour-associated protein found in melanomas which is delivered to the lymphatic system by **lipid nanoparticles**.

There are several types of cancer vaccines on trial:

- **Dendritic cell (DC) vaccines.** *Dendritic cells* are antigen-presenting cells (APCs) (see 'T cell activation', p. 87, and Figure 5.8, p. 87). In a laboratory, these cells are developed to carry tumour antigens. When given to the patient, they activate T cells to attack similar antigens present on the malignant cells (see 'Brain tumour vaccines', Chapter 14, p. 269).
- **Pluripotent stem cells (PSCs)**, for example, **human embryonic stem cell (hESC) vaccines**, are being developed, using whole stem cells, to increase immunity against tumours (see 'Stem cell therapy', Chapter 17, p. 314).
- **Viral vector vaccines** involve a virus that is rendered harmless which is used to carry a cancer antigen (a protein or nucleic acid) into the cells and thus boost immunity against that cancer. The virus becomes the *vector*, that is, the mechanism of transportation into the cell. An example is a vaccine in development for colon and endometrial cancer, using a viral vector.
- Apart from *viral vector vaccines*, **ancient viral DNA** that is present in the **human genome**, that is, the total DNA within human genes, is viral in origin. It amounts to about 8% of the genome and is derived from **retroviruses** that have implanted their DNA in humans a long time ago during human evolution. This is then replicated in all future generations. Some serve useful purposes, whilst others remain dormant. Cancer cells reactivate these dormant viral DNA remnants and make the malignant cells look like they are virally infected. This is often enough to trigger an immune response, with immune cells and antibodies produced specifically to kill the 'infected' cells, which are the cancer cells. Now this can be used as a basis for new vaccines which would boost the immune system to hunt for these ancient viral DNA remnants. This is similar to the *DNA and RNA vaccines* approach.
- **DNA and RNA vaccines** use fragments of cancer genetic material to stimulate the immune system. An example is a vaccine in development against the bacterium *Fusobacterium nucleatum* which will deliver messenger RNA (mRNA) from the bacterium into the body to strengthen the immune response against the organism. *Fusobacterium nucleatum* is a bacterial commensal of the mouth and is linked to drug-resistant colon cancer. mRNA housed in lipid nanoparticle

vaccines (mRNA-LNP) are proving effective. These nanoparticles can deliver the mRNA to the lymphatic system, where T cells gain their specificity, rather than to the liver (see 'T cell lymphocytes', Figure 5.7, p. 86). Another example is the vaccine in development for breast, ovarian, and prostate cancers using DNA antigen. Another future vaccine, called mRNA-4359, uses mRNA encapsulated in lipid nanoparticles (LNPs) to treat advanced melanoma, lung cancer, and other solid tumours, such as the breast and bowel. The mRNA in the vaccine produces multiple copies of the antigens PDL1 (see 'Monoclonal antibodies (MABs) known as immune checkpoint inhibitors (ICIs)', p. 104) and the catabolic enzyme indoleamine 2,3-dioxygenase 1 (IDO1),[10] both of which prime the immune system to destroy the cancer cells. Another vaccine is mRNA-4157 (V940), a personalised treatment developed from biopsy specimens taken from the patient. The mRNA is again encapsulated in lipid nanoparticles (LNPs) and shows promise in treating melanoma and possibly lung, bladder, and kidney cancers.

- **Protein vaccines** use proteins produced by the malignant cell to encourage the immune cells to seek out and destroy malignant cells. Some use very small proteins called peptides.

  Examples are vaccines in development for pancreatic cancer using a peptide antigen and for breast triple-negative cancer (see 'Triple-negative breast cancer', Chapter 11, p. 210) using a protein antigen.

- **Heat shock protein vaccines** are currently in development. They use certain tumour proteins called **heat shock proteins (HSPs)** to boost immunity against malignant cells (Figure 5.21). **Heat shock transcription factors (HSFs)** respond to stress factors from the cellular environment. HSFs are then moved to the nucleus, where they bond with **heat shock elements (HSEs)**. The binding of HSFs with HSEs begins the genetic transcription of HSPs.

Heat shock proteins are classified according to their molecular size, for example, HSP27, HSP40, HSP60, HSP70, and HSP90. They are found within all cells that are subjected to stress, where they assist other proteins to fold and function correctly in stress conditions. In tumour cells, they are often produced in greater numbers and moved to the external environment, where they are actively involved in malignant cell proliferation, differentiation, tissue invasion, and metastases. When HSPs are exposed on the cancer cell surface, or in the blood, various HSPs can trigger an immune response which the vaccines would boost. So HSPs can both promote cancer cell survival and promote the immune system to destroy cancer cells. They also act as biomarkers that demonstrate the stage of growth and how aggressive the tumour is. HSPs are also involved in the response to various treatments and, ultimately, the patient's prognosis.

Key points

Immunity

- There are two main types of immunity: innate (non-specific) and adaptive (specific).
- Innate immunity defends against the entry of non-specified unwanted foreign agents.
- Innate immunity consists of physical barriers (e.g. the skin), chemical barriers (e.g. gastric acidity), cellular barriers (e.g. phagocytes), and species differentiation, that is, some species cannot catch certain diseases.
- *Antigens* are foreign agents that invade the body, causing an immune response.
- Antigens are mostly proteins, for example, bacteria, viruses, and pollen, but they can be other substances, such as dust particles.

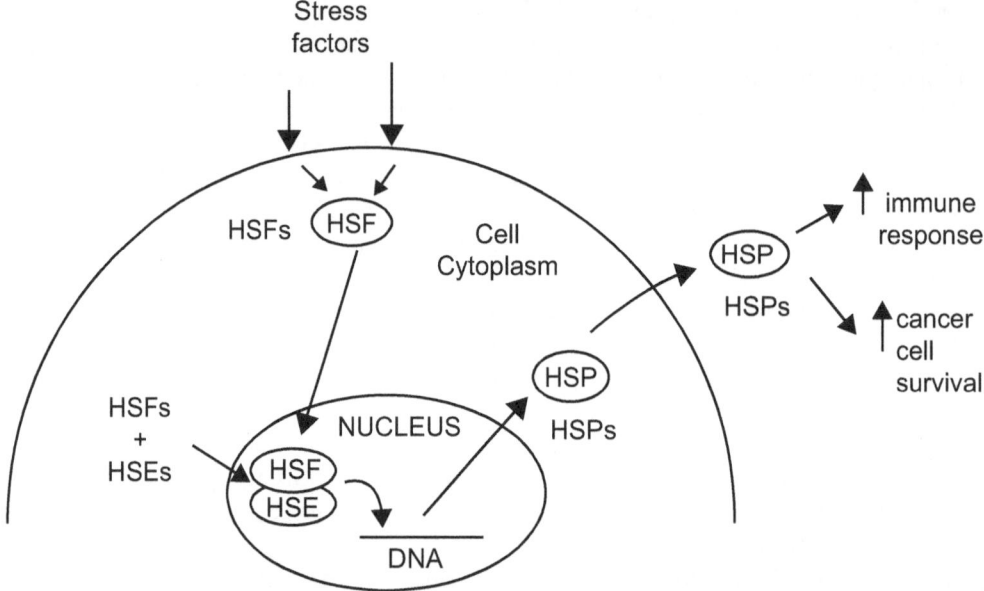

FIGURE 5.21   Production of heat shock proteins. When the cancer cell is subject to stress factors from outside, these stress factors interact with heat shock factors (HSFs), which then move to the nucleus. In the nucleus, they bind with heat shock elements (HSEs), and this triggers gene transcription of heat shock proteins (HSPs). HSPs are moved to the extracellular environment, where they may boost the immune response or promote cancer cell survival, depending on the environmental conditions.

- Adaptive immunity involves lymphocytes which respond to a specific antigen and not to any others.
- Two types of lymphocytes are B cells and T cells.
- Activation of B cell lymphocytes results in these cells being converted into plasma cells, which then release proteins called antibodies.
- Activation of T cell lymphocytes results in several forms of cells which are capable of killing antigens.

Antibodies

- Antibodies are also known as immunoglobulins (Ig) and occur in five classes: IgA, IgD, IgE, IgG, and IgM.
- Antibodies are 'Y'-shaped proteins with antigen-binding sites at the end of the two 'arms' and a site lower down for activating complement.
- In active immunity, the body produces its own antibodies in response to antigens, but in passive immunity, the body uses antibodies from an outside source, for example, from mother to child through breast milk or the placenta.
- *Natural immunity* means the antibody production is purely natural, that is, by the hand of nature, whilst *artificial immunity* is when antibody production is caused by human intervention, that is, vaccination.

Immune cells

- There are two major types of activated T cells: the T helper (T_H) and the T cytotoxic (T_C) cells.
- Activated B cells are called plasma cells.
- Both B cell and T cell lymphocytes produce memory cells when they are activated by antigen exposure.
- Natural killer cells (NK cells) are lymphocytes, or large granular lymphocytes (LGL), that kill cancer and infected cells.

Complement system

- The complement system consists of nine blood proteins that must be activated in a particular sequence in order to function.
- There are four main products of complement activation: (1) chemotaxins, which attract immune cells to where they are needed; (2) opsonins, which coat antigens for phagocytosis; (3) anaphylatoxins, which cause inflammation; and (4) the lytic complex, which kills antigens.

Cytokines

- *Cytokines* are small chemical molecules produced by a variety of cells in response to stimulation.
- They are cell-signalling agents, binding to either themselves (autocrine activity) or to other cells nearby (paracrine activity).

Immunotherapy

- Boosting the immune system to destroy cancer cells is called *immunotherapy*.
- It includes adaptive cell therapy, monoclonal antibodies (including immune checkpoint inhibitors), oncolytic viruses, small synthetic molecules, cytokines, and cancer vaccines.

Notes

1 It is tempting to think of something that has arrived in the stomach as having already entered the body. This is not the case. Contents of the entire digestive tract, from mouth to anus, are not strictly *inside* the body until they have been absorbed through the gut wall into the cells and blood. The inside of the gut lumen is an extension of the outside world. This concept allows bacteria and other organisms to thrive inside the gut without causing infections, and for toxic substances, such as faeces, to reside inside the colon without causing harm.
2 Remember the strong emphasis placed on washing hands during the Covid pandemic.
3 *Proteolytic enzymes* are those that break down and destroy proteins (*proteo* = protein; *lytic* = to break down).
4 *Cytoskeleton* is the protein internal structure that gives internal shape and support to the cell.
5 See 'Integrins', Chapter 6, p. 116.
6 **NHS Galleri Trial** aims to further develop a test that would detect DNA biomarkers in the blood from any of 50 different cancers in one test. If successful, the test could be adopted to run alongside other screening methods and would detect cancer signals at a very early stage in the disease development. The trial is currently in its final years.

7 GM-CSF can help suppress tumour growth by boosting some aspects of the immune response. Too much GM-CSF can also have the opposite effect by exhausting the immune response so it fails sooner.

8 *Multicentric Castleman disease* (MCD) is a rare disease of multiple lymph nodes causing fever, night sweats, enlarged liver, fatigue, oedema, and skin lesions. It also increases the risk of lymphoma. It may be caused by excessive production of Il-6 (Table 5.3, p. 95). Some cases are linked to herpesvirus 8 (HHV-8) infection (Figure 4.2, Chapter 4, p. 61).

9 This is because receptor expression may vary between cancer cell lines within the same tumour (see 'Cell lines', Chapter 1, p. 19).

10 Indoleamine 2,3-dioxygenase 1 (IDO1) is an enzyme that breaks down (catabolises) tryptophan.

6

METASTASES

- **Introduction**
- **Cellular adhesion molecules (CAMs)**
- **Other cell-to-cell junctions**
- **Metastases**
- **Key points**

Introduction

The largest proportion of normal cells in the solid tissues of the body are in fixed positions, where they are served with the requirements they need to survive and function. They form consortia of cells that are mostly identical in their structure, requirements, and function, that is, the organs and tissues. They often have a mixture of other cells present, all there to serve specific functions. Organs are surrounded by **basement membranes** made from an **extracellular matrix (ECM)** consisting of proteins, mostly **laminins, collagen**, and **proteoglycans**. Only blood cells are naturally free to travel in the circulation. Red blood cells (RBCs) are loose but are confined to circulation. They must be free for blood to behave as a fluid. White blood cells (WBCs) are free to pass through capillary walls into the tissues, and they need this ability to fight infection. Inflammation facilitates this freedom of movement for WBCs in and out of tissues during infection.

Cells that make up the tissues and organs are anchored together and fixed to the basement membrane, so they are unable to move. To achieve this, cells must have an internal structure which provides shape and support. This is the **cytoskeleton**, a protein framework inside the cell consisting of three elements:

1. **Microfilaments** (5 nm in diameter), made from a protein called **actin**
2. **Intermediate** filaments (10 nm in diameter), made from six different proteins
3. **Microtubules** (25 nm in diameter), made from two strands of a tubular protein called **tubulin**

DOI: 10.4324/9781003389125-6

Cellular adhesion molecules (CAMs)

Epithelial cells rest on a **basement membrane** which consists of glycoproteins,[1] such as **collagen, laminin, fibronectin**, and **proteoglycans**. Connective tissue cells bind to the **extracellular matrix (ECM)**, a mixture of proteoglycans and other glycoproteins (see 'Extracellular matrix', p. 124). Epithelial and connective tissue cells are therefore *anchorage-dependent* within a matrix of **cell adhesion glycoproteins**. Any cell that breaks free from anchorage would normally stop growing and would die, that is, the cell dies by triggering **anoikis**, a type of apoptosis, or cell death, occurring when normal cells become separated from anchorage.

The cell-to-cell attachment is through a combination of different groups of receptors called **cell adhesion molecules (CAMs)** (Pecorino 2021). CAMs are *transmembranous glycoproteins*, which means the molecular structure of the receptor extends right through the cell membrane, with one end facing the external environment for binding purposes, with the other end facing the internal environment, that is, the intracellular cytoplasm. Different CAM receptors have their own specific attachments.

One group of CAMs are **carcinoembryonic antigen-related cell adhesion molecules (CEACAMs)**. They are 12 highly glycosylated[2] immunoglobulins involved in cell adhesion, cell signalling, immune reactions, and numerous other cellular processes. They can be involved in modulating the immune reaction to cancer cells, and this makes them possible targets for ADC drug treatment (see 'Monoclonal antibodies (MABs) known as antibody–drug conjugates (ADCs)', Chapter 5, p. 105). An example is CEACAM5 in non-small-cell lung cancer, but also CEACAM1, CEACAM6, and CEACAM8 in other cancers.

The CAM receptor groups as a whole are **cadherins**, **integrins**, **selectins**, and **immunoglobulin-like** proteins.

Cadherins (CDH) (Figure 6.1)

These are a class of transmembranous glycoprotein cell surface receptors that provide extracellular cell-to-cell attachment using hook-like features. They have critical roles in tissue formation and in the function of epithelial barriers. Cadherins have letters and numbers associated

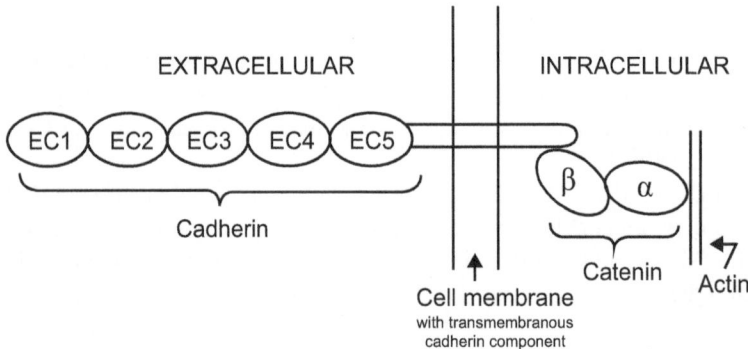

FIGURE 6.1   Classical cadherin and catenin molecule. The cadherin has an extracellular component, a transmembranous component, and an intracellular component that links to a catenin protein. Catenin has alpha (α) and beta (β) components linking to actin, part of the cell cytoskeleton.

with the tissue that produces them; for example, *E-cadherin* (CDH1) is from epithelial tissue, *N-cadherin* (CDH2) is from neuronal tissue, and *P-cadherin* (CDH3) is found in the basal layer of epidermis and many other tissues. The *intracellular* components of the cadherins interact with an internal protein called **catenin** from the cell cytoplasm. Catenin interacts with the microfilaments (actin) of the cytoskeleton, and they can influence gene expression.

Some cadherins are involved with cancers:

- CDH1 (E-cadherin) and CDH2 (N-cadherin) are involved in direct tissue invasion by cancer cells and spread of metastases.
- CDH3 (P-cadherin) is involved in tumour invasion and metastatic progression in many tissues, but in some cancers, for example, melanoma, it is down-regulated to allow the tumour to become more aggressive, so it may act as a tumour suppressor in those tissues.
- CDH5, also called VE-cadherin for *vascular endothelial*, is involved in angiogenesis.
- CDH17, also called LI-cadherin for *liver/intestinal*, is involved in liver cancers.
- CDH13, also called H-cadherin for *heart*, or T-cadherin for *truncated*, because it lacks the transmembranous and intracellular components seen in all other cadherins, is found largely in the heart but also in a range of other tissues. It is involved in various carcinomas.

These cadherins are some of those under investigation as potential anti-cancer drug targets: CDH1, CDH2, CDH6, CDH11, and CDH17 (Table 6.1).

TABLE 6.1 Cadherins under investigation as drug targets

Cadherin	Drugs in trial	Cancer
CDH1 (E-cadherin)	ADH-1 (see CDH2).	Various cancers, including gastric and colon.
CDH2 (N-cadherin)	ADH-1 inhibits CDH1 and CDH2 and prevents interaction with the cell cytoskeleton and other cell surface receptors, causing loss of cancer cell migration, invasion, and angiogenesis. GC-4 is a monoclonal antibody that prevents CDH2 binding.	Melanoma, ovarian, and pancreatic cancer; prostate, breast, and glioblastoma.
CDH6	HKT228, DS-6000, and PCA062 are drugs called ADCs (see 'Antibody–drug conjugates', Chapter 5, p. 105).	Solid tumours of the renal tract, ovarian cancer, and other metastatic cancers.
CDH11	PF-03732010 is a MAB (see 'Monoclonal antibody (MABs)', Chapter 5, p. 102).	Solid tumours of the renal tract and other metastatic cancers.
CDH17	Lic5 is a MAB (see 'Monoclonal antibody (MABs)', Chapter 5, p. 102). BI 905711 is an antibody that promotes apoptosis in cancer cells. VHH1-CAR T cell (see 'Adaptive cell therapy (ACT)', Chapter 5, p. 99).	Various cancers, including gastrointestinal and hepatocellular; colorectal and pancreatic cancers; neuroendocrine tumours; gastric, colorectal, and pancreatic cancers.

Integrins (Figure 6.2)

These are a group of transmembranous protein cell surface receptors that bind to components of the extracellular matrix (ECM). This prevents the cell from moving out of position. They are made from various combinations of alpha (α) and beta (β) protein elements. The alpha and beta combination determines which component of the ECM, that is, collagen, laminin, or fibronectin, it will bind to, for example, α1 = collagen, α2 = collagen, α3 = laminin, α4 = fibronectin, α5 = fibronectin, α6 = laminin, α7 = laminin, and α10 = collagen. These act in conjunction with several variations of beta strands, for example, β1, β2, β3, β5, and others.

Three amino acids, **arginine**, **glycine**, and **aspartame**, are regular components of the ECM that are involved in integrin binding. The binding of integrins to ECM promotes integrin clustering and further binding, which then strengthens the cell's adhesion to the extracellular matrix. Binding also promotes the assembly of elements of the cytoskeleton through intermediaries, such as actin-binding proteins and enzymes, for example, **focal adhesion kinase (FAK)**. Integrin, therefore, creates internal changes through external binding, that is, external to internal signalling. Similarly, signals are generated inside the cell and passed to the external component. These signals adjust the binding to regulate the affinity of the integrin binding site on the ECM. If integrin–ECM binding is reduced and the cell develops loss of adhesion to the ECM, integrins then have a role in triggering **anoikis**, that is, cell death, due to the cell breaking free. A lack of integrin–ECM binding causes the cell to produce **caspase-8**, a member of the **cysteine–aspartic acid protease (caspase)** family, and this triggers apoptosis. Cell survival is, therefore, dependent on integrin–ECM binding.

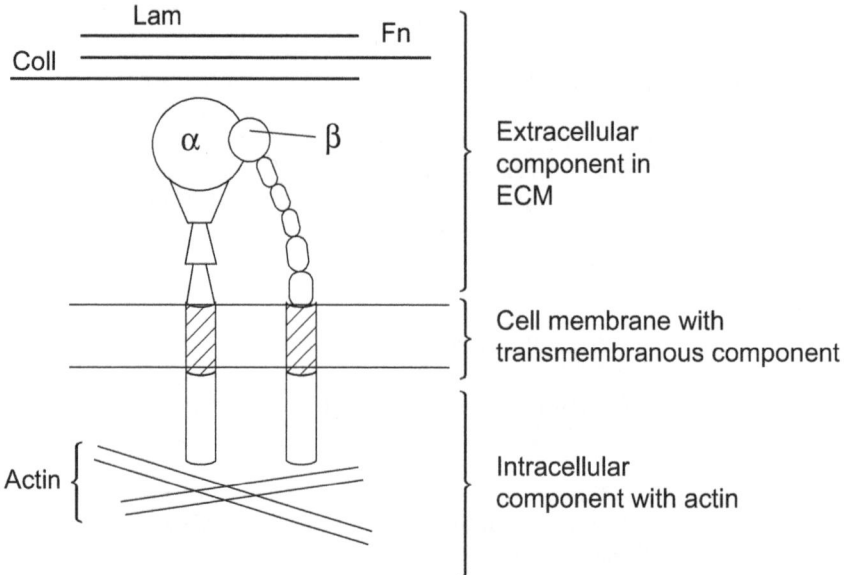

FIGURE 6.2   Integrin and ECM binding. The integrin molecule is composed of an alpha (α) and a beta (β) strand. It has an extracellular component extending into the ECM that binds to either collagen (Coll), fibronectin (Fn), or laminin (Lam). Which it binds to depends on the combination of different alpha and beta components present. The transmembranous component passes through the membrane, and the intracellular component interacts by focal adhesion with actin, part of the cytoskeleton, and signalling to the nucleus, affecting cell survival, migration, proliferation, and differentiation.

One important integrin is $\alpha_v\beta_3$ because it is involved in angiogenesis, that is, the creation of new blood vessels. It is found in endothelial cells lining blood vessel walls but is not found in normal epithelial cells. In tumours, it is critical for the formation of the new blood supply, which will serve the tumour with the blood it needs for survival. This makes it a prime target for drug therapy, which will stop the growth of the blood supply to the tumour.

Selectins

These are transmembranous glycoprotein CAM receptors that bind polysaccharides, also known as glycans, on the surface of neighbour cells. There are three types: E-selectin on endothelial[3] cells, L-selectin on leukocytes, and P-selectin on platelets. They function within the blood and vascular system and therefore interact with metastases that have gained entry to the circulation. They are also involved in cellular activity during inflammation, a process linked to cancer.

Immunoglobulin-like CAM proteins (IgCAMs)

These are a large family of cell surface molecules with immunoglobulin-like structures (called **domains**) in their extracellular component. These domains provide cell-to-cell adhesion and cellular signalling. They bind to other IgCAMs or integrins on the neighbour cells.

Carcinoembryonic antigen-related cell adhesion molecules (CEACAMs)

These are closely related cell surface glycoprotein CAMs that are vital during foetal development, but cells normally stop producing these CAMs at birth. They usually occur only in very low amounts in adulthood. Human cells have 12 different types of CEACAMs, that is, CEACAM1, 3, 4, 5, 6, 7, 8, 16, 18, 19, 20, and 21. Some solid tumour cells in adults often over-express these, especially CEACAM1, CEACAM5, and CEACAM6. They can then be identified as cancer biomarkers and sites for potential targets for the treatment of lung, colorectal, and pancreatic cancers. Blood levels of these CAMs can also be raised in heavy smokers.

Other cell-to-cell junctions

In addition to CAMs, other cell attachments exist. **Cell junctions** are points where epithelial cells touch, for example, tight junctions, gap junctions, and desmosomes (Figure 6.3). **Tight junctions** are a mesh of interlocking cell membrane proteins where nothing can pass between the cells. They are a fusion of the proteins in one cell membrane with the proteins of the neighbouring cell membrane. They play an important role in locking cells together. **Gap junctions** are where the membrane of one cell is very close to the neighbouring cell membrane but there is enough space to allow the passage of some substances between the cells. Openings (called **connexons**) between the two cells across the junction occur to allow movement of substances between the cells without having to pass via the extracellular fluid or the blood. **Desmosomes** are junctions that anchor one cell to the next. At specific sites across the two facing cell membranes, cadherins extend out across the extracellular space between the membranes and lock onto each other, without the membranes touching. These junctions are also attached to the intermediate filaments of the cytoskeleton on the inside of each cell. So effectively, this locks one cell cytoskeleton to the next and gives great strength to cellular adhesion. They are found in tissues subjected to mechanical stress, like the skin and heart muscle (Marieb and Hoehn 2022).

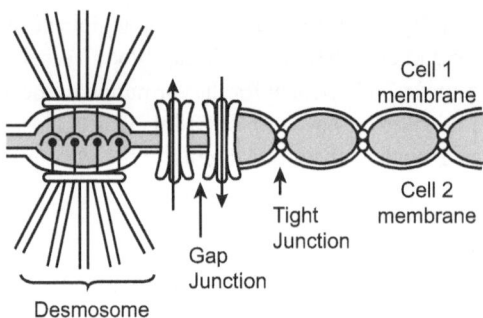

FIGURE 6.3 Cells junctions. Tight junctions, gap junctions, and desmosomes.

CD44 is an important cell surface glycoprotein adhesion receptor that is involved in cell-to-cell communications, cell adhesion, and cell migration of embryonic stem cells. It binds to some proteins in the extracellular matrix, for example, collagen and metalloproteinases.

Syndecans are transmembranous glycoproteins that bind to other protein components of the extracellular matrix and act as a co-receptor with integrins and cadherins. Inside the cell, they are linked to the actin cytoskeleton and are involved in cell migration, adhesion, junction formation, and differentiation.

Metastases

Metastases are malignant cells that have broken free from being *anchorage-dependent*, and having survived, they are able to continue to grow, that is, they are now *anchorage-independent*. Malignant metastases have overcome the apoptosis (**anoikis**) trigger to ensure their survival. They have broken away from the original tumour, called a **primary**, by severing the normal cell-to-cell adhesion, and they may cause another tumour, a **secondary**, to arise elsewhere in the body. Approximately 90% of cancer deaths are due to secondary tumours, that is, metastases. Cells that cause secondary tumours, or cause re-growth of a primary tumour after treatment, are sometimes called **high-relapse cells**.

Setting malignant cells free from anchorage results in cells acquiring three states:

1. Freedom to move from the place they were first located (primary tumour) to any other site in the body (secondary tumour)
2. Freedom to survive and replicate as independent units (part of **autonomy**)
3. Freedom to function regardless of the body's needs and natural control mechanisms of growth and cellular activity (the other part of **autonomy**)

Acquiring these states requires complex, interconnecting biochemical pathways (cell-signalling pathways) within the cancer cell. These are grouped broadly into four functions:

- **Mobility** pathways to achieve state 1.
- **Viability** pathways to achieve states 1, 2, and 3.
- **Proliferation** pathways to achieve state 2.
- **Differentiation** pathways to achieve states 2 and 3.

Each of these responds to extracellular factors that bind to receptors on the cancer cell surface. The study of the way cancer cells change and free themselves from the constraints of body needs, and of the way they spread, has shed much light on the natural history of this disease.

Epithelial–mesenchymal transition (EMT)

This is the gradual change in cell type as epithelial cells become mesenchymal cells (Figure 6.4). *Mesenchymal cells* are undifferentiated stem cells that can transform into any cells type. They normally form collections of loose connective tissue in early embryogenesis before becoming specific tissues. This process is also normally seen in wound healing. In cancer, however, the epithelial cells regress back to this undifferentiated state.

Mesenchymal cancer cells are characterised by:

- Loss of epithelial cell-to-cell adhesion
- Increase in cell motility and becoming invasive
- Change of cell shape
- Loss of apical–basal polarity, that is, the spatial orientation of the cell
- Reprogramming of energy sources and growth factors for their own gain
- Change from E-cadherin to N-cadherin, a mesenchymal protein usually found in neurons
- Avoiding apoptosis and the immune system
- Increase in stem cell qualities, for example, self-renewal and reproductive immortality, leading to **cancer stem cells (CSCs)**

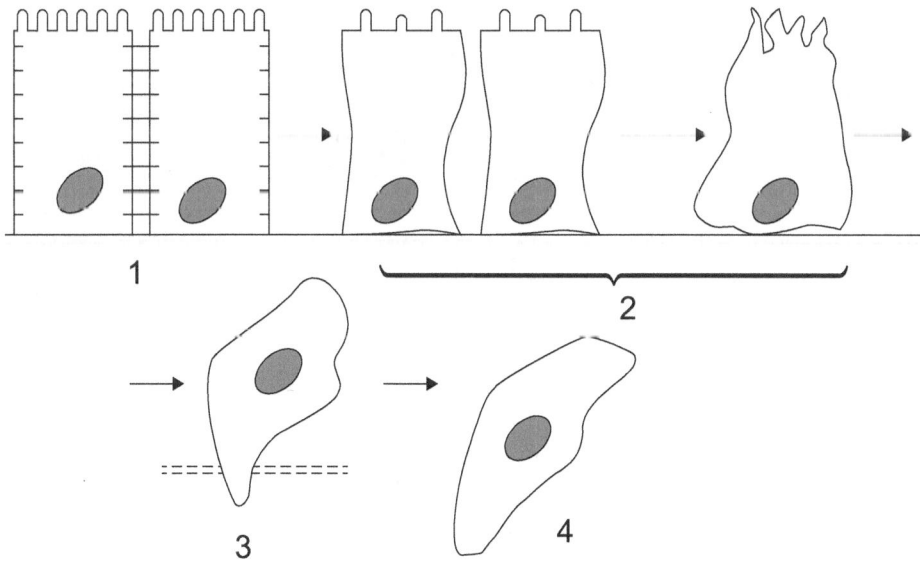

FIGURE 6.4   Epithelial–mesenchymal transition (EMT). This is a gradual, progressive process, and tissues going through this will show a mix of cells at all four stages: (1) epithelial cells → (2) early hybrid EMT cells → (3) late hybrid EMT cell → (4) mesenchymal cell. During the process, there is a complete loss of cadherin attachment and basement membrane, and the mesenchymal cell is free to move, that is, in cancer, this becomes a metastatic cell.

The tumour and its microenvironment

A tumour grows from CSCs within a carcinoma *in situ* (Figure 1.14, Chapter 1, p. 18). A great deal of modern research is based around the understanding of the composition of the inside and the immediate outside of a tumour: the **tumour microenvironment (TME)** (Figure 6.5). The reason for this is to see what factors are either promoting or inhibiting tumour progression and to target treatment to the best advantage. This means treatment that will block those factors that promote tumour growth, metastases, and immune evasion and will boost those immune factors that kill CSCs or inhibit their growth and spread (Anderson and Simon 2020).

Spatial transcriptomics is the study of positional data of cellular components, and their environments, within a tumour. When viewed at microscopic level in three dimensions, tumours show considerable diversity (**heterogeneity**) in their structure and contents. The microenvironment of tumours varies between different cancers, but typically it consists of more than just malignant cells. There are immune cells of all kinds and other cells, for example, stromal cells and fibroblasts; plus different proteins, for example, collagen and fibronectin; and other chemical agents, for example, cytokines and chemokines (Figure 6.5). Understanding these factors collectively is important for clinicians so they can identify the specific treatment the patient requires. It is a move away from the 'one treatment fits all' approach of the past to tailor-made therapy, leading to a better prognosis. Single-cell studies (see 'Single-cell multiomics', Chapter 1, p. 21) are a vital part of the picture. A holistic approach becomes necessary to recognise the cell within

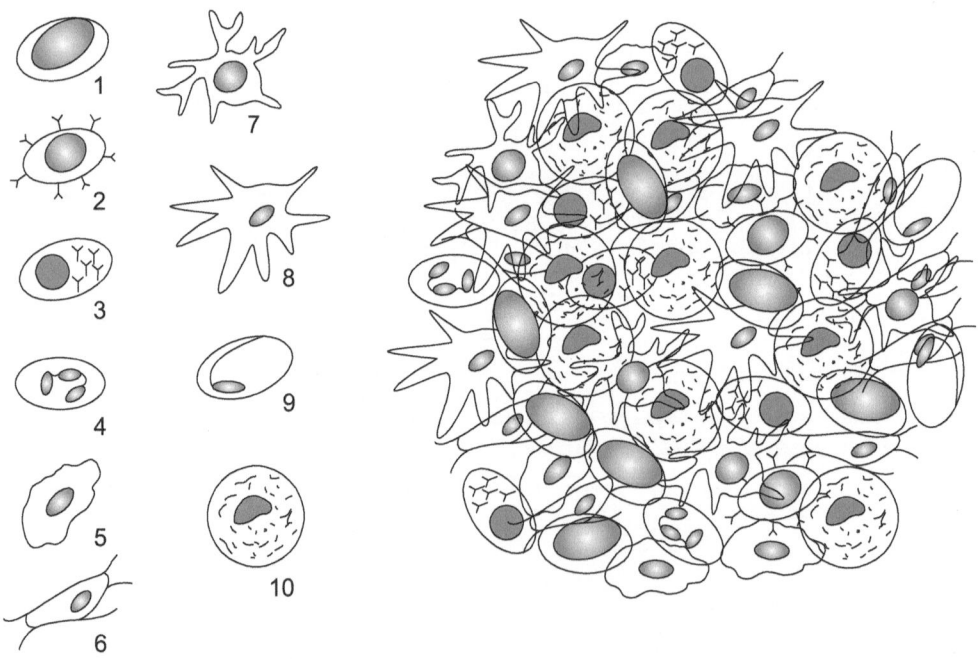

FIGURE 6.5   The tumour microenvironment (TME). The cells present, shown in the key (left), are threaded through with a framework of laminin, fibronectin, collagen, and blood vessels. Key: (1) T cell; (2) B cell; (3) plasma cell; (4) neutrophil; (5) NK cell; (6) fibroblast; (7) dendritic cell; (8) macrophage; (9) adipocyte; (10) cancer cell.

its TME, and the complex, dynamic interactions that take place between them. It can also help identify those factors that cause drug therapy resistance. Spatial transcriptomics have been applied to breast, lung, skin, colorectal, brain, and prostate cancers.

Inflammation involves vasodilation within the TME, and this brings more blood; therefore, it brings more immune cells that can kill tumour cells. Some pro-inflammatory cells and chemical agents that cause inflammation are often present for this reason. But contrary to this, it is worth remembering that tumours can develop from chronic inflammation caused by persistent infection in otherwise-normal tissues, notably liver, colorectal, and cervical cancers. So inflammation can be useful, especially within an established tumour, but in normal tissues, prolonged inflammation from infection may be detrimental.

Tumours may exist in any of three immunological states (Table 6.2).

The main cells and other factors involved in the tumour microenvironment are (Sounni and Noel 2013):

1. Immune cells

   - **Cytotoxic T cells** (T_C cells) that kill tumour cells and block new blood vessel growth, that is, they prevent angiogenesis by producing **interferon gamma** (**IFN-γ**). The presence of T_C cells in the TME is often associated with a good prognosis.
   - **Helper 1 T cells** (T_H-1 cells) work with T_C cells and produce **IFN-γ** and **interleukin 2 (IL-2)**. They are also pro-inflammatory.
   - **Regulatory T cells** (Tregs; previously known as suppressor T cells) are normally required to reduce the immune response back to a standby status. In the TME, these cells aid tumour advancement by reducing the anti-tumour immune response. They also secrete growth factors which promote tumour progression, and Il-2 that modulates natural killer (NK) cells.
   - **B cells** mostly accumulate in the tumour margins and in lymph nodes local to the tumour. They produce anti-tumour antibodies and act as **antigen-presenting cells** (**APCs**) (Figure 5.8, Chapter 5, p. 87). They can also show pro-tumour activity by the production of cytokines, such as **transforming growth factor beta** (**TGF-β**) and **interleukin 10 (Il-10)**, that promote the immunosuppressive activity of macrophages, neutrophils, and Tc cells.
   - **Macrophages** are phagocytes derived from monocytes (see 'Tissue invasion: macrophages', p. 125).
   - **Neutrophils** infiltrate the TME and release cytokines to induce inflammation. Early in the process, they cause tumour cell death (apoptosis), but later, they promote tumour cell progression through various means, including releasing **vascular endothelial growth factor** (**VEGF**), which promotes angiogenesis (tumour's blood supply), and producing **metalloprotease-9** (**MMP-9**) (see 'Tissue invasion', p. 123). They also increase their

TABLE 6.2 The three immunological cell profiles of different tumour microenvironments

Immune infiltrated	*Immune excluded*	*Immune silent*
Immune cells are distributed throughout the tumour.	Immune cells are positioned outside of the tumour.	No immune cells involved in the tumour.

Source: After Anderson and Simon (2020).

own length of survival and start to cause immunosuppression. This transformation from anti-tumour to pro-tumour cells is the result of changes made to the neutrophil epigenetics whilst inside the TME (see 'Epigenetics', Chapter 2, p. 36). Under cellular stress conditions, neutrophils release small pieces of DNA which form **neutrophil extracellular traps** (**NET**s), that is, sticky, web-like structures. Stress raises the glucocorticoid level, and this triggers the neutrophil to release the DNA. In stress from infections, NETs help trap and kill the microorganisms. In cancer stress, NETs can provide an environment that benefits the malignant cells, so future drugs may be able to prevent NET formation as part of the cancer treatment regime.

- **Natural killer cells** (**NK cells**) are most active in the blood circulation, where they are effective in killing tumour metastases and blocking their invasion into other tissues. They also kill virally infected cells. Their activity inside tumours is less effective.
- **Dendritic cells** are antigen-presenting cells (Figure 5.8, Chapter 5, p. 87). They are in the skin (called **Langerhans cells**) (see 'Structure and function of skin: Langerhans cells', Chapter 13, p. 243) and in the blood and the mucous lining of the digestive and respiratory tracts. They migrate to lymph nodes, where they interact with T cells and B cells. In a tumour, they initiate a T cell–specific response to the tumour cells, but eventually, the TME produces cytokines that may, or may not, succeed in causing dendritic cells to accept the presence of tumour cells.

2. **Stromal cells**, also called **mesenchymal**[4] **stroma cells** (**MSC**), are connective tissue cells that support the **parenchymal** (or functional) cells of the organs. A common type of stromal cell are fibroblasts, but stroma also includes vascular endothelial cells, adipocytes, and stellate cells. In the TME, the interaction between stomal cells and the tumour cells is very important for tumour growth and progression:

   - **Cancer-associated fibroblasts** (**CAF**s) are abundant in the TME. They are mostly derived from fibroblasts present before the tumour but can also be formed from other cell types. Once converted to CAFs in the TME, they produce growth factors and cytokines to promote tumour proliferation and metastasis development, angiogenesis, immunosuppression, and to make changes in the ECM in favour of tumour spread. They produce TGF-β, which is required for angiogenesis and epithelial–mesenchymal transition (EMT) (Figure 6.4). They also produce MMP-3, which breaks down E-cadherin to aid cancer cell invasion.
   - **Stellate cells** are liver and pancreatic stromal cells. Normally they are inactive but become activated by pathological changes, and they transform into **myofibroblasts**. Cancer of the liver activates **hepatic stellate cells** (**HSC**s). Active HSCs promote angiogenesis and modifies the ECM in favour of tumour growth. In the pancreas, activated stellate cells modify the ECM to allow proliferation and migration of tumour cells.
   - **Adipocytes** are fat cells of adipose tissue. Tumours that develop in tissues rich in adipocytes, such as breast cancers, form a critical relationship with fat cells. Lipids are broken down to release fatty acids for tumour cells usage, such as an energy supply and formation of tumour cell membranes. Adipocytes also release **metalloproteins**, for example, MMP-1, MMP-7, MMP10, MMP-11, and MMP-14 (see 'Tissue invasion', p. 123), which modify the ECM in favour of tumour invasion. Adipocytes also produce the hormone **leptin**, which activates macrophages and promotes breast cancer cell proliferation. For these reasons, overweight is a risk factor that increases the chance of several types of cancers (Figure 3.3, Chapter 3, p. 47).

Glucose-regulating protein 78 (GRP78)

GRP78 is normally a protein resident in the endoplasmic reticulum (ER) of the cell cytoplasm (see Table 1.1, Chapter 1, p. 5). It is known as a **chaperone protein**, that is, it is involved in the folding, unfolding, and assembly process of other proteins. Under cellular stress conditions, such as viral infection of the cell, or the cell becoming malignant, GRP78 relocates to the nucleus and changes its role to interfering with gene transcription. It promotes activity in the gene EGFR, which encodes a growth factor receptor (see 'Chromosome 7', Addendum, p. 348). This results in the cell becoming more mobile and invasive. Another protein is ID2, which normally prevents excessive gene transcription, leading to excessive gene over-expression, including EGFR, but GRP78 binds to ID2, making it unavailable to carry out its task. Therefore, GRP78 promotes tissue invasion and metastases by over-expressing EGFR and by blocking ID2 in lung, colon, pancreatic, and breast cancers. It may become a target for drug treatment in the future.

Tissue invasion

CSCs invade surrounding tissues as **collective cell migration** or **individual cell migration**. In order to cross the basement membrane, the CSCs must produce several families of **proteolytic enzymes**, that is, enzymes that break down proteins. Two such enzyme families are **serine proteases** and **metalloproteinases** (**MMPs**) (Figure 6.6). There are three main groups of these enzymes in the metalloproteinase family, the **collagenases**, which break down collagen; the **gelatinases** (MMP-2 and MMP-9), which break down a range of different proteins; and the **stromelysins**, which break down stromal elements. The activity of the gelatinases appears to be particularly important for the invasiveness of CSCs. Gelatinase is involved not only in the destruction of proteins but also in embryonic growth and development, tumour spread through

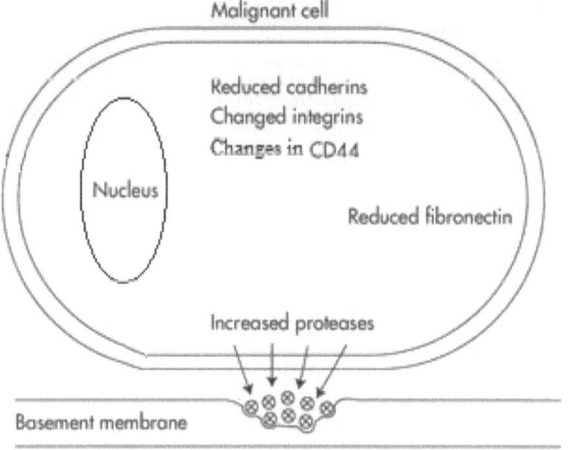

FIGURE 6.6   Changes in a malignant cell to become a metastatic cell. The cancer cell's ability to break through the basement membrane requires reduction of the level of cadherins and fibronectin. There is also a change to a variant CD44, and metalloproteinases are released in exosomes. There also has to be down-regulation of those genes responsible for blocking metastasis formation (see 'Metastatic suppressors', p. 127).

the tissues, angiogenesis,[5] and inflammation. Carcinomas have a greater tendency to invade the lymphatic system, whilst sarcomas have a greater affinity for invading the bloodstream.

To pass through other tissues successfully, malignant cells must have *very low* E-cadherin levels. E-cadherin is therefore down-regulated, meaning, that the gene that codes for E-cadherin is 'switched off'. Malignant cells also reduce the amount of **fibronectin** from their cell surface. Fibronectin is also found in basement membranes. Normally, it is active in cell-to-cell adhesion, so this loss again helps free the cell.

Invasive cancer cells must also maintain cell-to-cell communication, as this improves their chances of survival. Collectively, cancer cells can create the processes that prepare the tumour microenvironment (TME) for cellular invasion and distribution.

The change to metastatic cells at a cancer primary site marks the development from carcinoma *in situ* to *invasive carcinoma*. Invasive carcinoma is the generation of metastatic cells that have penetrated the basement membrane (Figure 1.14, Chapter 1, p. 18).

Several factors affect the survival and spread of metastases:

- **Telomeres** are lengths of non-coding, repeating DNA sequences located at the end of the chromosome that protect the chromosome and prevent it from tangling. Telomeres shorten after each cell cycle. At a critical short length, the telomere prevents further cell divisions and triggers apoptosis, or cell death. In cells that reproduce rapidly, the telomere would shorten quickly and the cell would have a very short existence. In this case, an enzyme called **telomerase** rebuilds some of the telomere so it shortens at the same rate as other cells. The telomere is maintained by protein products from three genes, *TERT* (see 'Chromosome 5', Addendum, p. 347), *ACD* (see 'Chromosome 16', Addendum, p. 356), and *POT1* (see 'Chromosome 7', Addendum, p. 349). Cancer cells cannot allow apoptosis to happen, so they overcome this by mutations of these genes. In this way, cancer cells achieve immortality.
- The **extracellular matrix** (**ECM**) is an important component of the TME. It consists of a glycoprotein framework, that is, collagen, fibronectin, and laminin, with the protein elastin, within which cells exist. Some solid tumours have up to 60% of their mass as ECM. CAFs secrete the bulk of the proteins that constitute the ECM. MMPs break down the ECM framework to allow tumour cells to progress and form metastasis. **ECM stiffness** is an important factor. For any metastatic cell to spread through the ECM, that ECM must be stiff. Soft matrix provides a difficult environment for cancer cells to penetrate and survive. Any enzyme that softens the matrix is suppressed by the cancer cell, and it will increase any other factors that make the ECM stiffer. A stiff ECM promotes factors in favour of the tumour cells, notably:

  1. Uncontrolled cell proliferation
  2. Angiogenesis, forming new blood vessels for tumour growth
  3. Immunosuppression
  4. Further metastases
  5. Drug therapy resistance

- **Extracellular exosomes** are microvesicles, or membrane-bound pockets of cytoplasm, which can leave the cell. They may contain enzymes, RNA, DNA, lipids, and transcription factors. **Cancer-derived exosomes** (**CDEX**s) can contain many diverse pro-tumour factors to aid the cancer cells to survive and spread. These include proteins, such as proteolytic enzymes, growth factors to promote angiogenesis, factors promoting inflammation and tumour progression, factors to evade immunity, and nucleic acids (mRNAs). CDEXs also facilitate cell-to-cell communication between the tumour cells and other cells, including vascular endothelial cells, mesenchymal cells, and even immune cells.

- **CD44** (see 'CD (cluster of differentiation) system', Chapter 5, p. 90) changes from standard CD44 (sCD44) to variant CD44 (vCD44) in cancer cells promoting invasion and migration of CSCs into the surrounding tissues. It is highly expressed in many CSCs and moved to the cell surface. sCD44 is reduced (down-regulated) in colon, ovary, and prostate cancers, but vCD44 is increased (upregulated) in melanomas.
- **Macrophages** are cells of the immune system which are derived from blood monocytes, and their role is to ingest antigens[6] and destroy them. They also present antigens to T cells to activate the T cell response. They are then called **antigen-presenting cells** (**APCs**) (Figure 5.8, Chapter 5, p. 87). Two types of macrophages exist, the **M1** and the **M2**. M1 are *classically activated*, meaning, they are provoked into action by bacteria or *pro-inflammatory* **cytokines** and carry out phagocytosis. M2 are *alternatively activated*, which means they are activated by different *anti-inflammatory* cytokines. They reduce inflammation and have a role in tissue repair and healing. In cancer, both are found in tumours, but the TME supports mostly the M2 type by the presence of cytokines, such as interleukin 4 (Il-4), and this promotion of M2 cells favours tumour progression. M1s reduce tumour growth by triggering apoptosis and autophagy[7] in CSCs, and they promote other anti-tumour responses. M2 can promote tumour growth by increasing angiogenesis, tissue invasion, and immunosuppression. High levels of macrophage infiltration in a tumour are often linked to unfavourable prognosis in certain cancers, such as gastric, lung, and breast cancers. M1 versus M2 can have consequences for the outcome of cancer therapy. Macrophages also accumulate in the TME blood supply, where they promote angiogenesis by releasing **vascular endothelial growth factor** (**VEGF**).

Once metastatic cells have invaded the tissues, they can spread (Figure 6.7):

- *By direct invasion* into tissues surrounding the tumour
- *Via the lymphatic system*, involving first local, then distal lymph nodes
- *Via the blood* to any part of the body
- *Transcoelomic*, that is, malignant cells moving through a body cavity after they have invaded through the wall of the organ that contains the primary tumour

Metastatic cancer cells in the blood, also known as **circulating tumour cells** (**CTCs**), often form clusters. The blood is not a good place for CTCs. They are washed along under pressure by the blood flow with little control over their destiny. Estimates indicate that only about 0.01% of individual CTCs in the blood can establish a new (secondary) tumour away from the primary tumour. But as clusters, they increase their chances of success by 50 times.

The reasons for CTC mortality in circulation are:

1. Malignant cells are removed and destroyed by the body's immune cells (see 'Natural killer cells', Chapter 5, p. 91).
2. They are destroyed by **proteolytic enzymes**, that is, enzymes that break down their proteins.
3. They die from mechanical stresses, for example, they get damaged by high arterial pressure and by trying to squeeze through the microscopic holes in the walls of the smallest blood vessels.

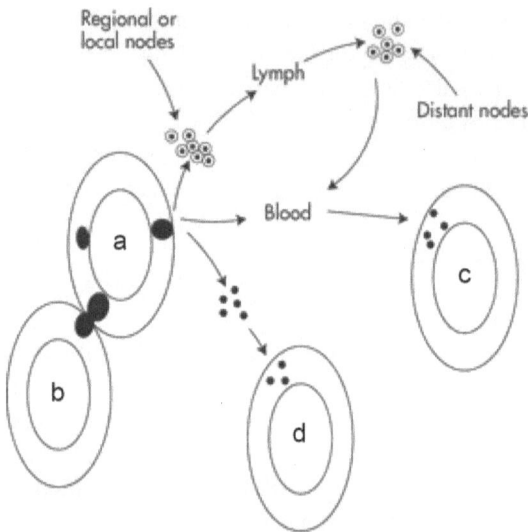

Regional or local nodes

Lymph

Distant nodes

Blood

a

b

c

d

FIGURE 6.7 The spread of tumours. The tumour in organ (a) can undergo direct spread locally and infiltrate into the next organ (b). Metastases can move into the local (regional) lymph nodes, then on to distant lymph nodes. From there they can pass into the blood. Direct metastatic spread into circulation can lead to secondary growths in distant organs (c). Metastases from the primary tumour can sometimes spread across a body cavity (transcoelomic) to separate organs within that cavity (d).

4. They become coated with **platelets** (see 'Blood cell types: group 4', Chapter 7, p. 132), and this makes them larger and stickier. They are then more likely to become jammed in the next downstream capillary bed.

When a CTC does arrive at another tissue, they may still face problems. The new tissue is very different from the tumour they left, and it is effectively a harsh and hostile environment. Some fail because they were unable to establish a new blood supply for themselves, that is, failed angiogenesis. Others may die due to the absence of vital factors, for example, growth factors, in the microenvironment of the new location, that is, factors required for survival and replication. Many secondary tumours occur in the lung, the liver, and the bones, and these sites may offer better opportunities for metastatic cells to meet their needs.

To invade the tissues, CTCs must first stop at a particular site, then pass through the blood vessel wall. It could be that certain CAMs (see 'Cellular adhesion molecules (CAMs)', p. 114) on the blood vessel epithelium surface 'capture' malignant cells from the blood.

Metastases in the lymphatic system may adhere to the lymphatic wall and grow along the lymphatic vessels. Malignant cells in the lymph have a somewhat-easier time than in the blood, until they arrive at a lymph node. Here they accumulate and are attacked by activated **lymphocytes** (see 'Innate (non-specific) immunity', Chapter 5, p. 78). Lymph nodes containing malignant metastases are sometimes called *seeded*, and the node may become overwhelmed by cancer cells, where they form a focus for malignant growth. Naturally, the nearest lymph nodes to the tumour are the first to be affected, particularly if they directly drain lymph from the tissues containing the tumour. Lymph nodes that are more distant from the primary site can also become seeded over time. Ultimately, the lymph will drain into the blood (see Figure 7.7, Chapter 7, p. 142), and malignant cells may enter the circulation via this route.

Metastatic suppressors

These are naturally produced proteins that slow or prevent the development of metastases. Some may promote the metastatic cancer cell's death, called **anoikis**, that is, apoptosis caused by breaking free from the cells' anchored location. Others may decrease the cells' ability to pass through the extracellular matrix (ECM) or interfere with signal transduction. In many tumour cells, the genes encoding metastatic suppressor proteins are deactivated, or *down-regulated*, as much as possible to give the metastatic cell a chance to survive (Table 6.3). It is hopeful that drugs can be developed to enhance the activity of these genes and therefore increase the proteins that prevent the formation of secondary growths. Some chemical agents are already known to do this.

Since tumour growth is dependent on the development of a blood supply, called angiogenesis, drugs that block angiogenesis are a useful branch of tumour treatment. However, many tumours become resistant to these drugs, and therefore, they often become useful only in the short term.

Another approach involves identifying the genes that code for metastatic suppressors. Drugs that improve transcription of these genes may be a way forward, and work to develop these drugs is ongoing. The challenge for the future resides in the clinical trials. Drugs that kill tumours show a distinct and measurable outcome, indicating the drug's success or failure. However, drugs preventing the formation of metastases would result in nothing tangible to measure in the clinical setting. The need for different forms of clinical trials becomes evident.

TABLE 6.3 Some metastatic suppressor genes which are down-regulated in these cancers

Metastatic suppressor gene	Gene location	Protein	Cancer involved
NME1	17q21.33	NME/NM23 nucleoside diphosphate kinase 1	Melanoma, breast, and colon
MAP2K4	17p12	Mitogen-activated protein kinase kinase 4 (MKK4)	Prostate and ovary
GAS1	9q21.33	Growth arrest specific 1	Melanoma
CD82	11p11.2	CD82 molecule	Prostate and breast
KISS1	1q32.1	KISS-1 metastasis suppressor (KISS1)	Melanoma and breast
MED23	6q23.2	Cofactor required for SP1 transcriptional activation, subunit 3 (CRSP3)	Melanoma
TXNIP (VDUP1)	1q21.1	Thioredoxin-interacting protein (vitamin D– upregulating protein 1)	Breast, liver, gastric, bladder, and lung
BRMS1	11q13.2	Breast cancer metastasis repressor 1 (BRMS1)	Breast and melanoma
SDPR	2q32.3	Caveolae-associated protein 2 (cavin-2)	Breast
DRG1	22q12.2	Developmentally regulated GTP-binding protein 1	Lung, breast, and larynx

Cancer of unknown primary (CUP)

About 3–5% of metastatic cancers are CUP, that is, they cannot be traced back to a primary tumour. These tend to result in a poor outcome. A recently developed artificial intelligence (AI) machine learning classifier called OncoNPC (oncology next generation sequencing [NGS]–based primary cancer-type classifier) is significantly improving the outcome for this difficult group of cancers (see 'Artificial intelligence (AI) in cancer management', Chapter 17, p. 320).

Key points

Cell attachment

- Most cells remain locked in their correct position within the tissues.
- The *cytoskeleton* is a protein framework of the cell consisting of microfilaments, intermediate filaments, and microtubules.
- Cell adhesion molecules (CAMs) are transmembranous glycoprotein receptors, and they provide anchorage between cells (e.g. E-cadherin).
- Cells also have tight junctions, gap junctions, and desmosomes between them.

Metastases

- The change to metastatic cells in a cancer is a change from carcinoma *in situ* to invasive carcinoma.
- Malignant cells can become free from anchorage, that is, they become anchorage-independent.
- Malignant tumours can spread by direct invasion, via the lymph or blood and via transcoelomic spread.
- To invade other tissues successfully, malignant cells must try to avoid the immune system.
- The most common secondary tumours sites are the bones, lung, liver, and brain.

Notes

1 *Glycoproteins* are proteins with one or more sugars attached. This is an example of structural sugars, that is, sugars used in a framework rather than in metabolism.
2 Highly glycosylated, that is, having a large number of sugar molecules attached.
3 Endotheliums are smooth, pavement-like cells that line the inside of blood vessels.
4 Mesenchymal cells are multipotent (Chapter 7. Figure 7.1, p. 130) stem cells capable of becoming any of several types of connective tissue.
5 Anti-angiogenesis is a good possibility for drug treatment in order to starve the tumour of its blood supply.
6 *Antigen* is a harmful foreign entity that has entered the body, such as a bacterium or virus. They are often, but not always, proteins. Metastatic cancer cells can be considered as antigens.
7 *Autophagy* is the orderly degradation and recycling of cellular components, resulting in the death of the original cell.

7

BLOOD AND LYMPHATIC CANCERS

- Blood cellular differentiation
- Bone marrow cancers
- The lymphatic system
- Lymphatic cancers
- Blood transfusion
- Key points

Blood cellular differentiation

Chapter 1 introduced the basic biology of blood (see 'Blood tissue', Chapter 1, p. 13) and identified blood cells as of three main types: **erythrocytes** (**red blood cells, RBC**), **leukocytes** (**white blood cells, WBC**), and **thrombocytes** (**platelets**). All these are derived from the same cells, called bone marrow **stem cells**, or more specifically, **haemopoietic stem cells** (*haem* = blood; *poiesis* = forming), which are found in **bone marrow**.

Stem cells are **undifferentiated**, that is, they are at the earliest stages of cell formation and have not yet, at that point, started to become a specific cell type. The move towards cell specialisation is called **differentiation**. It is useful to remember differentiation by the fact that specialised cells, for example, brain and muscle cells, are different than each other. They carry out very different functions and are normally incapable of reverting back to their former primitive condition. At much earlier stages of development, all cells are derived from the same cell cluster, which is formed from the fertilised ovum. The terms **totipotent** (*potent* = able to do), **pluripotent** (*pluri* = more), and **multipotent** (*multi* = many) **stem cells** are often used to reflect the different stages of stem cell development (Figure 7.1), where totipotent cells are capable of becoming any one of the 216 different body cell types, that is, they are cells of the very early cell mass after fertilisation. Cells then move on from totipotent to multipotent by *switching off* genes in the nucleus, leading to increasing specialisation (or differentiation). Ultimately, the stem cells remaining in adult life are only those there to replace the fully differentiated cells that are lost by depletion, are damaged, or are simply at the end of their lifespan. Such is the usual outcome for blood cells.

DOI: 10.4324/9781003389125-7

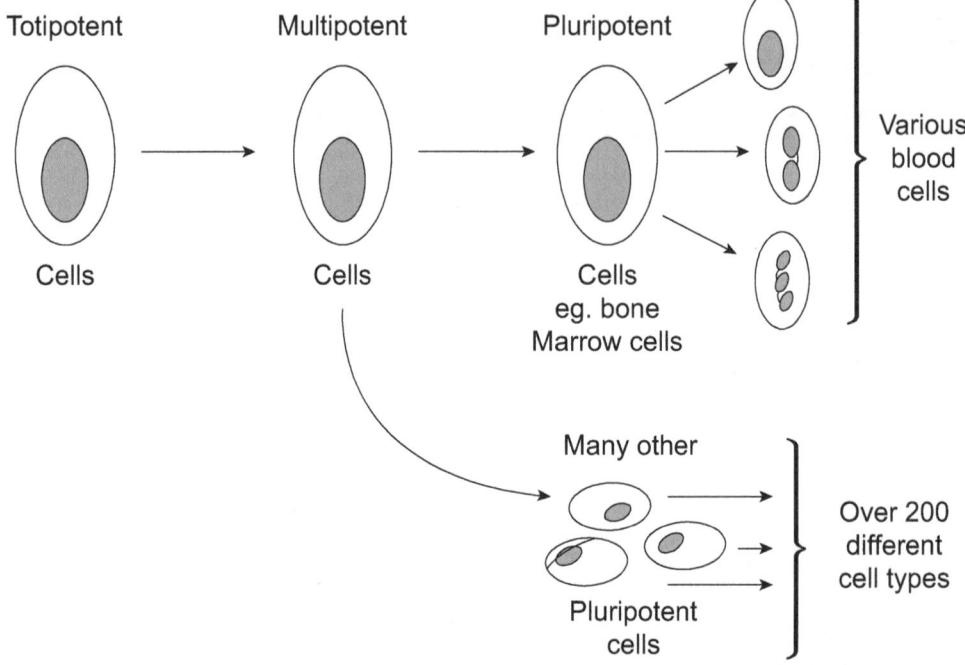

FIGURE 7.1 Sequence of cell development. Totipotent cells are derived from the fertilised ovum, and they are the starting point for 216 different cell types in the body. Multipotent cells have switched some genes off, so they are becoming more specialised. Pluripotent cells (e.g. bone marrow cells) are a further specialisation, by deactivating more genes. They give rise to over 200 types of highly specialised cells, for example, blood cells.

Blood cell formation

Haemopoietic stem cells develop into any one of four major types of blood cells, called **cell lineages**:

1. **Myeloid**, the granulocytes, also known as **polymorphonuclear cells** and mononuclear cells
2. **Lymphoid**, the lymphocyte lineage
3. **Erythroid**, the erythrocyte lineage
4. **Megakaryocytes**, the platelet lineage

The development of mature blood cells from stem cells in bone marrow involves several stages for each cell line. Figure 7.2 shows the cells involved at the various stages of development (or differentiation) from haemopoietic stem cells. They are:

1. *Myeloid* cell lines develop first to **myeloid stem cells**, and these can become either (a) **myeloblasts**, which then develop into **myelocytes** and, finally, any of the granulocytes, or (b) **monoblasts** and, finally, **monocytes**. Notice the term *blast* indicates a primitive cell type.
2. *Lymphoid* cell lines develop first to **lymphoid stem cells**, and these become **lymphoblasts**, which then develop into lymphocytes.

3. *Erythroid* cell lines develop first to **pro-erythroblasts**, and these become **erythroblasts**, which then develop into erythrocytes.
4. **Megakaryocytes** are the precursor of the thrombocytes (or platelets).

Blood cell types

Group 1, the myeloid lineage, includes the **polymorphonuclear cells**, or **polymorphs** for short (*poly* = many; *morph* = shape, that is, the cells with many-shaped nuclei). These same cells are also known as **granulocytes** because they also have granules in their cytoplasm (Figure 7.2). There are three types of granulocytes (polymorphs), called **neutrophils**, **basophils**, and **eosinophils**.

Neutrophils are by far the commonest of the white blood cells (WBCs) in circulation, accounting for about 60–70% of adult WBCs, and the commonest of the granulocytes, that is, over 95% of circulating granulocytes. They are short-lived phagocytes, surviving

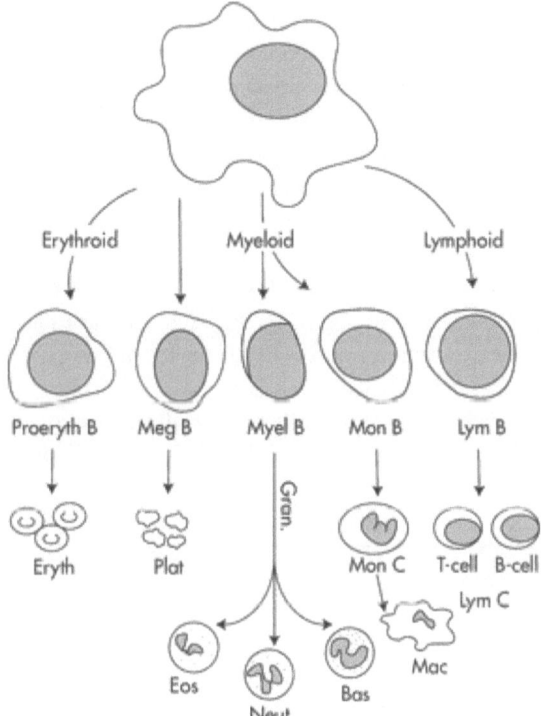

FIGURE 7.2 Blood cell lineages. The four lineages branch from bone marrow stem cells. They are erythroid, leading to red blood cells (erythrocytes); megakaryoblasts, leading to mega-karyocytes and on to platelets; myeloid, splitting into two lines, one leading to granu-locytes (Gran.), the other leading to monocytes; and lymphoid, leading to lymphocytes. *Bas* = basophils; *Eos* = eosinophils; *Eryth* = erythrocytes; *Lym B* – lymphoblasts; *Lym C* = lymphocytes; *Mac* = macrophages; *Meg B* = megakaryoblasts; *Mon B* = monoblasts; *Mon C* = monocytes; *Myel B* = myeloblasts; *Neut* = neutrophils; *Plat* = platelets; *Pro-eryth B* = pro-erythroblasts.

Source: Redrawn from Blows (2024, Figure 4.8).

about five and half days before being replaced. A **phagocyte** is any cell that engulfs and destroys unwanted foreign substances (known as **antigens**), such as bacteria and viruses, that may enter the body, and these cells are therefore extremely valuable in our defences against infections.

Basophils (Table 7.1) have cytoplasmic granules that contain inflammatory agents, such as histamine, and when these are released, they trigger an inflammatory response. This is valuable in aiding the immune defence against certain antigens but is also the cause of allergic responses, that is, inappropriate immune responses.

Eosinophils occur in small numbers in blood (Table 7.1). They also have cytoplasmic granules, but this time the granules contain, amongst other things, antihistamine, and this helps settle any inflammatory response. These cells also appear to act in defence of the body against parasitic infections.

The other cells included in the myeloid lineage are the **mononuclear cells**, or **monocytes**. These are the largest white cells and are important phagocytes that can migrate out of circulation into the tissue fluid (called **extracellular fluid**, or **ECF**). On moving from the blood to the ECF, monocytes change their nature and are then known as **macrophages**. They are very important in our defences against bacterial and viral infections and in lymphocyte activation.

Group 2, the lymphoid lineage, consists of two types of **lymphocytes**, B cells and T cells (see 'Specific immunity', Chapter 5, p. 81).

Group 3, the **erythrocytes** (or **red blood cells, RBC**), contains **haemoglobin**, necessary for oxygen transportation around the body. They have no nucleus, that is, they are **anucleated** (*a* as a prefix = without, that is, without a nucleus) and therefore only survive about 120 days, after which they are destroyed and must be replaced from bone marrow. They have a shape described as a *bi-concave disc*, that is, they are round with two flattened surfaces, both of which are dented slightly in. This shape allows for ease of passage through capillaries and provides the best possible surface area for the exchange of gases. Erythrocytes are more numerous than any other cell group (Table 7.1).

Group 4 are platelets (thrombocytes), which are critical in preventing blood loss by two mechanisms. Small holes in capillaries can be physically blocked by platelets until a repair is

TABLE 7.1 Normal blood cell and haemoglobin values

Blood cell	*Cell count (in blood)*
Erythrocytes	Male: 4.6–$6.2 \times 10^6/\mu l$ (SI = 4.6–$6.2 \times 10^{12}/L$) Female: 4.2–$5.4 \times 10^6/\mu l$ (SI = 4.2–$5.4 \times 10^{12}/L$)
Lymphocytes	$1,000$–$4,800/\mu l$ (SI = 1.0–$4.8 \times 10^9/L$)
Monocytes	0–$800/\mu l$ (SI = 0.0–$0.8 \times 10^9/L$)
Eosinophils	0–$450/\mu l$ (SI = 0–$0.45 \times 10^9/L$)
Basophils	0–$200/\mu l$ (SI = 0–$2 \times 10^9/L$)
Neutrophils	$1,800$–$7,000/\mu l$ (SI = 1.8–$7.0 \times 10^9/L$)
Thrombocytes	$150,000$–$400,000/\mu l$ (SI = 0.15–$0.4 \times 10^{12}/L$)
Haemoglobin (in erythrocytes)	Male: 13.5–18.0 g/dl (SI = 2.09–2.79 mmol/L) Female: 12.0–16.0 g/dl (SI = 1.86–2.48 mmol/L)

Note: *g* = grams; *dl* = decilitre; *SI* = Système International; *mmol* = millimole; *L* = litre; *μl* = microlitre.

complete. For larger damage to major vessels, platelets initiate the blood clotting mechanism. Platelets are the body's own method of **haemostasis**, or the control and prevention of blood loss (Blows 2024).

Blood groups

There are several different ways for the grouping of blood, but two methods are of particular importance: the **ABO system** and the **rhesus system**. In the *ABO system*, the red blood cells have any combination of two antigens on their surface: **antigen A** and **antigen B**. If the red cells have only antigen A, this is blood group A; cells with only antigen B produce blood group B; antigens A and B together produce blood group AB; and no antigen A or B on the red blood cell surface is blood group O. Present in the plasma are **antibodies**. Table 7.2 indicates which antibody is in each blood group. Individuals do not have the antibodies to react with their own antigen. However, they do have the antibodies that can react with antigens of a different blood to their own.

The *rhesus system* is a second type of RBC surface antigen, the **D factor**, or the **Rhesus factor**. If the D factor is present, the blood is **rhesus (Rh) positive** and the plasma has no **anti-D antibody**. If the D factor is absent, the blood is **rhesus (Rh) negative** but the plasma has anti-D antibody. Any of the four ABO groups can be either Rh-positive or Rh-negative, that is, a total of eight blood groups.

Blood cancers

Blood cancers are classified into leukaemia and myeloma. Some classifications add lymphoma to this list, but here they are considered separately (see 'Lymphatic cancers', p. 143).

Leukaemia

This is a group of diseases involving malignant changes to white blood cells in the bone marrow. The haemopoietic stem cells of the bone marrow show a lack of ability to differentiate normally into the range of blood cells expected. Instead, the bone marrow stem cells incline towards the production of white cells in large numbers, with a corresponding lack of red cells or platelets. Worse still, the white cells that are produced appear to enter circulation and exist at an immature stage of their production, that is, 'blast' cells, and therefore do not function fully. The result is an abnormal blood picture showing a mix of excessive immature white cells with a lack of red cells and platelets due to their abnormal development in the bone marrow. Much less common is the condition of **aleukaemic leukaemia** (*a* = without), showing low levels of immature blast cells with a corresponding low WBC count.

TABLE 7.2 The ABO blood group system

Blood group	Antigen on RBC	Antibodies in plasma
A	A	Anti-B (reacts with B antigen)
B	B	Anti-A (reacts with A antigen)
AB	A and B	Neither anti-A nor anti-B are present
O	Neither A nor B	Anti-A + anti-B (reacts with both)

Leukaemia exists in various forms, depending on which cell lineage is predominant in the peripheral blood. Then each type can be further divided into a rapidly developing severe leukaemia with blast cells in peripheral blood (the *acute* form) or a slowly developing, less-severe leukaemia with some mature cells in peripheral blood (the *chronic* form).

Acute leukaemia is the result of two abnormal processes going on simultaneously. These are:

1. *Excessive growth expansion*, where the growth of new blood cells has accelerated well beyond the requirements of the blood
2. *Failure of differentiation and maturation*, where the stem cells have failed to become the normal range of mature red cells, white cells, and platelets, instead becoming mostly of one immature type (i.e. white cells)

Chronic leukaemia tends to be less severe than the acute disorders partly because mature cells do appear in the blood, reducing the symptoms of the disease. They also mostly occur in the older age group.

The four forms of leukaemia are:

1. **Acute lymphocytic (or lymphoblastic) leukaemia (ALL)**
2. **Chronic lymphocytic leukaemia (CLL)**
3. **Acute myelocytic** (or **myeloblastic) leukaemia (AML)**
4. **Chronic myelocytic** (or **myeloid) leukaemia (CML)**

This classification is a little simplistic but covers most of the cases seen. The symptoms of both the acute and chronic leukaemia are found in Table 7.3.

Acute lymphocytic (or lymphoblastic) leukaemia (ALL)

This form of leukaemia is the most common cancer seen in children, accounting for about 80% of childhood cancers, and is found in boys more than girls. Half of all cases have an age of onset from 2 to 5 years old, peaking between 3 and 4 years old. The other half of the cases occur at any age, but again, the majority of these are before 15 years of age. The cause of ALL indicates the strongest links are with radiation and chemical exposure.

The white cells in this disease develop rapidly, but most do not progress to become mature cells, that is, 60–100% of the WBCs remain as immature blast cells. They accumulate in the bone marrow and suppress the differentiation of any remaining normal stem cells. The result is a shortage of red cells (anaemia), whilst normal mature white cells and platelets are also low, and this causes most of the symptoms and complications of the disease (Table 7.3).

A classification of ALL is as follows:[1]

1. Precursor B cell ALL. This is the most common type in adults.
2. Precursor T cell ALL. This is more likely to affect young adults and men.
3. Mature B cell ALL (Burkitt-type ALL). This is identified by specific genetic changes.

Precursor B cell ALL

B cell ALL is a fast-growing form producing excess immature B lymphoblasts. Various forms of B cell ALL exist based on genetic changes, such as too many chromosomes. One example

TABLE 7.3 The symptoms of leukaemia

Acute leukaemia	Chronic lymphocytic leukaemia (CLL)	Chronic myeloid leukaemia (CML)
• Rapid onset of symptoms • Fatigue, pallor, and breathlessness due to the anaemia, a lack of haemoglobin in circulation, caused by the low red cell count • Infections and fever due to low mature white cell count • Bleeding due to low platelet count, for example, petechiae, dark-red spots of bleeding into the skin or mucous membrane; ecchymoses, that is, bruising due to bleeding into the skin; epistaxis (nosebleeds); or bleeding from the gums • Bone pain due to bone marrow expansion • Lymphadenopathy, that is, disorder of lymph nodes; splenomegaly (enlarged spleen); and hepatomegaly (enlarged liver), all due to the spread of leukaemic cells to these organs • Headache and vomiting due to central nervous system involvement	• Often asymptomatic (*a* = without, that is, no symptoms), especially at first • Vague symptoms of fatigue, weight loss, and anorexia, that is, loss of appetite • Anaemia (see under 'acute leukaemia') • Increased risk of infections • Lymphadenopathy, hepatomegaly, and splenomegaly (see under 'acute leukaemia') • Unlike CML, conversion to an acute form by 'blast crisis' rare (see under 'CML')	• Slow onset of symptoms and slow progress of the disease • Fatigue, weight loss, weakness • Anorexia (see under 'CLL') • Extreme splenomegaly (see under 'acute leukaemia'), causing a dragging feeling in the abdomen • After an unpredictable period, half of patients entering a gradual *accelerated stage* with increased symptoms, especially anaemia; failure in response to treatment, leading to a 'blast crisis', that is, many immature cells in circulation, similar to acute myelocytic leukaemia (AML) • Other half developing 'blast crisis' quickly

is the **Philadelphia chromosome–like ALL (Ph-like ALL)**. It is a precursor B cell ALL with a 9–22 translocation forming the Philadelphia chromosome (Figure 7.3) (see 'Chromosome 9', Addendum, p. 350), which is present in 20–30% of adult ALL and 5% of child ALL.

Precursor T cell ALL

T cell ALL is a fast-growing form producing excess immature T lymphoblasts. One type of T cell ALL producing very early lymphoblasts is linked to a poor prognosis.

Mature B cell ALL (Burkitt type)

Mature B cell ALL (also called Burkitt leukaemia) is a rare disorder that has the same genetic errors and the same cell surface markers as Burkitt lymphoma, a type of non-Hodgkin lymphoma (see 'Lymphatic cancers', p. 143). The difference is the course of the disease. Burkitt leukaemia follows a similar course to other ALLs, and Burkitt lymphoma follows a disease course similar to those of other lymphomas.

The treatment of ALL has improved enormously, and prognosis is good for many children, although some children, and particularly adults with this disease, have a less-favourable outcome.

Chronic lymphocytic leukaemia (CLL)

CLL accounts for about 30% of leukaemia in the Western world but remains rare in Asia. It affects mostly people over the age of 50 years. The cancer is that of B cell lymphocytes in most cases, only about 5% being T cell lymphocyte in origin.

The B cells involved do not respond to activation by antigens, causing a low antibody count in the blood and a corresponding increased risk of infection. About 15% of cases show antibody production against red cells, causing the RBCs to break down, that is, a **haemolytic anaemia** (*haemo* = blood; *lysis* = breakdown). Abnormal B cells migrate from the bone marrow into the blood and infiltrate many other tissues, including lymph nodes.

Half of the patients have abnormalities of their **karyotype** (see Figure 1.5, Chapter 1, p. 6), of which the most characteristic abnormality is **trisomy 12** (three number 12 chromosomes instead of the normal two). Unfortunately, this karyotype abnormality carries a poor prognosis. They may also show abnormalities of chromosomes 11 or 14.

Acute myelocytic (or myeloblastic) leukaemia (AML)

This is a group of diseases affecting mostly adults, the incidence increasing with age. The group, also called **acute nonlymphocytic leukaemia**, arises from various origins, including multipotent stem cells or monocyte–granulocyte precursor cells (Figure 7.2).

Previously, eight different disorders were recognised by the **French–American–British (FAB)** system (Table 7.4).

The resulting blood picture is different in each case, depending on which cell line is most affected, and that depends on which precursor or stem cell is involved in the malignancy. Classes M6 and M7 (Table 7.4) are unusual subtypes since they involve erythrocyte and platelet cell lines, respectively. Hence the reason for the term *non-lymphocytic*, that is, involving all the cells except lymphocytes. Class M3 involves a **translocation** between chromosomes 15 and 17, that is, t(15:17) (see 'Mutation of genes', Chapter 2, p. 27, and 'Chronic myelocytic leukaemia (CML)', p. 137). The new translocated combination involves the retinoic acid receptor gene *RARA alpha* on chromosome 17 (see 'Chromosome 17', Addendum, p. 356). Retinoic acid is an active metabolite of vitamin A (Devlin 2010), and the

TABLE 7.4 French–American–British (FAB) system of classifying AML

Class	Name	Notes
M0	Undifferentiated acute myeloblastic leukaemia	AML with no differentiation in the stem cells
M1	Acute myeloblastic leukaemia with minimal maturation	AML with very little differentiation in the stem cells
M2	Acute myeloblastic leukaemia with maturation	AML with differentiation present in the cells
M3	Acute promyelocytic leukaemia (APL)	AML affecting promyelocytes (see text)
M4	Acute myelomonocytic leukaemia	AML affecting the myeloid (myelocyte and monocyte) cell lines
M4 eos	Acute myelomonocytic leukaemia with eosinophils	AML affecting the myeloid (myelocyte and monocyte) cell lines
M5	Acute monocytic leukaemia	AML subtype affecting mostly monocytes
M6	Acute erythroid leukaemia	AML subtype affecting mostly erythrocytes
M7	Acute megakaryoblastic leukaemia	AML subtype affecting mostly platelets

translocation of the gene blocks myeloid differentiation. This can be treated with high doses of retinoic acid.

A second system of AML classification is proposed by the World Health Organization (WHO) (Table 7.5).

Chronic myelocytic leukaemia (CML)

This disorder affects mostly adults between the ages of 25 and 60 years, peaking in incidence between 40 and 50 years of age. It accounts for about 20% of all cases of leukaemia. The genetic basis for this disease lies with the formation of the **Philadelphia chromosome (Ph^1)** (Figure 7.3). Ph^1 is a **translocation** (see 'Mutation of genes', Chapter 2, p. 27) occurring between chromosomes 9 and 22, that is, t(9:22). Chromosome 9 has the *ABL* gene, and chromosome 22 has the *BCR* gene (see 'Chromosome 9' and 'Chromosome 22', Addendum, p. 350 and 359).

The translocation involves a small portion of the long arm of chromosome 22 (the q arm, that is, 22q), which breaks off, leaving the gene *BCR* behind. This 22q fragment swaps places with a tiny fragment that has broken off from the q arm of chromosome 9 containing the *ABL* gene. The 9q fragment joins onto chromosome 22, and the two genes (*BCR* and *ABL*) come together (*BCR-ABL*). This is known as the Philadelphia chromosome (Ph^1) (Figure 7.3).

The break occurs in the *BCR* gene (short for *breaking point cluster*) on chromosome 22 and the *ABL* gene on chromosome 9. The new combination on chromosome 22 creates an **oncogene**

TABLE 7.5 WHO classification of AML

Name	Notes
AML with certain genetic abnormalities	AML can be associated with chromosomal translocations and inversions. The list includes translocations t(8:21), t(16:16), t(9:11), t(6:9), and t(3:3)[2] and inversions inv(16), inv(3).[3] Gene mutations are *NPM1* (see 'Chromosome 5', Addendum, p. 347), *CEBPA* (see 'Chromosome 19', Addendum, p. 352), and *RUNX1* (see 'Chromosome 21', Addendum, p. 359).
AML with myelodysplasia-related changes	AML with more than 20% immature blasts in the blood or bone marrow. These cells fail to function properly. The number of immature cells gradually increases as the disease progresses.
AML related to previous chemotherapy or radiation (t-AML)	t-AML is part of treatment-related myeloid neoplasms (t-MN) induced by treatment for a separate underlying tumour.
AML not otherwise specified	Includes FAB classifications M0, M1, M2, M4, M5, M6, and M7, plus acute basophilic leukaemia and acute panmyelosis with fibrosis.
Myeloid sarcoma (granulocytic sarcoma or chloroma)	Tumour consisting of myeloid blast cells situated at a site outside of the bone marrow.
Myeloid disease linked to Down syndrome	Down syndrome (trisomy 21) increases the risk of myeloid leukaemia.

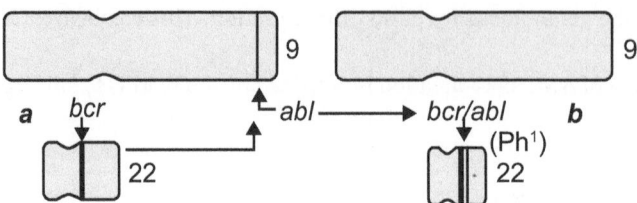

FIGURE 7.3   The Philadelphia chromosome (Ph¹): (a) Before the translocation, the gene *BCR* (thick line) is on chromosome 22, and the gene *ABL* (thin line) on chromosome 9. During translocation, some genetic material from 22 is swapped to chromosome 9 (left open-headed arrow), but leaving *BCR* on 22. (b) Genetic material from chromosome 9, including gene *ABL*, is swapped to chromosome 22 (right open-headed arrow). The new combination results in *BCR* and *ABL* coming together on chromosome 22, creating the Philadelphia chromosome (Ph¹), that is, the combined *BCR-ABL* oncogene.

('BCR-ABL', Chapter 2, p. 27) that leads to cancerous changes in the bone marrow since it causes uncontrolled cell growth in affected cells (Nussbaum et al. 2015). About 95% of patients with CML have the Philadelphia chromosome, but the presence of the Ph¹ chromosome is not diagnostic by itself, since this genetic error is also sometimes seen in acute myeloblastic leukaemia (AML) and acute lymphoblastic leukaemia (ALL).

The blood picture for CML shows a large increase in the numbers of leucocytes, which are mostly granulocytes of the neutrophil type, but also eosinophils and basophils. There appears to be no block to the maturation of these cells, so the cells in the blood are mature, but mostly of the granulocyte type. The bone marrow shows a large increase in the myeloid stem cell mass.

Multiple myeloma, also called **plasma cell myeloma**, or **myeloma**, is a rare cancer of the plasma cells within bone marrow. Plasma cells are normally activated mature B cells that produce antibodies (see 'Specific immunity', Chapter 5, p. 81). It can occur in multiple sites within the bones (hence the name *multiple*), causing bone pain in the skull, chest, ribs, pelvis, or spine. Other symptoms include nausea, fatigue, weight loss, bone fractures (known as **pathological fractures**), spinal cord compression, anaemia, raised blood calcium, dyspnoea, bleeding, bruising, kidney problems, and frequent infections. There is a link between multiple myeloma and a blood disorder called **monoclonal gammopathy of undetermined significance (MGUS)** in those who are overweight (see 'Obesity', Chapter 3, p. 45). During the early stages of the multiple myeloma, it may be without symptoms, that is, **asymptomatic**. It affects mostly males over 60 years of age, and mostly African Americans. The abnormal plasma cells grow in large numbers in the bone marrow, crowding out other blood cell production, for example, erythrocytes, causing the anaemia. The abnormal plasma cells also produce an abnormal antibody, called **M protein (monoclonal protein)**, which attacks other structures, such as the kidney, causing further problems. About 60–70% of patients have M protein which is **IgG kappa**, that is, two IgG heavy chains with two purely kappa light chains (Figure 7.4). About 20% of patients have M protein which is IgA kappa (Figure 7.4c).

The lymphatic system

The **lymphatic system** is a tissue fluid drainage system which serves several functions, mainly to return excess tissue fluid to the blood and to filter and destroy unwanted **antigens**, for example,

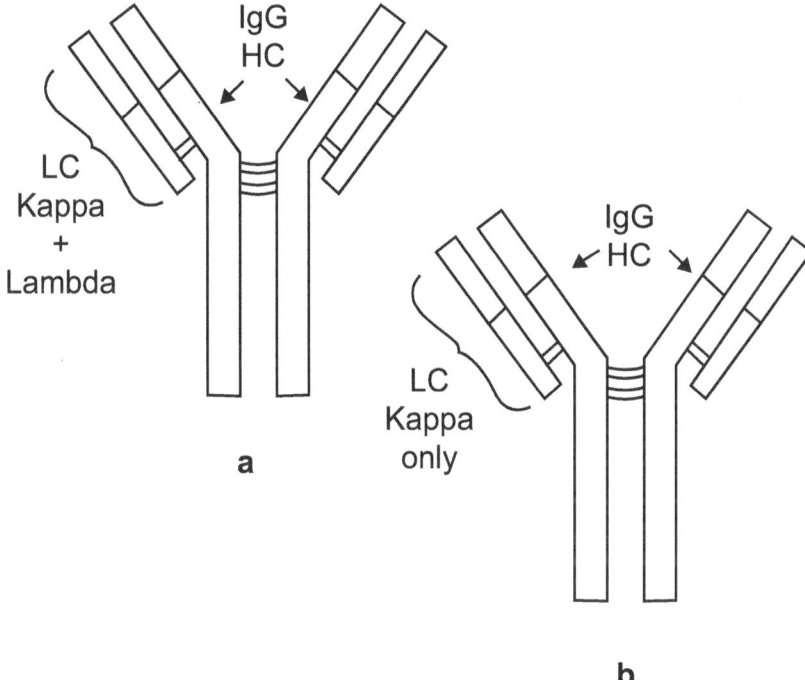

FIGURE 7.4 Multiple myeloma M protein IgG kappa antibodies: (a) The normal IgG. The heavy chain is HC. The light chains (LC) are half kappa and half lambda, which is the case for the light chains of all five classes of normal antibodies (see Chapter 5, Figures 5.3 and 5.5, p. 83). (b) IgG kappa M protein seen in 60–70% of multiple myeloma patients. The light chains are entirely kappa. The same occurs in IgA, that is, IgA kappa M protein, where again the light chains are entirely kappa. This is found in 20% of multiple myeloma patients. Overall, ten variations of M proteins are possible in multiple myeloma, but most are rare: IgA kappa, IgA lambda, IgG kappa (shown in *b*), IgG lambda, IgD kappa, IgD lambda, IgE kappa, IgE lambda, IgM kappa, IgM lambda. 'Light chain only' is a rare type of myeloma where the heavy chain is lost completely.

bacteria or viruses. Lymph is water derived originally from blood plasma which has already formed **tissue fluid** (also called **extracellular fluid**, or **ECF**) (Figure 7.5). Some ECF returns to the blood, but excess ECF drains away as lymph. Tissue fluid enters blind-ended lymphatic capillaries in the tissues, and the fluid is then called lymph. This drains towards the **lymph nodes** in **afferent vessels** (*afferent* = towards), which have non-return valves.

Lymph nodes (Figure 7.6) are small (most are less than 2.5 cm long), and they contain several compartments. In the **cortex** (or outer layer), the compartments contain **follicles** of densely packed B cell lymphocytes. Surrounding the B cell core of these follicles are T cells, which migrate in and out of the node and extend into the inner layer of the node (the **medulla**). The medulla also has many macrophages and plasma cells present.

Lymphocytes are originally derived from the bone marrow, and they find their way into lymph nodes via the blood and ECF. T cells spend some time in the **thymus gland** prior to relocating in the lymph nodes (see Chapter 5, Figure 5.7, p. 86). The thymus gland is in the chest, above the

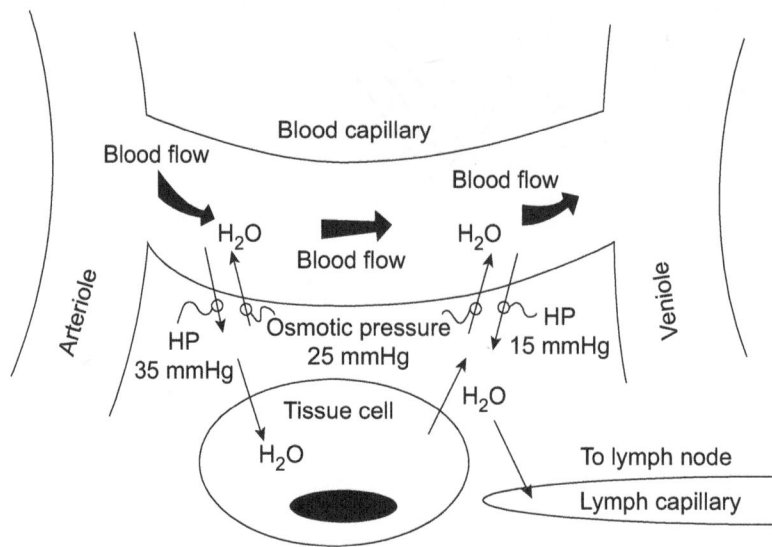

FIGURE 7.5 The formation of extracellular (tissue) fluid. The hydrostatic pressure (HP, the equivalent of blood pressure) forces water (H_2O) out of the capillary. This is higher at the arterial end of the capillary (35 mmHg) than at the venous end (15 mmHg). The osmotic pressure is caused by plasma proteins in the blood attracting water back into the capillary at 25 mmHg pressure throughout. The net flow of water is 35–25 (= 10 mmHg) *out* of the capillary at the arterial end, and 25–12 (= 13 mmHg) *into* the capillary at the venous end of the capillary. Lymph is formed from the excess tissue fluid collected by the lymphatic capillaries.

heart (see Chapter 5, Figure 5.6, p. 86), and it is the site of T cell maturation, where these cells gain their specificity. The lymph nodes are the site where many of these cells will reside and may meet with antigens. Specific antigens will trigger a response, that is, activate T cell and B cell conversion to plasma cells to produce antibodies. Lymph glands become a hive of activity and swell up when infections occur. Macrophages, the phagocytic cells, also collect within the lymph nodes. They remove and engulf any invading antigens, such as bacteria and viruses, that are passing through the gland.

Lymph glands are also the sites where circulating malignant cells, that is, **metastases**, become trapped after they have entered circulation from a malignant tumour, and these also provoke an immune response. Lymph nodes are often the first line of defence against metastases, and these glands can become overwhelmed and heavily involved in the cancer. Surgical removal or radiation of lymph nodes involved in the cancer is usually an important component of the treatment.

On leaving the nodes, the lymph drains back towards the blood via **efferent vessels** (*efferent* = away from), which then empty into one of two main **lymphatic ducts**.

1. The left lymphatic duct is the largest and extends from the abdomen to the left shoulder. This returns lymph to the blood of the left **subclavian vein**, the lymph having come from the legs, the left arm, and most of the left side of the trunk and head.

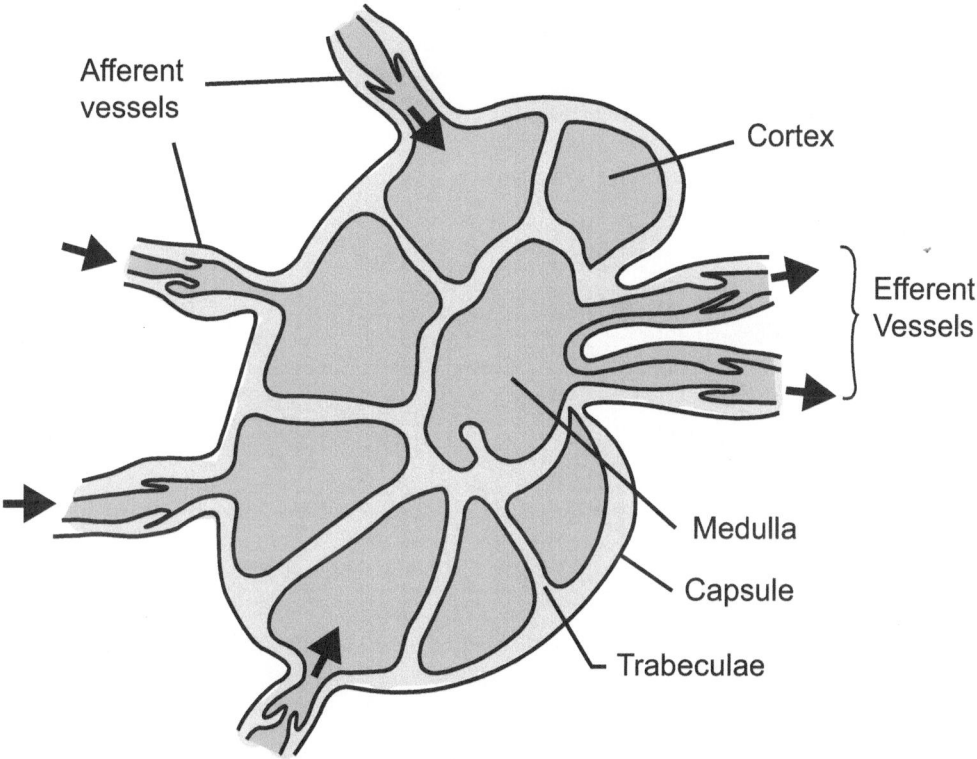

FIGURE 7.6   Cross section of a lymph node. There is a cortex surrounding an inner medulla. The cortex is divided into compartments by walls called trabeculae. Lymph flows into the node via several afferent (= towards) vessels and passes through channels called sinuses. Lymph then leaves via two efferent (= away from) vessels, the lymph ultimately returning to the blood. The outer cortex consists of follicles where dividing B cell lymphocytes occur. The deeper cortex houses T cell lymphocytes, which are constantly interchanging with the blood. The medulla contains both lymphocyte types.

2. The much smaller right lymphatic duct returns lymph to the blood in the right subclavian vein, the lymph having drained from the right side of the head, the right arm, and the right side of the chest (Figure 7.7).

The drainage of lymph becomes more problematic when the lymph nodes become involved in a cancer, and often when they are removed as part of the treatment. This slows down lymphatic drainage, with the potential for the pooling of lymph in the tissues, causing a swelling known as **lymphoedema**. Normally, proteins do not easily escape from the blood capillaries, so tissue fluid is usually low in proteins. When proteins do get into the tissue fluid, the only way for them to get back into the blood is via the lymphatic drainage. Lymphoedema prevents the proteins from returning to the blood, and the tissue fluid becomes richer in protein, that is, sometimes up to 30 g/L. These proteins attract more water out of the blood capillaries, and the tissues swell further.

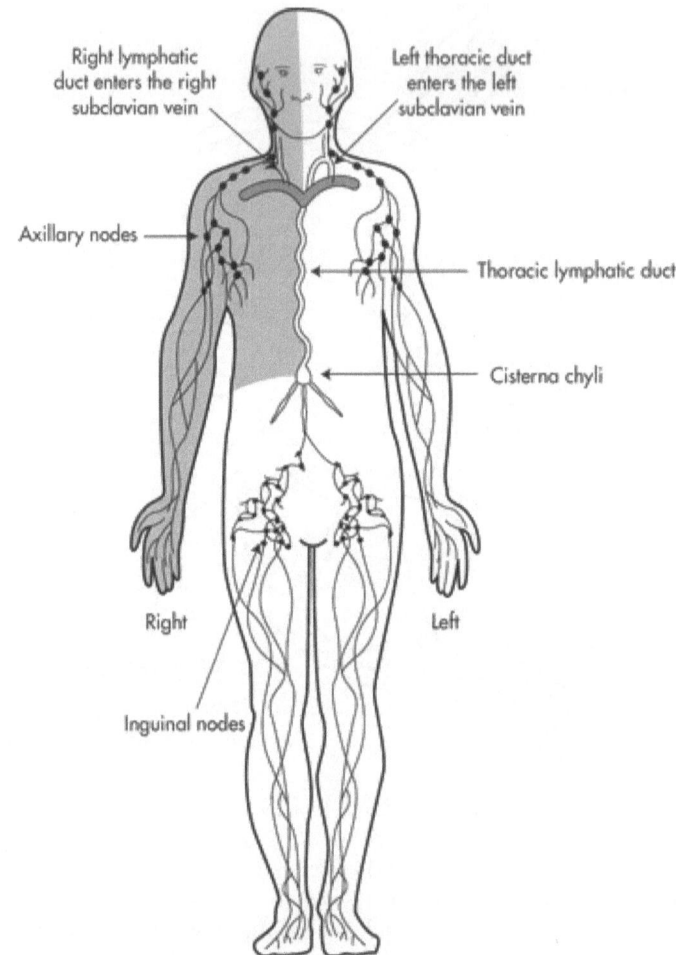

FIGURE 7.7 The drainage of lymph back to the blood. The shaded area on the right of the body is drained by the short right lymphatic duct into the right subclavian vein. The unshaded area on the left side and lower parts of the body is drained by the long thoracic duct, which starts at the cisterna chyli in the upper abdomen and empties into the left subclavian vein. Some lymphatic nodes form clusters in certain areas, for example, the axillary and inguinal nodes (as shown). This drainage pattern is important to know which nodes are likely to be involved in a particular cancer, depending on the site of that cancer.

Source: Redrawn from Marieb and Hoehn (2022).

Some larger, specialised lymphatic nodes form specific organs, for example, the **tonsils** (in the throat) and **adenoids** (in the nose) and **Peyer's patches** (associated with the digestive tract) are all important components of the lymphatic system. The **spleen** (in the abdomen) is not strictly a lymph node. It has a blood circulation and lymphatic drainage but filters blood rather than lymph.

It carries out functions very similar to lymph nodes, as follows:

1. It filters and destroys old, damaged, and abnormal red blood cells, helping control the number of healthy red cells and platelets in circulation.

2. It detects and filters bacteria and viruses directly from the blood. In the event of an infection, the spleen initiates immune responses by increasing the number of lymphocytes that fight that infection in circulation.
3. It stores a pool of blood cells which can be released into circulation if required.
4. It produces substances that promote inflammation and healing.
5. It can provide a defence against metastases, that is, loose cancer cells in circulation from a cancer somewhere else. It does this by producing lymphocytes and anti-cancer chemicals.

Cancer of the spleen itself is usually a *secondary* growth, that is, derived from a leukaemia or a lymphoma (the *primary* growth). Removal of the spleen is known as **splenectomy**, a surgical procedure done either as an emergency, due to internal abdominal haemorrhage associated with trauma of the spleen, or more selectively, because of splenic involvement in diseases such as cancer. Whilst it is true that an individual can live without a spleen, the loss of the spleen is potentially a problem in the long term and should be avoided if possible. Splenectomy patients may suffer more future infections due to the presence of blood-borne bacteria, and they also show abnormally old red cells remaining in circulation, as well as an increased platelet count.

Lymphatic cancers

Cancers of the lymphatic system fall into two categories, *primary* tumours that arise from the lymphatic system itself, and more often, *secondary* tumours, which are delivered to the lymphatic nodes in the form of metastases from primaries arising elsewhere.

Lymphomas are primary tumours of lymph nodes. Thomas Hodgkin was a pathologist at Guys Hospital, London, who first described lymphomas in the early 1800s, and now lymphomas are classified into either **Hodgkin lymphoma** or **non-Hodgkin lymphoma**, depending on the tissue pathology of the tumour. Lymphocytes are residential cells in lymph nodes, and most lymphomas arise from malignancy of one of the lymphocyte types, that is, either B cells or T cells.

B cell lymphomas sometimes stem from a translocation between chromosomes 14 and 18, that is, t[14;18], involving the *BCL2* gene (see 'Chromosome 18', Addendum, p. 357). *BCL2* normally suppresses and regulates apoptosis, helping control the correct number of healthy B cell lymphocytes. The translocation moves *BCL2* from chromosome 18 to chromosome 14, where it meets with a stronger promoter, causing overproduction of the gene protein. Apoptosis is then abnormally and excessively suppressed, allowing survival of too many abnormal B cell lymphocytes, which go on to form B cell lymphoma. *BCL2* is part of a family of genes, most of which are linked to cancers. The protein p53 helps regulate genes of the *BCL2* family, and cancers involving mutations of the *BCL2* family often involve mutations of the *TP53* gene (see 'Chromosome 17', Addendum, p. 356).

Hodgkin lymphoma (HL)

This disease is derived from B cell lymphocytes and causes swollen, often painless lymph nodes usually at sites close to the axis of the body, that is, the trunk. These frequently start in the cervical (neck) region and go on to involve the axillary and inguinal nodes, spreading by *contiguity*, that is, by contact with neighbouring cells. Tissues outside the nodes are not often involved. The cause and pathology of this disease are not fully known. It can spread to the nodes serving other tissues, including the liver, lungs, spleen, and bone marrow. As Hodgkin disease progresses, it causes anorexia, weight loss, anaemia, and weakness. A fever (known as **Pel–Ebstein fever**) is also seen, where the temperature rises and falls in a cyclic manner. Hodgkin disease is characterised by the presence of abnormal cells called **Hodgkin cells** and **Reed–Sternberg cells**, collectively known as **HRS cells**. These are giant malignant cells derived from lymph node germinal centre B cell lymphocytes. Hodgkin cells have a single nucleus, whilst Reed–Sternberg cells have two nuclei.

The disease occurs twice as often in men as in women and peaks in incidence between the ages of 15 and 35 years, then again between 55 and 75 years. The two main types of this disease are:

1. Classic Hodgkin lymphoma (CHL)
2. Nodular lymphocyte-predominant Hodgkin lymphoma (NLPHL)

Classic Hodgkin lymphoma has four subtypes, totalling about 90% of cases (Table 7.6).

Nodular lymphocyte-predominant Hodgkin lymphoma (**NLPHL**) is a rare disease (10% of cases of HL) which is distinct from classic HL. It is slow-growing and affects B cell lymphocytes, which then resemble popcorn and dominate the tissues. It affects men more than women between the ages of 30 and 50 years.

Non-Hodgkin lymphoma

This term is used to describe a collection of lymphomas, all of which show an *absence* of Hodgkin and Reed–Sternberg cells. There are more than 30 subtypes classified by the lymphocytes involved (B cells or T cells) and if they are fast-growing (aggressive) or slow-growing (indolent).

The highest incidences occur between the ages of 50 and 70 years, with men more frequently affected than women.

Non-Hodgkin lymphoma involves more peripheral nodes in the limbs than Hodgkin lymphoma and spreads by *non-contiguity*, that is, not directly to neighbour cells but spreads over distance. It also spreads more to tissues outside the nodes than Hodgkin lymphoma does.

Table 7.7 shows some of the subtypes of non-Hodgkin lymphoma.

TABLE 7.6 Subsets of classic Hodgkin lymphoma (CHL)

Subset	Notes
Nodular sclerosis 60–70% of cases	Most common of the subtypes, with large nodules containing HRS cells surrounded by lymphocytes, eosinophils, activated B cells (plasma cells), and fibrosis. Sclerosis (scaring) present.
Mixed cellularity About 20–25% of cases	Relatively common subtype, with HRS cells mixed in with lymphocytes, eosinophils, and plasma cells. No sclerosis. Often linked with Epstein–Barr virus (EBV) infections in HRS cells (Chapter 4, Figure 4.2a, p. 61).
Lymphocyte-rich 4–5% of cases	Rare subtype with good prognosis. Scattered HRS cells surrounded by many small lymphocytes.
Lymphocyte-depleted About 1% of cases	Very rare subtype, with several different HRS cells and few lymphocytes.

TABLE 7.7 Some subtypes of non-Hodgkin lymphoma

Subtype	Aggressive	Indolent	Notes
Burkitt's lymphoma	√		Usually in African children. It is a lymphoma starting in B cell germinal centres of lymph nodes, often in the abdomen. The cause is unknown but may be linked to cases of malaria, *MYC* gene mutations, and Epstein–Barr virus (EBV) infections.
Mantle cell lymphoma	√		Mostly in older men. It forms from B cells in the mantle zone of lymph nodes, and B cells accumulate to form painless swellings of the neck, axilla, and groin.
Follicular lymphoma		√	Mostly in the elderly. It forms from B cells which grow slowly in groups, forming nodules in lymph nodes and organs.
Small lymphocytic lymphoma (SLL)		√	Mostly in the elderly. It is almost the same as *chronic lymphocytic leukaemia (CLL)* (p. 136), except B cells grow in the lymph nodes, whilst in CLL they grow in the blood and bone marrow.
Diffuse large-cell lymphoma	√		Children and the elderly. It is a lymphoma of abnormal and enlarged B cells dispersed in a diffuse manner.
Lymphoblastic lymphoma	√		Mostly in children. It is a lymphoma of abnormal immature T cells causing painless swelling of nodes in the neck, axilla, and groin and affects the thymus gland.
MALT (mucosa-associated lymphoid tissue) lymphoma		√	Mostly in older men. It is a rare lymphoma starting in mucosal linings of organs outside of lymph nodes, for example, the digestive system.

Key points

Blood

- Stem cells are undifferentiated, meaning, they have not yet become a specific cell type, and can become RBCs, WBCs, or platelets.
- The four major types of blood cell lineages are myeloid (the granulocytes or polymorpho-nuclear cells and the mononuclear cells), lymphoid (the lymphocyte lineage), erythroid (the erythrocyte lineage), and megakaryocytes (the platelet lineage).
- Three types of granulocytes (polymorphs) exist, namely, neutrophils, basophils, and eosinophils.
- Neutrophils are the commonest of the white blood cells in circulation.
- Neutrophils are phagocytes, that is, a cell that engulfs and destroys antigens.
- Monocytes are large phagocytic cells that can migrate out of circulation into the tissue fluid, where they change their nature and are known as macrophages.
- Two types of lymphocytes occur, T cells and B cells.
- Erythrocytes are red blood cells (RBCs) containing haemoglobin, which carries oxygen around the body.
- Platelets are the body's own method of haemostasis, that is, the control and prevention of blood loss.

Blood cell formation

- Myeloid cell lines develop first to myeloid stem cells, which can become either myeloblasts (becoming myelocytes and, finally, granulocytes) or monoblasts (becoming monocytes).
- 'Blast' indicates a primitive cell type.
- Lymphoid cell lines develop first to lymphoid stem cells, becoming lymphoblasts, then lymphocytes.
- Erythroid cell lines develop first to pro-erythroblasts, becoming erythroblasts, then erythrocytes.
- Megakaryocytes become thrombocytes (platelets).

Blood groups

- In the ABO blood grouping system, red blood cells have combinations of two antigens, A and B.
- Only antigen A on the RBC surface is blood group A, only antigen B is blood group B, antigens A and B together form blood group AB, and no antigen A or B on the red blood cell surface is blood group O.
- The rhesus system means the D factor is either on the RBC surface (Rh-positive) or is missing (Rh-negative).
- The plasma of Rh-positive blood has no anti-D antibody.
- The plasma of Rh-negative blood has anti-D antibody.

Blood cancers

- *Leukaemia* is a group of diseases involving malignant changes to bone marrow cells.
- The types of leukaemia are acute lymphocytic (or lymphoblastic) leukaemia (ALL), chronic lymphocytic leukaemia (CLL), acute myelocytic (or myeloblastic) leukaemia (AML), and chronic myelocytic leukaemia (CML).
- Acute leukaemia causes abnormal blood with excessive immature white cells and a lack of red cells and platelets.
- Chronic leukaemia has more normal mature cells in circulation and affects the elderly more than the young.

Lymphatic system

- The lymphatic system returns excess tissue fluid back to the blood and filters out and destroys bacteria and viruses.
- Lymph is derived from blood plasma, which first forms extracellular fluid, then lymph.
- Lymph nodes have compartments in the cortex containing follicles of densely packed B cell lymphocytes with T cells surrounding.
- The inner layer of the node is the medulla, with macrophages and plasma cells.
- Lymph nodes are the sites where many malignant cells (metastases) from the malignant tumour become trapped, and these provoke an immune response.
- Removal of lymph nodes involved in cancer often makes the drainage of lymph more problematic, that is, it slows down, causing pooling of lymph in the tissues and swelling (lymphoedema).

- The spleen acts like a lymph node attached to the blood circulation.
- Splenectomy (removal of the spleen) may result in more infections due to blood-borne bacteria and abnormally old red cells remaining in circulation, with an increased platelet count.

Lymphatic cancers

- *Lymphomas* are primary tumours mostly of lymph nodes and are classified into either Hodgkin disease or non-Hodgkin disease.
- Hodgkin disease causes swollen, painless lymph nodes, anorexia, weight loss, anaemia, fever, and weakness and is characterised by the presence of Hodgkin and Reed–Sternberg cells.
- *Non-Hodgkin disease* is a term used to describe a collection of lymphomas, all of which show an absence of Hodgkin and Reed–Sternberg cells.

Notes

1 A previous classification, the French–American–British (FAB) classification of ALL, may still be found in the literature, and possibly in clinical practice. It is L1, small uniform cells; L2, large varied cells; L3, large varied cells with vacuoles (small spaces within the cytoplasm). This FAB classification of ALL must not be confused with the FAB classification of AML (Table 7.4).
2 The small 't' is *translocation*, that is, some genes have moved from one chromosome to another. The chromosomes involved are shown in the brackets.
3 The 'inv' means *inversion*, meaning, some genes have become back-to-front (inverted) on the chromosome that is noted in the brackets.

8

CANCERS OF THE DIGESTIVE SYSTEM

- **The digestive system**
- **Neoplastic disease of the upper digestive tract**
- **Pancreatic cancers**
- **Colorectal neoplasms**
- **Liver**
- **Liver cancers**
- **Key points**

The digestive system

The digestive tract is essentially a tube made from **smooth muscle** which functions automatically, that is, without conscious control. It is very different from skeletal muscle (see 'Muscle tissue', Chapter 1, p. 13). The muscle of the gut wall contracts and pushes food along the tube. This wave of contraction is called **peristalsis**, and other muscular contractions ensure that food is well mixed and broken down with the digestive enzymes. The inner lining of the tract is **mucous membrane** (see 'Epithelial tissues', Chapter 1, p. 9), and this is important because not only does it prevent digestion of the muscle layer by the enzymes, but it also contains many glandular structures. These glands are often the site where tumours of the digestive tract arise.

The digestive system (Figure 8.1) begins in the mouth. Here, the twin mechanical actions of chewing and churning use the teeth and tongue to mix food with the saliva to form a **bolus**, which is then swallowed.

Saliva contains the enzyme **amylase**, which breaks down **starch**, a complex carbohydrate, into sugars called **disaccharides**. A swallowed bolus enters the **oesophagus**, a muscular tube that drives food towards the stomach. Like all the digestive tract, the oesophagus is lined by mucous membrane. In the stomach, more mechanical churning of food is also accompanied by chemical activity (Figure 8.2). About 1 to 3 L per day of **hydrochloric acid (HCl)** is produced by **parietal** (also called **oxyntic**) cells in the stomach mucosal wall lining. HCl is acidic, having a pH value of about 1.5, the acid end of the **pH scale**, which is a measure of *hydrogen ion concentration* in a liquid (Blows 2024). The low pH of HCl is essential for the conversion of the

DOI: 10.4324/9781003389125-8

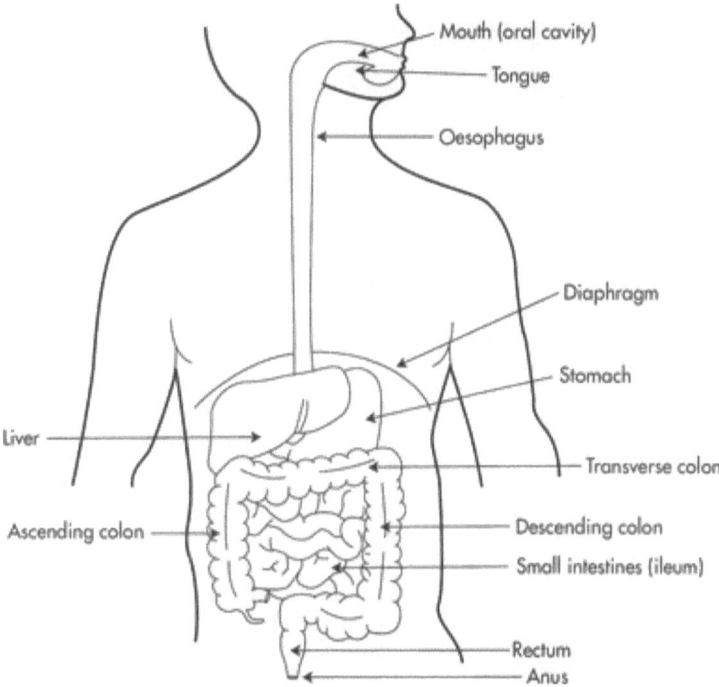

FIGURE 8.1   The digestive system. It is essentially a long tube with accessory organs, the liver and the pancreas (not shown here) (see footnote 1, p. 180).

protein-digesting enzyme **pepsinogen** to an active state called **pepsin**, and this can then start the process of breaking down proteins into **peptides**, that is, small proteins. Pepsinogen comes from the **chief** (or **zymogenic**) cells of the mucosal stomach wall lining. HCl production is increased by the action of two secretions:

1. **Histamine** produced by **enterochromaffin-like (ECL)** cells (see footnote 2, p. 180)
2. **Gastrin** from G cells

Both cell types are present in the gastric mucosal lining. What leaves the stomach is **chyme**, an acidic mix of broken-down food particles and digestive chemicals. This enters the **duodenum** through the **pyloric sphincter** (Figure 8.2).

In the duodenum, bile enters from the liver via the biliary apparatus, that is, two hepatic ducts beneath the liver join to form a common bile duct, which then joins the duodenum (Figure 8.3).

The cystic duct leads to the gall bladder, which stores and concentrates bile (Figure 8.3). Bile emulsifies fats, that is, allows fats to blend with water, a vital step for lipase activity (Table 8.1). Bile also converts the acidity of chyme back to alkaline, as it was in the mouth, a vital step for amylase activity.

Also joining the duodenum is the pancreatic duct, bringing enzymes that will continue the digestive process (Figure 8.4, Table 8.1). Both ducts, the bile duct and the pancreatic duct, join together just prior to the point where the duct joins the duodenum: the **ampulla of Vater**. An *ampulla* is a small nipple-like protrusion that extends a short way into the lumen of the

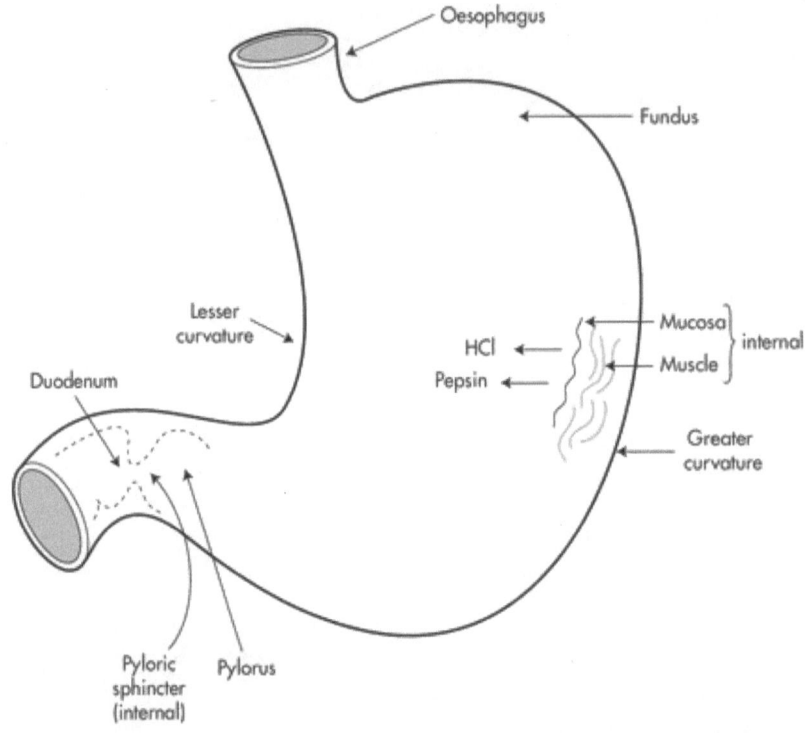

FIGURE 8.2 The stomach. The internal wall structure consists of multiple layers of smooth muscle, providing mechanical movement, and mucosa, secreting hydrochloric acid (HCl) and the enzyme pepsin.

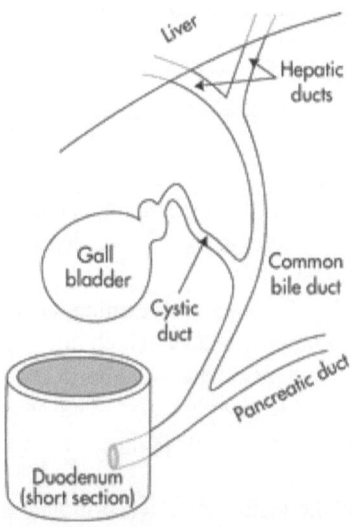

FIGURE 8.3 The biliary system. The common bile duct joins the liver to the duodenum. Bile can be stored in the gall bladder, which connects with the common bile duct via the cystic duct.

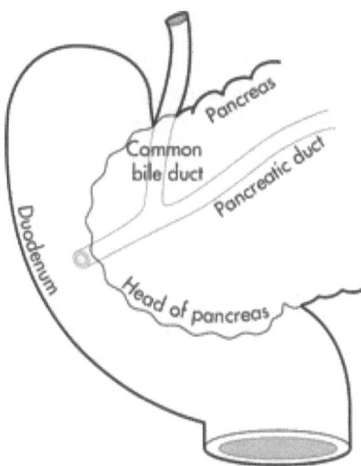

FIGURE 8.4 The duodenum and the head of the pancreas. The pancreatic and common bile ducts join just prior to entry into the duodenum.

TABLE 8.1 The main substances in the duodenum

Substance	From	Function	Notes
Bile	The liver	Emulsifies fats (i.e. combines fats with water) and changes the acid conditions from the stomach back to base (alkaline).	Drains into the duodenum from the bile duct, part of the biliary apparatus from the liver.
Pancreatic amylase (an enzyme)	The pancreas	Continues the conversion of starch to sugars.	Salivary amylase is destroyed by the stomach acid, but in the alkaline of the duodenum (see 'Bile'), pancreatic amylase continues this function.
Lipase (an enzyme)	The pancreas	Breaks down fats from triglyceride form to fatty acids and monoglyceride.	Fats must be emulsified by bile.
Trypsinogen (a pro-enzyme, that is, not yet activated)	The pancreas	As trypsin, it breaks down proteins to amino acids.	Must be converted to the active form trypsin in the duodenum.
Chymotrypsinogen (a pro-enzyme, that is, not yet activated)	The pancreas	Chymotrypsin breaks down proteins to amino acids.	Must be converted to the active form chymotrypsin in the duodenum.

bowel. The bile and pancreatic enzymes arrive in the duodenum together because the pancreatic enzymes amylase and lipase are dependent on bile. Bile consists largely of bile salts, bile pigments, and water, and it is also an important excretory mechanism from the liver. Substances arriving in the bowel via the bile can either be reabsorbed and recycled via the liver or become incorporated into the faeces for excretion.

The **jejunum** is a continuation of the duodenum leading to the small bowel (the **ileum**). In the ileum, the final stages of digestion take place, followed by the absorption of nutrients into the blood. Table 8.2 identifies the events and the enzymes involved. Lipids are also absorbed from the ileum in fatty acid and monoglyceride form (Table 8.1), only to be reconstructed as triglycerides again after absorption. Minerals, vitamins, and water are all absorbed without prior digestion.

After passage through the ileum and absorption is complete, the bowel contents consist mostly of the indigestible fibre content of the diet and water. This enters, first, the **caecum** (also the site of the **appendix**), then the **colon** (the large bowel). The colon is divided into several sections, first the **ascending colon**, then the **transverse colon**, the **descending colon**, and finally, the **sigmoid colon**. The whole digestive system ends at the **rectum** and the **anus**. The colon absorbs water, making the contents dryer and more solid.

Intestinal flora (microbiota or microbiome)

The human digestive system is home to a huge collection of microorganisms (bacteria, fungi, and viruses[1]) which together form the **intestinal flora**, also called the **microbiome** or **microbiota** (Table 8.3). Of these, the bacteria alone account for about 10^{14} (one hundred trillion, or 100,000,000,000,000) organisms. The microbiota of the digestive system is not equally distributed throughout the bowel. The levels of organisms are low in the stomach and duodenum and only rise slightly in the jejunum. The reason for this includes gastric acidity, which destroys microorganisms, and the waves of peristalsis which push the microbiota away from the stomach towards the large bowel. Levels increase within the ileum (small intestines) but reach a peak in the colon and rectum, where the conditions are right to support a huge colony of organisms. The appendix, long thought of as a vestigial organ, may have the important role of replenishing the microbiome should the gut organisms be destroyed, for example, following oral antibiotic therapy.

In relation to immunotherapy for cancer, some patients show greater resistance to this treatment than do others. Those responding well to immunotherapy may be found to have great numbers of specific microorganisms in their bowel compared with those who are resistant to treatment.

Several species of gut bacteria within the microbiome are known to down-regulate a molecule called **repulsive guidance molecule B** (**RGMb**). RGMb binds to the surface

TABLE 8.2 The main enzymes and their products active in the ileum

Nutrient from duodenum	Acted on by (enzyme)	End product for absorption
Maltose	Maltase	Two glucose molecules per single maltose molecule
Sucrose	Sucrase	One glucose and one fructose per single sucrose molecule
Lactose	Lactase	One glucose and one galactose per single lactose molecule
Peptides	Aminopeptidase	Amino acids
Peptides	Carboxypeptidase	Amino acids
Peptides	Dipeptidase	Amino acids
Peptides	Tripeptidase	Amino acids

TABLE 8.3 Organisms and their locations within the human microbiota

Organisms	Prevalence	Usual location	Notes
Bacteria			
Bacteroides sp. (B)	Very common	Ileum, colon	Mostly anaerobic, that is, they
Enterococcus faecalis (F)	Very common	Stomach, ileum, colon	can survive without oxygen;
Escherichia coli (*E. coli*) (P)	Very common	Colon	oxygen is fatal to them.
Enterobacter sp. (P)	Common	Colon	Around 100 trillion bacteria in
Klebsiella sp. (P)	Common	Colon	the gut, mostly in the colon.
Bifidobacterium sp. (A)	Common	Colon	These are some of the
Staphylococcus aureus (F)	Common	Colon	species present.
Lactobacillus sp. (F)	Common	Stomach, ileum, colon	They are commensals, that is,
Clostridium perfringens (F)	Moderate	Colon	they are harmless to man
Proteus mirabilis (P)	Moderate	Colon	whilst in the gut, and many
Clostridium sp. (F)	Infrequent	Ileum, colon	provide a valuable function.
Pseudomonas (P)	Rare	Colon	They can be pathogenic if
Salmonella enterica (P)	Rare	Colon	they get into the blood or
Faecalibacterium (F)	Not known	Colon	a wound.
Peptostreptococcus sp. (F)	Not known	Stomach, colon	These bacteria are severely
Peptococcus sp. (F)	Not known	Colon	decimated by antibiotic
Streptococcus (F)	Not known	Stomach, ileum	therapy.
Coprobacillus sp. (F)	Not known	Ileum, colon	
Viruses (e.g. bacteriophages)	Not known	Variable and widely distributed	Bacteriophages normally prey on bacteria, but in the gut, they reside in harmony with them and may have a controlling or modifying function over the bacteria.
Fungi	Dependent mostly on diet, that is, ingested with food	Variable and widely distributed	Mostly intransient whilst passing through the gut en route from mouth to anus, for example, *Saccharomyces* (a yeast in bread and beer).

Note: A = Actinobacteria (Actinomycetia); B = Bacteroidetes; F = Firmicutes (Bacillota); and P = Proteobacteria.

receptor **PD-L2 (programmed cell death 1 ligand 2)** (see 'Monoclonal antibodies (MABs) known as immune checkpoint inhibitors (ICIs)', Figure 5.18, Chapter 5, p. 104), an **antigen-presenting cell** (**APC**, also called a **dendritic cell**) receptor, and this binding inhibits the immune system response. Healthy gut organisms cause reduced expression of PD-L2, which links with the T cell surface receptor PD-1, and this binding reduces T cell killing function. Higher levels of PD-L2 will enable tumour cells to evade the T cell immune response; therefore, reduction of PD-L2 by the healthy gut organisms improves the immune response. *Coprobacillus cateniformis* (Table 8.3) is one such bacterium that reduces PD-L2 and, by combining this effect with drugs that block PD-1, gives a better therapy response than using PD-1-blocking drugs alone. Drugs blocking RGMb also improve the response to immunotherapy.

Vitamin D is known to encourage the growth of the gut organism *Bacteroides fragilis* (Table 8.3, *Bacteroides* sp.). This bacterium provides better immunity to fight cancer and also improves the anti-cancer response to immunotherapy. Vitamin D deficiency may increase the risk of developing cancer.

Neoplastic disease of the upper digestive tract

Malignancy of the digestive tract carries with it the problem of **malnutrition**. Poor nutrition is discussed in Chapter 18 (see 'Nutritional considerations in cancer', Chapter 18, p. 324). Digestive cancers can cause malabsorption by obstructing the digestive tract and by causing **anorexia**, that is, poor or no appetite. Cancers of the bowel can induce nausea, vomiting, constipation, and diarrhoea. Maintaining nutrition in patients with digestive disorders becomes a major healthcare challenge.

Cancers of the mouth (oral cancers)

Smoking and alcohol are often major contributors to the cause of cancers involving the mouth, tongue, lips, and jaw. Smokers have 2 to 4 times greater risk of oral cancers than non-smokers, and if smoking is combined with regular alcohol consumption, the risk rises to 6 to 15 times that of the non-smoker and non-drinker. Tobacco is the most important factor, with higher incidence of the disease in individuals who chew tobacco and those who smoke a pipe. Males are as much as 10 times more often affected than females, especially with lip cancer, that is, the site where cigarettes and pipes are held. Oral cancer affects the elderly more often, being rare before 40 years of age but showing a sharp increase in cases over 70 years of age. Mouth cancer is on the rise, with increasing death rates, in the UK and elsewhere.

About 95% of cases of oral cancers are **squamous cell carcinomas** (see 'Epithelial tissues', Chapter 1, p. 9, for squamous epithelium cells) (Kumar et al. 2022). Over 50% of the cancers of the mouth occur on the undersurface of the tongue and floor of the mouth. Spread can be local, into the deeper tissues of the jaw, creating a major problem for complete surgical removal and resulting in extensive disfigurement if the jaw and tongue are removed. Lymph node spread is also a problem and is often present at first consultation. The first involved are usually the lymph nodes beneath the lower jaw, that is, the **submandibular** nodes, followed by more distal spread to the lungs, the bones, or the liver.

Cell **biomarkers**, that is, organic molecules derived from the tumour, including genes, can be measured in affected tissue, blood, or saliva. They give a good indication regarding diagnosis, treatment response, and prognosis. Examples of these biomarkers are:

- Proteins that are changed by the cancer (**proteomic biomarkers**), for example, **cytokeratins** and **annexins**. Cytokeratins are produced by keratinising cells, that is, cells that produce keratin in the cytoplasm. Annexins are a family of proteins normally found inside many human cells.
- Microbes (bacteria and viruses) linked to oral cancers, for example, Epstein–Barr virus (EBV) and human papillomavirus (HPV) (p. 60).
- Genomic changes related to oral cancers include loss (deletion) of chromosome 3p (*p* is the short arm), *EGFR* gene amplification (see 'Chromosome 7', Addendum, p. 348), *TP53* gene mutations (see 'Chromosome 17', Addendum, p. 356), *CDKN2A* gene mutations (see

'Chromosome 9', Addendum, p. 350), and *CYP1A1* mutations (see 'Chromosome 15', Addendum, p. 355). This suggests that there is an important role for gene mutations in the cause of this disease.

Symptoms of oral cancers are:

1. Swelling of the face, the neck, and under the jawline
2. Ulceration of the lips and gums that is not healing
3. White or red patches in the mouth
4. Sore gums and dental pain
5. Swelling or ulcerative changes to the tongue, roof, or floor of the mouth, or to the mucosa inside the cheeks
6. Persistent sore throat for more than two weeks
7. Persistent blocked ears or earache

Many of these will be non-cancerous lesions, but they should be checked by a doctor or dentist at an early stage.

Ameloblastoma

This is a rare tumour of the odontogenic epithelium tissue. Ameloblasts are the outer cells covering the enamel of teeth during tooth development. These tumours are more common in the lower jaw rather than the upper jaw. There are four types of ameloblastoma:

1. Conventional
2. Unicystic
3. Metastasising
4. Peripheral

Ameloblastomas cause a large swelling in the jaw and face. They can be either cystic or solid, and although most are benign, some can become aggressive and infiltrative. They are linked to mutations of the *KRAS*, a member of the *RAS* gene family (see 'KRAS, chromosome 12', Addendum, p. 353).

Salivary gland cancer

Tumours of the salivary glands are either benign or malignant. There are numerous subtypes of each:

Mucoepidermoid carcinoma is the commonest malignant salivary cancer. These cells line the salivary glands, and tumours start with very small mucus-filled cysts. They are mostly within the parotid glands but can start in any of the glands (Figure 8.5). They are mostly slow-growing, but occasionally they can grow quickly. They consist of a painless, solid mass with cystic patches filled with mucus.

Adenoid cystic carcinoma (ACC) is a subtype of *triple-negative breast cancer* (**TNBC**). These tumours are negative for ER, PR, and HER2 (see Table 11.2 and 'Triple-negative

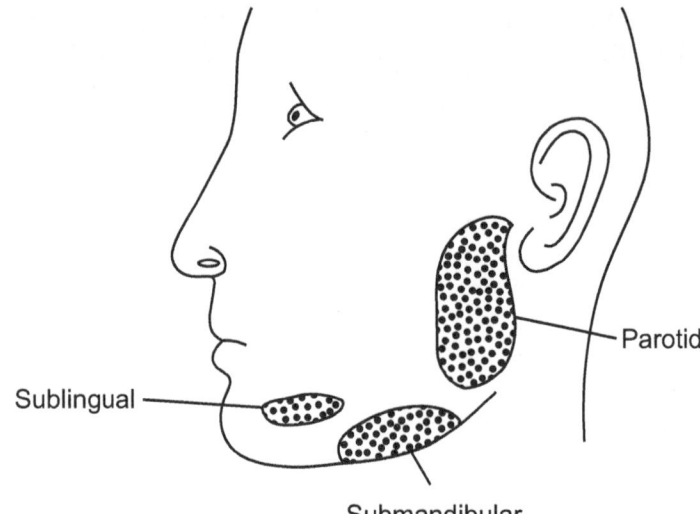

FIGURE 8.5 The salivary glands. These are the parotid gland, the largest gland, occurring in the cheek region; the submandibular gland, below the lower jaw; and the sublingual gland, below the tongue. They occur as bilateral pairs.

breast cancer', Chapter 11, p. 210). ACC is an important cause of salivary gland cancers, but it is also a rare type of breast cancer.

A chromosomal translocation t(6:9) (Chapter 2, p. 33) occurs between two genes, *MYB* (6q22–23) and *NFIB* (9p23–24), and this forms a *MYB–NFIB* fusion gene on chromosome 6. This is linked to ACC of the head, neck, breast, and salivary glands. *MYB–NFIB* gene fusion promotes cell proliferation and cell cycle progression. A similar t(8:9) translocation is also identified in ACC. It occurs between the proto-oncogene *MYBL1* (8q13.1) and *NFIB* (9p23.24) and forms a *MYBL1–NFIB* combined gene on chromosome 8.

Oesophageal cancer

More than half of cancers of the oesophagus are adenocarcinomas arising from the glandular components of the mucous membrane. Squamous cell carcinomas arising from squamous epithelium account for the next largest number. Between them, adenocarcinoma and squamous cell carcinoma account for more than 95% of cases. Small-cell carcinoma, arising from neuroendocrine cells, is a very rare type found mostly in elderly males.

Factors influencing the onset of oesophageal carcinoma are chronic inflammation of the oesophagus;[2] alcohol and tobacco use, retarded passage of food through the oesophagus, and dietary factors, such as vitamin or mineral deficiency and high nitrate content of food.

Genetic factors are involved as well. Close to 50% of squamous cell carcinomas involve the genetic error of the *Tp53* gene (see 'Tp53, chromosome 17', Addendum, p. 356). About 50% of them arise in the central one-third of the oesophagus, 30% in the lower (distal) third, and 20% in the upper (proximal) third.

An adenocarcinoma may arise from what is called **Barrett's oesophagus**, which is an abnormal change in the squamous epithelium lining due to varying degrees (or grades) of cellular dysplasia (see Figure 1.14, Chapter 1, p. 18). The cause of the dysplasia is chronic gastric acid regurgitation, causing repeated heartburn over a long period. This affects at least 3 cm of the distal end (stomach end) of the oesophagus but could involve the whole tube. Barrett's oesophagus increases the risk of developing oesophageal cancer.

Oesophageal cancers can spread locally into the wall and beyond into the lower respiratory tract, the lung itself, and the **mediastinum**, that is, the space between the lungs that contains the heart. The heart and aorta are rarely involved. Because the disease comes on gradually and with few or no early symptoms, it is often the case that spread has occurred before diagnosis is made, making treatment more difficult and the prognosis poorer. Symptoms are **dysphagia** (difficulty or pain in swallowing), **anorexia** (poor appetite), weight loss, and fatigue as the oesophagus begins to become obstructed by the tumour. Pain also occurs associated with the passage of food. Acid reflux causing 'heartburn' and a cough that does not improve sometimes occur. If the tumour can be detected early enough before spread occurs, surgical excision and replacement by an artificial tube may be an option.

Gastric cancer

Cancer of the stomach (**gastric adenocarcinomas**) occurs in two forms, **cardia** and **non-cardia**, according to site or origin. *Cardia cancers* arise in the upper regions of the stomach, around the oesophageal–gastric junction, and they share similar causation to oesophageal cancers. Non-cardia cancers arise in the lower distal parts of the stomach and are more common than cardia cancers.

Two different cell types are seen in gastric cancer. They are described as either **intestinal** or **diffuse**. **Intestinal** cancer arises from gastric mucosa that has first undergone chronic inflammation, that is, **chronic gastritis**, followed by changes in the cell type, from cells typical of the stomach to cells that resemble those of the small or large intestines. This change of cell type is called **intestinal metaplasia**. The intestinal form is the commonest stomach cancer seen.

The **diffuse form** is an aggressive cancer arising from the **enterochromaffin-like cells**[3] of the stomach mucosa and is associated with excessive gastrin stimulation. This form of stomach cancer is not associated with chronic gastritis. It is linked to having **blood group A**, with about 50% of the patients having this blood type. The onset of the disease is often before 50 years of age, and most cases are linked to mutations of the *CDH1* gene (see 'CDH1, chromosome 16', Addendum, p. 356).

Gastric carcinoma generally occurs more frequently in elderly males and more often in developed countries rather than in non-developed countries. A high incidence of the disease occurs in Latin America and Eastern and Central Asia, with the highest incidence in South Korea (Rawla and Barsouk 2019).

An important risk factor in the cause of intestinal carcinoma is nitrites in the diet derived from nitrates in food, which may be changed to **nitrosamines** and **nitrosamides** (Figure 8.6).

Other risk factors include the eating of smoked foods, since the smoking process puts coal combustion carcinogenic agents on the food (see 'List of carcinogen chemicals: coal combustion products', Chapter 3, p. 43); eating pickled vegetables and a *high* salt diet; a *low* intake of green vegetables; chronic gastritis, especially if the organism *Helicobacter pylori* is present (Rawla and Barsouk 2019); and **pernicious anaemia** (deficiency of vitamin B$_{12}$).

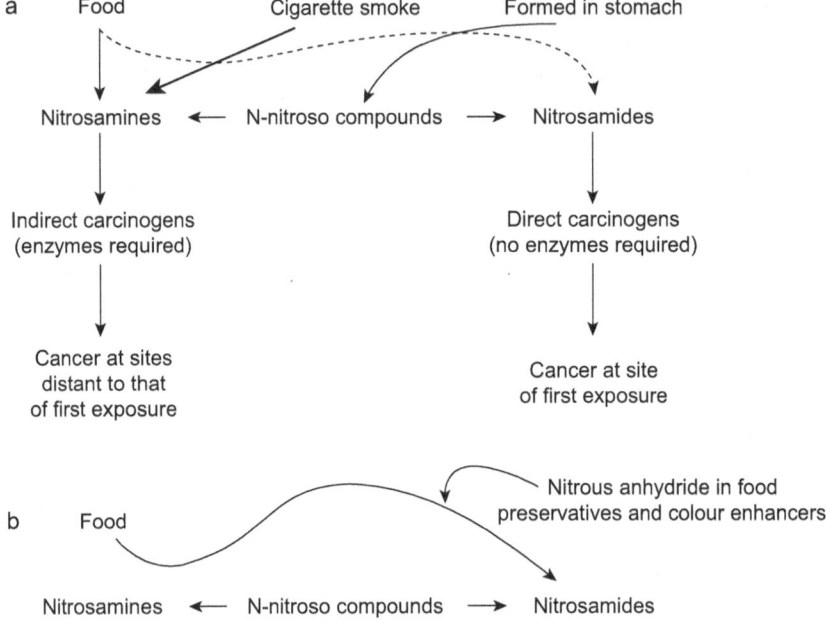

FIGURE 8.6 The N-nitroso compounds: nitrosamines and nitrosamides formation. (a) Most nitrosamines come from smoking or chewing tobacco, with far less coming from food or
produced in the stomach. There is very little nitrosamides normally found in food. Nitrosamines are indirect carcinogens (they need enzymes), so they cause cancers beyond
the first site of exposure. Nitrosamides are direct carcinogens (no enzymes needed),
so they cause cancer directly at the site of first exposure. (b) The addition of nitrous
anhydride in food preservatives or food colour enhancers converts nitrosamines to
nitrosamides.

Helicobacter pylori is a bacterium which is an important cause of acute gastritis, resulting in
80% of gastric ulcers and 90% of non-cardia cancers. Conversely, *H. pylori* has been found to
reduce acidity in the cardia (upper) region of the stomach and, as such, helps protect against the
cardia forms of cancer.

Gastric carcinoma usually begins insidiously and may show vague, obscure symptoms or
even be asymptomatic (without symptoms) at first. This makes early detection very difficult,
and those persons at high risk should be screened regularly for signs of the disease. Symptoms
include nausea and vomiting, **anorexia** (loss of appetite), weight loss, indigestion, **dysphagia**
(difficulty swallowing), gastric bleeding associated with **iron deficiency anaemia**, fatigue, acid
reflux, and upper abdominal pain.

The degree by which the cancer has infiltrated into the stomach wall is the important factor,
that is, the *depth of invasion*, as it determines how advanced the disease is and the likelihood of
spread outside of the organ, and thus the potential outcome. Growth occurs in three main types:

1. **Exophytic**, where the tumour extends out from the wall and into the stomach lumen
2. **Flat** (or **depressed**), where the tumour is not easily identified within the mucosa
3. **Excavated**, where the tumour erodes into a crater extending into the stomach wall

Treatment of gastric cancer is often surgery, to remove as much of the tumour as is possible: a partial or total **gastrectomy**. Postoperatively, the patient may experience **dumping syndrome**, which occurs mostly after partial gastrectomy of the distal portion of the stomach and joining (**anastomosis**) of the stomach stump with the **jejunum** or **duodenum** (Figure 8.7). Dumping syndrome occurs when a food **bolus** passes too quickly from the stomach into the duodenum or jejunum. The bolus attracts water from the blood into the intestines, which then become dilated with fluid. Bowel movements, that is, bowel **motility**, are increased. The symptoms of dumping syndrome occur about 5 to 30 minutes after eating and include nausea and vomiting, cramping pain in the stomach (**epigastric**) area, and loud active bowel sounds (called **borborygmi**). Later symptoms are those associated with disturbance of blood glucose levels. The blood sugar rises, and this triggers a large insulin release, which in turn results in **hypoglycaemia** (low blood sugar level). **Tachycardia** (fast pulse rate) and a period of low blood pressure may occur, with corresponding dizzy spells. Dumping syndrome will eventually correct itself after a year or so following surgery, but it is unpleasant. The symptoms can be reduced by eating smaller, more frequent meals and by allowing more time to eat the meal. The patient should be encouraged to break up the food into small portions. It may help separate the consumption times of fluids from food, increase the fats and protein in the diet, and reduce carbohydrates, especially the sugar content of the food. Resting after the meal in a **semi-recumbent** (partly upright) position for 30 minutes after the meal can help.

Gastrectomy can also cause **pernicious anaemia** due to the loss of **intrinsic factor** in the formation of vitamin B$_{12}$ (Figure 8.8). *Intrinsic* factor is produced by the stomach in response to the consumption of *extrinsic* factor in the diet. The combination of the two factors results in **B12 complex**, which is then absorbed into the **terminal ileum**, that part of the bowel where the small intestine joins the large intestine. Removal of the stomach means that B$_{12}$ complex cannot be formed or absorbed. Vitamin B$_{12}$, which is needed for the formation of **haemoglobin**, is normally stored in the liver and will now need to be given by injection for life to keep the liver stores topped up.

Also, following gastrectomy, the patient may develop poor absorption of **folic acid, calcium**, and **vitamin D**. Weight loss, seen in nearly 50% of gastrectomy patients, is due to the

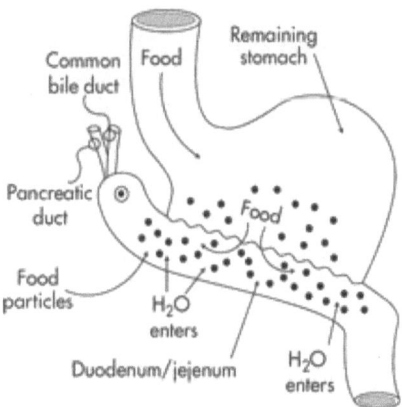

FIGURE 8.7 Dumping syndrome. After a gastrointestinal anastomosis, food passes quickly into the intestine, causing water to enter and swell the bowel.

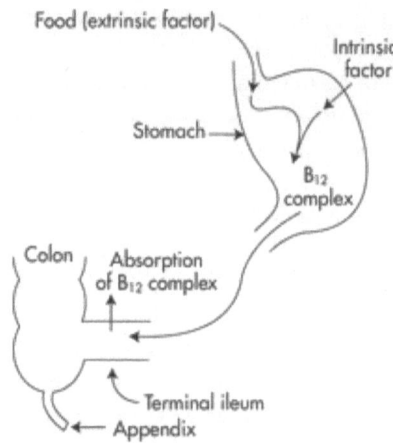

FIGURE 8.8 Vitamin B$_{12}$ synthesis and absorption. Extrinsic factor in the diet meets intrinsic factor in the stomach to form the B$_{12}$ complex. This complex is absorbed in the terminal ileum.

combination of reduced meal size involving poor calorie intake, with nutrient malabsorption. Dietary adjustments involving the advice of the dietician are needed to improve the patient's nutritional status (see 'Nutritional considerations in cancer', Chapter 18, p. 324).

Cancer of the small bowel

Small bowel cancers, that is, those of the duodenum and ileum, are uncommon, being 40 to 60 times *less frequently* encountered than those of the colon. In total, they account for only 5% of tumours of the digestive tract. About 45% of them are **adenocarcinomas**, about 30% are **carcinoid tumours**, and a further 10% are small bowel **lymphomas**. The remainder are of connective tissue origin, that is, **sarcomas**.

Adenocarcinomas arise from the glandular component of the internal mucosal lining. Approximately 40% occur in the duodenum around the **ampulla of Vater** (see 'The digestive system: ampulla of Vater', p. 149). Many of these tumours are found in association with **Crohn's disease**, also called **regional ileitis**, a chronic inflammatory condition affecting mostly the small bowel. Digestive cancers are often linked to chronic inflammatory diseases of the mucosa (see 'Polyps: ulcerative colitis', p. 164). **Small-cell**, or **oat cell**, **carcinoma** is similar to the small-cell carcinoma of the lung (see Table 9.1, Chapter 9, p. 187) that consists of small round or oval cells producing and secreting small proteins called peptides. These tumours are prone to invasion and spread widely from the point of origin, resulting in a poor prognosis.

Carcinoid tumours are a subset of neuroendocrine tumours derived from neuroendocrine cells (see footnote 2), which are located throughout the mucous membrane of various organs, especially the digestive system. These tumours occur most frequently in the appendix and less frequently in the ileum. Together, the appendix and ileum account for about 60–80% of all carcinoid tumours. The others occur in the colon and rectum (10–20% of the total) and the oesophagus, stomach, and duodenum. Carcinoid tumours of the appendix are rarely aggressive and are often discovered on routine appendicectomy (removal of the appendix). The ileum and the colon are sites of the most aggressive carcinoid tumours that invade and spread easily. Generally, these aggressive tumours are slow-growing but highly invasive and produce metastases which spread to the liver and local lymph nodes. They can be the cause of **carcinoid syndrome**, a systemic reaction to a massive release of active compounds from tumour cells into the circulation. The effects of carcinoid syndrome include wheezing, **hypertension** (high blood pressure), palpitations, flushing of the face and chest, watery diarrhoea, and right-sided heart failure.

Small bowel **lymphomas** account for only about 10% of the total of small bowel tumours (see 'Lymphomas', Chapter 7, p. 143). They are diffuse and poorly differentiated and are important particularly in children as non-Hodgkin lymphomas. Small bowel lymphomas are often derived from B cells of the lymph node tissue that occur in the mucosa, that is, **mucosa-associated lymphoid tissue** (**MALT**) (see Table 7.6, Chapter 7, p. 144). The activation of this lymph tissue is a result of inflammation.

Sarcomas of the small bowel are relatively rare and are mainly **leiomyosarcomas** (*myo* = muscle), which are malignancies of the smooth muscle wall of the bowel (Tobias and Hochhauser 2014). They are aggressive and usually spread by metastases to other parts of the body. The other neoplasm of the smooth muscle is the **leiomyoma**, a benign tumour that forms as fibroid growths in the small bowel wall.

Cancer of the pancreas

Pancreatic cancer is one of the most difficult cancers to diagnose early, remaining asymptomatic until quite advanced, and this is the reason there has been a poor outcome, with around 9,000 deaths per year in the UK. Often, it is only amenable to palliative treatment. Most cases are sporadic, with only a few inherited, or familial, episodes recorded. In the UK, 48% of cases are female, 52% are male, and the overall incidence is increasing. The disease often starts in the seventh decade of life, with the highest peak occurring in the 85–89 years old.

One possible reason this appears to be a disease of the elderly may be age-related cells called fibroblasts (see 'Stromal cells', Chapter 6, p. 122) which are present in pancreatic tissue. Fibroblasts in older people, that is, 55+ years old, secrete a protein called **growth/differentiation factor 15** (**GDF-15**), which fibroblasts in younger people, that is, less than 35 years old, do not do. GDF-15 activates the AKT cell signalling pathway (see 'AKT1, chromosome 14', Addendum, p. 354) and promotes tumour cell growth and metastases. Inhibiting GDF-15, or the AKT pathway, in the elderly with pancreatic cancer could become part of the drug therapy for this disease. In addition, pancreatic cancer could use an enzyme called **uridine phosphorylase 1** (**UPP1**), which allows tumour cells to use **uridine** as an emergency energy source should it become deprived of sugars. Blocking this process could also become part of the treatment.

The symptoms of pancreatic cancer are:

- Pain in the abdomen, arms, or back
- Jaundice (yellow colour to the skin and whites of the eyes)
- Dark urine
- Anorexia, nausea, vomiting, and weight loss
- Asthenia (abnormal energy loss), weakness, feeling tired
- Itching of the skin
- Bowel function and bowel content changes

- Fever and shivering
- Indigestion, acid reflux, and sickness

Two forms are recognised: **ductal** (around 95% of cases) and **non-ductal** (around 5% of cases).

Pancreatic ductal adenocarcinoma (PDAC) is an aggressive cancer derived from glandular epithelium of the ducts. It accounts for most of the pancreatic tumours, and two-thirds of them arise from the head of the gland, where the pancreatic duct and common bile duct enter the duodenum (Figure 8.4). A tumour here can obstruct either or both ducts. Biliary duct obstruction blocks bile flow from the liver and causes **jaundice**, a yellow skin colour due to bile pigment deposits in the tissues. Abdominal pain is a feature of later-stage disease, often when surgery is no longer an option. Spread of the disease into the local lymph nodes, and then the liver, occurs. Survival rate is very poor – only around 2% of patients are alive after five years.

Causative factors are environmental and genetic. Environmental factors include smoking, which is now known to be a strong link, and perhaps viral infections. Genetic mutations can cause inherited (familial) or sporadic pancreatic cancer. The ductal form is often associated with genetic mutations more than the non-ductal type. There are several genes associated with the inherited form, called **familial pancreatic cancer (FPC)** (Table 8.4), and mutations of one gene, called *KRAS* (see 'KRAS, chromosome 12', Addendum, p. 353), which is strongly linked to as many as 90% of sporadic pancreatic cancer cases (Figure 8.9). One mutation of *KRAS* is G12D, a **missense substitution** (see 'Mutation of genes', Chapter 2, p. 27), where the amino acid glycine (G) is replaced by another amino acid, aspartate (D), at position 12 of the protein. *KRAS* G12D is the most common gene mutation found in pancreatic cancer, occurring in about 39% of cases, but other mutations do occur (Figure 8.9). This is linked to drug resistance, and therefore, it becomes very difficult to treat and is one of the reasons pancreatic cancers have carried a very poor prognosis. Now, a 'small molecule' treatment, called MRTX1133, a *KRAS* G12D blocking agent, has shown promise in treating pancreatic cancer caused by this mutation during early trials.

An experimental drug called **RMC-7977** inhibits a range of mutated *RAS* genes in pancreatic cancer, with few side effects, although its use in humans has yet to be tested. It may also be useful against other cancers caused my *RAS* mutations.

Normally, if pancreatic cells are damaged, they can switch back to a *dedifferentiated* state, that is, less differentiated than the mature cell, and this allows for damage repair prior to a return to the fully differentiated mature state. In pancreatic cells with *KRAS* mutations, any damage to the cell results in irreversible cancerous changes involving a communication loop between the cell and the immune system. This communication loop includes signalling interleukin Il-33 from the pancreatic cell and Il-4 from T cells.

A new treatment for pancreatic cancer is also showing good results in clinical trials. It involves a triple-therapy approach, targeting two checkpoint proteins, 41BB and LAG3 (see 'Immune checkpoint inhibitors' and Figure 5.18, Chapter 5, p. 105), and the protein CXCR2, which is a G protein–coupled receptor (see Figure 2.2, Chapter 2, p. 28) that binds a chemokine (see 'Chemokines', Chapter 5, p. 96). The first two are highly expressed in T cells within the tumour immune microenvironment (TIME) (see 'The tumour and its microenvironment', Chapter 6, p. 120). CXCR2 promotes suppression of the immune response and is involved in recruiting immunosuppressive cells. It therefore aids the tumour to grow and spread. The triple therapy involves using a 41BB agonist, a LAG3 antagonist, and a CXCR2 inhibitor (for agonist and antagonist, see 'Pharmacodynamics', Chapter 16, p. 295).

TABLE 8.4 Some genes linked to familial pancreatic cancer (FPC)

Gene	Locus	Gene	Locus	Gene	Locus
BRCA1	17q21.31 (p. 356)	BRCA2	13q13.1 (p. 354)	PALB2,	16p12.2 (p. 356)
CDKN2A	9p21.3 (p. 350)	ATM	11q22.3 (p. 352)	MLH1	3p22.2 (p. 344)
MSH2	2p21–p16.3 (p. 344)	MSH6	2p16.3 (p. 344)	PMS2	7p22.1 (p. 348)
SPINK1	5q32 (p. 347)	EPCAM	2p21 (p. 344)	TP53	17p13.1 (p. 356)

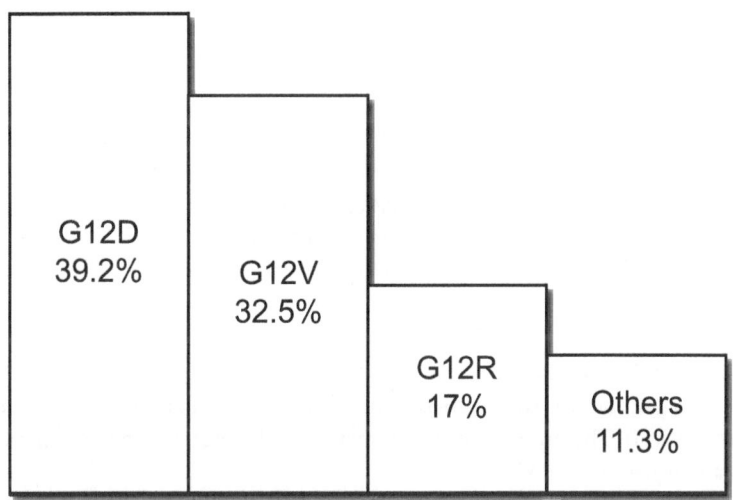

FIGURE 8.9 The prevalence of *KRAS* gene mutations in pancreatic cancer. The main ones are *KRAS* G12D (39.2%), where the normal glycine *G] at position 12 on the protein is replaced by aspartate [D]; *KRAS* G12V (32.5%), where the glycine is replaced by valine [V] at position 12; and *KRAS* G12R (17%), where the glycine is replaced by **arginine** [R]. All other mutations add up to 11.3%.

Vitamin B_6 could be a future target for pancreatic cancer. Vitamin B_6 is required by both the cancer cells and the NK cells that destroy cancer cells (see 'Natural killer (NK) cells', Chapter 5, p. 91). In the battle over limited vitamin B_6 resources, the cancer cell usually wins and the NK cells decline. To reverse this, a three-part therapy is being researched: (1) block the uptake mechanism of vitamin B_6 in cancer cells with drugs, (2) supply more vitamin B_6, and (3) provide therapy that boosts NK cell activity. The results in pancreatic cancer are promising.

A pancreatic cancer test is showing good results in picking up early-stage pancreatic tumours. It is based on a liquid biopsy analysis of micro-DNA from blood, plus high levels of a protein called CA19-9, which is known to be derived from pancreatic cancer.

Colorectal cancers

These are a group of diseases that include:

- Polyps
- Adenomas
- Adenocarcinomas

Polyps

Non-malignant (benign) and *non-neoplastic* (no malignant potential) **polyps** of the large bowel are growths arising from the mucosal or submucosal lining of the gut wall, and they extend into the lumen of the bowel. Although they are benign, they are problematic in themselves because they can obstruct the lumen and prevent normal bowel function. About 35–50% of adults have benign polyps in their colon.

These polyps can be classified into various types:

- **Hyperplastic polyps** are commonly found in more than 50% of the over 60 age group. They are *not* **pre-malignant**, that is, they do not become a malignant tumour, and consist of hyperplasia (Chapter 1, Figure 1.14, p. 18) of normal mucosal cells. They are mostly small (up to 5 mm in diameter) and mostly asymptomatic. **Papillary** is another term that means benign epithelial growths consisting of mucosal glandular tissue.
- **Juvenile polyps** are sporadic polyps most frequently found near the rectum in children under 5 years of age. They range from 1 to 3 cm in diameter and are pedunculated. Polyps generally may be **pedunculated** (i.e. on a stalk) or **sessile** (i.e. having no stalk) (Figure 8.10).
- **Inflammatory polyps** found in association with **inflammatory bowel disease (IBD)**. IBD is essentially two disorders, **Crohn's disease** (mostly of the small bowel) and **ulcerative colitis** (of the large bowel). The presence of inflammation of the digestive mucosa increases the risk of neoplastic disease at that site.

Adenomas

Adenomas are *neoplastic* tumours, that is, new growths with malignant potential, derived from the glandular epithelial components of the mucous membrane lining of the bowel. The new growth of tissue is a benign dysplasia (Chapter 1, Figure 1.14, p. 18), but as such, it can become malignant. Such a move to malignancy results in an **adenocarcinoma**. Adenomas may be:

- **Villous** (1%), large sessile growths, slow-growing, soft and spongy, with frond-like projections. They are potentially malignant.
- **Tubular** (5–10%), small growths made from tubular glands becoming pedunculated.
- **Tubulovillous** (over 90%), a mix of the previous two (Figure 8.11).

The potential for malignancy in adenomas is based on:

1. Tumour size, that is, large adenomas carry the greatest risk.
2. The **histology**, the nature of the tissue from which the tumour is made, that is, the greater the degree of dysplasia present, the higher the risk.

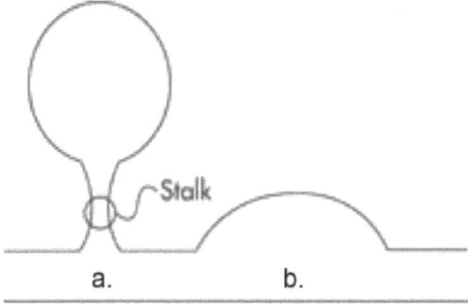

FIGURE 8.10   Polyps: (a) pedunculated (on a stalk), (b) sessile (no stalk).

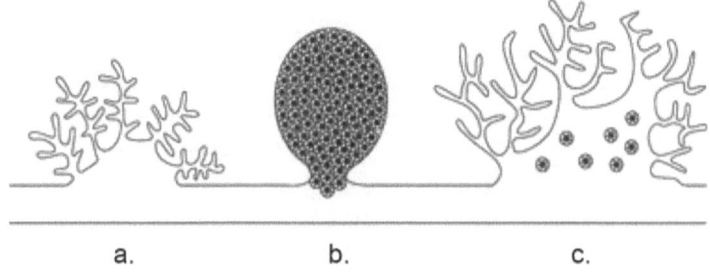

FIGURE 8.11   Adenoma polyps: (a) villous, (b) tubular, (c) mixed tubulovillous.

Because adenomas have a long pre-invasive phase and grow slowly – that is, they double their size in about ten years in most cases – there is an opportunity for early detection and removal, which is the only real safe treatment option. They may be asymptomatic for long periods, making routine screening for 'at risk' individuals the only means of detection. Patients may present with:

1. **Anaemia** due to bleeding at the adenoma site
2. **Occult blood** in the faeces, that is, the blood cannot be seen in the stool and must be detected by chemical tests
3. **Partial obstruction** of the bowel

Adenocarcinomas

Adenocarcinoma is the malignant growth of the bowel, that is, cancer of the small or large bowel. Adenocarcinoma was discussed in relation to the small bowel (see 'Cancer of the small bowel', p. 160), but here, its relevance to the large bowel is considered. The vast majority (98%) of colon cancers are adenocarcinomas.

This disease occurs mostly in the older-age population, with a peak age between 60 and 70 years. Less than 20% of cases exist below the age of 50 years. Men suffer about 20% more cases than women, and the underlying lesion is thought to be a pre-existing adenoma. The disease is unequally distributed geographically, with high incidence in the 'developed' countries, notably Europe, Australia, and North America, and low incidence in Africa, Asia, and South

America. The incidence correlates well with dietary factors, in particular, the presence of meat in the diet. A high level of meat consumption is associated with higher incidence of the disease, and this may be due to the higher levels of saturated fatty acids that come with the meat. High levels of saturated fatty acids in the diet are linked to a greater output of bile acids in the faeces, and these can be converted to dangerous carcinogens by the intestinal flora (see 'Intestinal flora (microbiome)', p. 152). Some organisms in the gut microbiota have been associated with certain colon cancers:

- The presence of *Ruminococcus bromi* improves life expectancy.
- *Coprobacillus cateniformis* boosts immunity against cancer by regulating PD-L2 (see 'Monoclonal antibodies (MABs) known as immune checkpoint inhibitors (ICIs)', Chapter 5, p. 104).
- Gut organisms, such as *Carnobacterium maltaromaticum*, have been shown to produce vitamin D and suppress colorectal cancers in animal models.

A bacterium called *Fusobacterium nucleatum*, an organism that causes dental plaque and gum infections, has been found to populate colorectal cancers. About 29% of people with this disease have this bacterium in their faeces, compared with only 5% of people without the disease. Those with high levels of this bacterium in their tumours have a poorer prognosis, with low response to chemotherapy and a higher incidence of relapse.

There are other risk factors, such as a low level of vegetable fibre, low levels of protective micronutrients, and high consumption levels of refined carbohydrates in the diet.

Low dietary fibre reduces the faecal bulk in the colon, which in turn increases the transit time, that is, how long faeces are held in the colon. Faeces that are held in the colon for a long time create a greater opportunity for the development of harmful carcinogens, which are then exposed to the colonic mucosa for longer periods. Faeces must be transported to the rectum and eliminated in reasonable time to excrete the dangerous carcinogens from the bowel.

Low dietary micronutrients, such as vitamins A, C, and E, reduce the antioxidants in the bowel, that is, chemicals which neutralise the harmful effects of **free radicals**. *Free radicals* are highly reactive chemicals which damage cells, including DNA, and cause gene mutations. Antioxidants protect the mucosa from the harm of free radicals, for example, one vitamin E molecule can neutralise two free radicals. An absence of micronutrients increases the free radicals in the bowel, and therefore the risk of genetic mutations.

High dietary refined carbohydrates, such as sugars, can lead to the formation of harmful toxic products by the intestinal flora, and these can damage mucosal cells, especially when the faecal transit time is increased due to low dietary fibre. These factors work together to cause the disease.

Genetic factors

Genetic factors also have a major role to play in the causation of this disease. **Familial adenomatous polyposis coli (APC)**, **Gardner syndrome**, and **Turcot syndrome** are examples of genetically inherited disorders that include a distinct increase in the risk of colon cancers (Table 8.4).

The tumour suppressor gene involved in APC and Gardner syndrome is found at 5q22.2 (see 'APC, chromosome 5', Addendum, p. 346). APC occurs as multiple pre-malignant adenoma polyps in the colon. There can be more than 100, and sometimes as many as 5,000, of such polyps. Sporadic (non-familial) cases of colon cancer often demonstrate a mutation in the *APC* gene at an early stage. Excision of the affected part of the bowel is the only preventative measure to stop progression to malignancy.

Other genetic errors in colorectal cancers include *KRAS* (see 'KRAS, chromosome 12', Addendum, p. 353), **DCC (deleted in colon cancer)** (see 'DCC, chromosome 18', Addendum, p. 357), and *TP53* (see 'TP53, chromosome 17', Addendum, p. 356). *KRAS* mutations are found in 50% of adenomas over 1 cm across and in half of all colon cancers. *DCC* is thought to be a tumour suppressor gene that is involved in over 70% of colon cancers and in 50% of large adenomas. This deletion gives a poorer prognosis, with a major drop in the five-year survival rate. *Tp53* is found to be mutated in 70–80% of colon cancers.

Mutations of the gene *TLR2* (see 'TLR2, chromosome 4', Addendum, p. 346) are linked to several colorectal cancers, notably one called **colitis-associated cancer (CAC)**. As the name suggests, this is a complication of **inflammatory bowel disease (IBD)**, a disease often referred to as **colitis**. CAC is usually detected at an advanced stage, by which time it has spread locally and produced metastases. The *TLR2* gene can activate an immune response to invading organisms and damaged host cells, thus helping prevent cancers. But on the other hand, *TLR2* has been overexpressed by some cancers, notably colorectal cancers, and this has increased their ability to promote the progression of those cancers. These conflicting activities in relation to cancer place this gene as both friend and foe, and its true place in the story of cancer is under further investigation (see 'Stages and treatment of lung cancer', Chapter 9, p. 189).

The gene *SOX17* (see 'SOX17, chromosome 8', Addendum, p. 350) is expressed during foetal development but is normally inactive (or silenced) in the adult intestinal epithelium. During the early stages of colorectal cancers, this gene may be activated and cause immune suppression, allowing the cancer to progress. Future drugs could be targeted to block this gene in colorectal cancers and therefore allow the immune system to attack the tumour.

TABLE 8.5 The major syndromes involving increased risk of colorectal cancer

Syndrome	Notes
Familial adenomatous polyposis coli (APC)	Pre-malignant collection of multiple polyps of the colon and duodenum, carcinoid tumours of the ileum, papillary tumours of the thyroid, and increased incidence of brain tumours. Familiar APC has an autosomal *dominant* inheritance pattern (Figure 2.5 left, Chapter 2), resulting in the loss of the tumour suppressor gene *APC*. An association of APC with brain tumours is called **Turcot syndrome**.
Gardner syndrome	Cysts of the epidermis, dermoid cysts (cysts containing hair, hair follicles, and sebaceous glands), and increased risk of colon cancer. Gene involved is also the tumour suppressor gene *APC*, inherited in an autosomal *dominant* pattern (Figure 2.5 left, Chapter 2).
Peutz–Jeghers syndrome	Gastrointestinal cancer with ovarian and testicular cancers. An autosomal *dominant* inheritance pattern resulting in a loss of the tumour suppressor gene *STK11* (see 'STK11, chromosome 19', Addendum, p. 358).
Hereditary non-polyposis colorectal cancer (HNPCC) (Lynch syndromes I and II)	Lynch syndrome type I: HNPCC involving cancer of the colon and rectum only. Lynch syndrome type II: HNPCC involving cancer of the colon and rectum with increased risk of cancer of the ovary, endometrium, and pancreas. An autosomal *dominant* inheritance syndrome involving the loss of any of several DNA repair genes.

About 50% of large bowel cancers occur in the rectum, that is, within 15 cm of the anus, and in the sigmoid colon closest to the rectum (Figure 8.12). From here, rectal tumours can spread through the rectal wall into the prostate in men or the vagina in women. Systemic and pulmonary metastases can occur from malignant cells getting into the **inferior vena cava**, the major vein returning blood to the heart from the lower parts of the body.

Other sites for cancers within the bowel and their frequencies at each site can be seen in Figure 8.13.

Staging and grading of colorectal cancers

Staging of colorectal cancers is important for two reasons: to make decisions with regards to the treatment and to assess the patient's prognosis. There are several different ways to stage the disease.

The **TNM (tumour, nodal, metastasis)** staging method (Table 8.6) uses letters to indicate variations in the nature of the three main components, that is, T = how far the tumour has spread; N = to what degree is there spread to lymph nodes; M = any spread of metastases to other organs.

Staging is a combination of these three letters:

Stage 0 = Tis, N0, and M0
Stage 1 = T1, N0, and M0, or T2, N0, and M0
Stage 2 = T3, N0, and M0, or T4, N0, and M0
Stage 3 = Any T number, N1, and M0, or any T number, N2, M0
Stage 4 = Any T number, any N number, and M1

Another staging system is the **Duke classification,** as follows:

Duke A: The tumour remains within the bowel wall, that is, no spread to lymph nodes.
Duke B: The tumour has grown through the bowel wall but has not involved lymph nodes.
Duke C: The tumour has involved at least one lymph node close to the bowel.
Duke D: The tumour has spread to involve metastases in distal organs.

The grading system categorises the nature of the cancer cells involved:

Grade 1 (or low-grade) cells look similar to normal, that is, well-differentiated, and they grow slowly.
Grade 2 (or moderate-grade) cells look more abnormal.
Grade 3 (or high-grade) cells are grossly abnormal, that is, poorly differentiated and grow quickly.

Grade 1 cancers are the least likely to spread. Grade 3 cancers will spread quickly.

Symptoms of bowel cancer

Colorectal cancers may possibly be asymptomatic for years. When symptoms do arise, they include bowel habit changes, for example, **dyschesia**[4] or diarrhoea, fatigue, weakness, weight loss, anaemia due to bleeding into the bowel, abdominal pain and discomfort, progressive bowel obstruction, and **hepatomegaly**, that is, enlarged liver due to metastases.

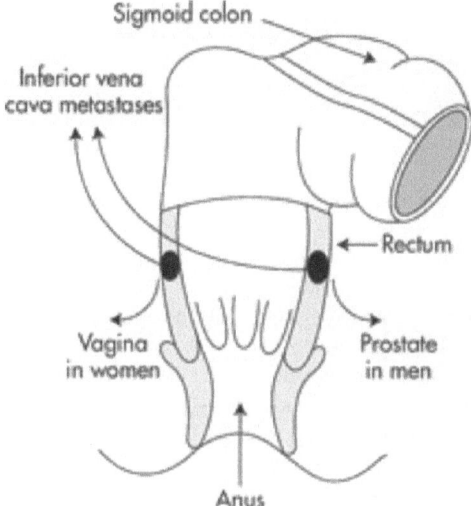

FIGURE 8.12 Rectal carcinomas. The tumours are shown in black. They can spread into the vagina in women, into the prostate in men, and cause metastases in the inferior vena cava in both sexes.

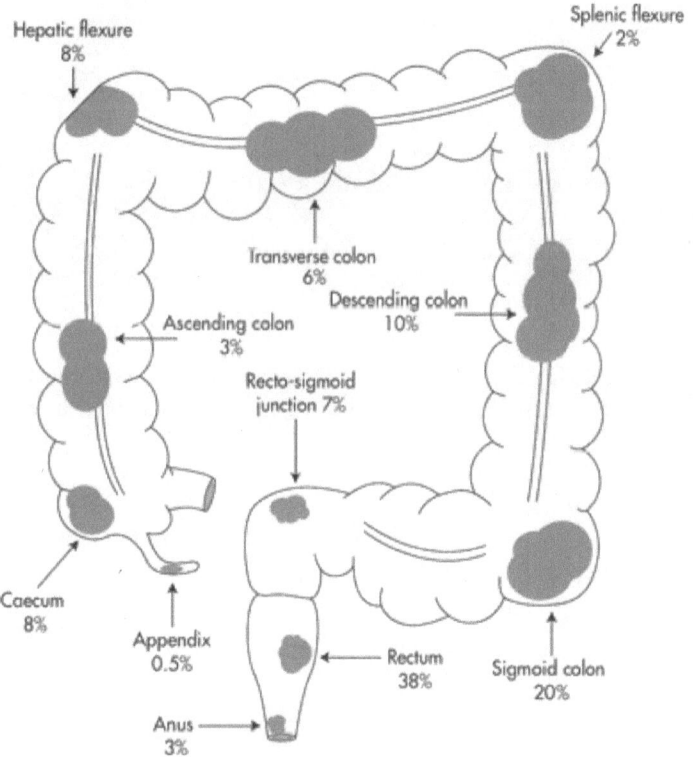

FIGURE 8.13 The sites and frequency of colorectal carcinomas.

Source: Redrawn from Tobias and Hochhauser (2014).

TABLE 8.6 TNM staging for colorectal cancer

Stage	Notes
T0	No primary tumour found.
Tis	Primary tumour in situ.
T1	Tumour has invaded the submucosa.
T2	Tumour has invaded the **muscularis propria**, a layer of muscle that separates the mucous membrane from the serosa in the colon wall (Figure 8.13).
T3	Tumour has invaded through the muscularis propria or into tissues surrounding the colon or the rectum (without entering the peritoneum).
T4	Tumour has entered the peritoneum and invaded other organs.
N0	No regional lymph node metastases.
N1	Cancer cells in one to three lymph nodes around the colon or rectum.
N2	Cancer cells in four or more lymph nodes around the colon or rectum.
N3	Cancer cells in any lymph node along the course of a local blood vessel.
M0	No distal metastases.
M1	Distal metastases found in other organs.

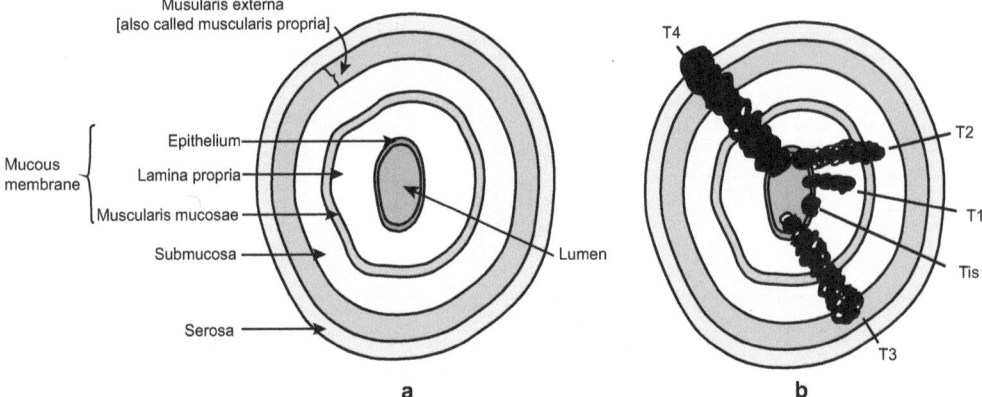

FIGURE 8.14 Section through the colon: (a) The layers of the colon wall showing the muscularis propria. (b) Various stages of a cancer (black) (see 'Staging and grading of colorectal cancers', p. 168).

Symptoms are also dependent on the site of the cancer within the bowel. In the **ascending colon**, tumours are often large and bulky, hence can bleed, causing dark-red blood *mixed with* stools and anaemia. They can ulcerate, causing pain. A palpable mass can be felt in the right side of the abdomen. Spread is to the liver via the **portal vein**, which runs from the gut to the liver.

Tumours in the **descending colon** start as small button-like elevated masses and eventually ulcerate centrally, causing some pain. They can obstruct the lumen as they grow circumferentially, that is, around the tube, to form a ring that then closes across the lumen. They can cause vomiting and constipation. Abdominal distension can occur, and bleeding causes bright-red blood *on* the stool surface. Spread is via the lymph nodes in the abdomen and pancreas, then to the liver via the **mesenteric veins**, which are part of the venous drainage of the abdomen.

Symptomology: Nausea and vomiting

Nausea and vomiting are common symptoms of most gastrointestinal disorders. *Nausea* is the condition of feeling sick. *Vomiting* (or **emesis**) is a complex series of coordinated activities involving muscles of the digestive and respiratory systems and the muscles of the abdominal wall. The **vomit centre** that controls these events is in the **medulla** of the brainstem, close to the **respiratory centre** and the **cardiac centre**. Near the vomit centre also is the **chemoreceptor trigger zone** (Figure 8.15) that is sensitive to chemical stimuli and the site where anti-emetic drugs act. Stimulation of the chemoreceptor trigger zone by emetic drugs, that is, those that cause vomiting, for example, morphine or cytotoxic agents; other chemicals, for example, toxins in the blood; unusual movements, for example, seasickness; bad sight; or unpleasant smells causes activation of the vomit centre. Whilst a single bout of vomiting is not especially harmful, persistent vomiting for hours, or even days, is not only unpleasant but can also cause **dehydration**; **hypokalaemia** (low blood potassium levels) and **hyponatraemia** (low blood sodium levels), that is, an electrolyte imbalance; **alkalosis**, that is, blood pH higher than the normal level of 7.4; **malnutrition**; reduced effectiveness of oral medication; and a risk of inhalation of vomited matter. Drug treatment, that is, anti-emetics, is often the only effective way of relieving vomiting.

Surgery and stomas

The treatment of colorectal cancers usually involves surgery, often **resection** of the affected part of the bowel, with or without the formation of a **stoma** (*stoma* = hole or opening). Surgery saves lives and improves the quality of life by reducing symptoms. Complications can occur, however, both physically and mentally. A complication of bowel surgery is **paralytic ileus**, that is, paralysis of **peristalsis**. The content of the bowel does not flow, and therefore, the patient is unable to eat or drink, may feel nausea and may vomit, and will become malnourished if this continues.

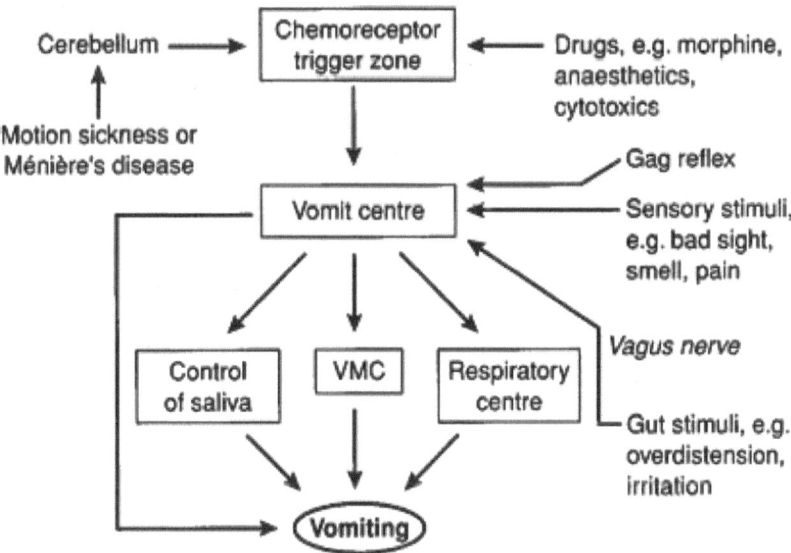

FIGURE 8.15 The vomit centre in the brainstem.

This problem normally corrects itself as the **autonomic nervous system**, which drives bowel movements, begins to function again.

Openings into the bowel are **colostomy** (colon) and **ileostomy** (ileum) for the collection of faeces into a bag worn on the abdomen. Stomas are either temporary, as may be in inflammatory bowel disease (IBD), or permanent. A colostomy can be sited anywhere along the colon, for example, an **ascending, transverse, descending**, or **sigmoid colostomy** (Figure 8.16). Owing to the water absorption function of the colon, the site of the colostomy will affect the nature of the faecal material eliminated from it. Ascending and early transverse colostomies are likely to eliminate more fluid faecal matter since the organ has had little opportunity to absorb the water. Colostomies sited further along the organ will produce progressively more solid faecal matter. Ileostomies eliminate the contents into a bag prior to reaching the colon, so the stoma bag is likely to contain liquid drainage, at least at first.

The liver

The liver is a complex organ. Excluding the skin, it is the largest organ inside the body. It is situated in the upper abdominal cavity on the right-hand side, beneath the diaphragm (Figure 8.1, p. 149).

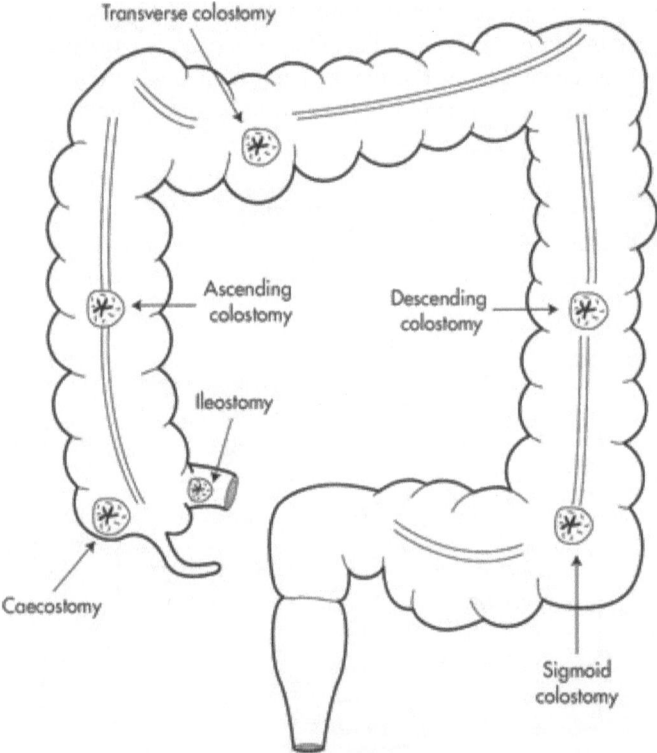

FIGURE 8.16 The sites for various stomas.

Liver cells (called **hepatocytes**) are packed in communities called **lobules** (Figure 8.17), with numerous lobules occurring throughout the gland. A single liver lobule consists of a connection to the central blood vessel, which is a branch of the **hepatic vein**. From this central vein, tiny vessels, called **sinusoids**, extend outwards, radiating similar to the spokes of a wheel from a central hub. The hepatocytes are lined up along each side of the sinusoid similar to houses along a street. From the outside of the lobule, blood is supplied to the sinusoids from branches of both the **hepatic artery** and the **hepatic portal vein**. The hepatic artery branch has brought blood from a main branch of the **abdominal aorta**. The hepatic portal vein conveys blood rich in the nutrient products of digestion from the bowel to the liver. The sinusoid is therefore getting a rich mix of arterial blood containing oxygen and hepatic portal blood containing nutrients. The hepatocytes can carry out their function using these materials delivered to them until the blood drains into the central hepatic vein and leaves the liver. The hepatocytes also produce **bile**, which drains from the liver via the small **biliary ducts** into the larger **common bile duct** outside the liver.

The functions of the liver are:

1. **Deamination** of excess amino acids from the diet. *Deamination* is the removal of an amine group, containing **nitrogen**, from the amino acid, leaving the non-nitrogenous component, which can be converted to glucose. This is **gluconeogenesis**, the creation of new glucose from a non-carbohydrate source. The amine group is further converted by the liver, first, to **ammonia (NH_3)**, then to **urea** for excretion.

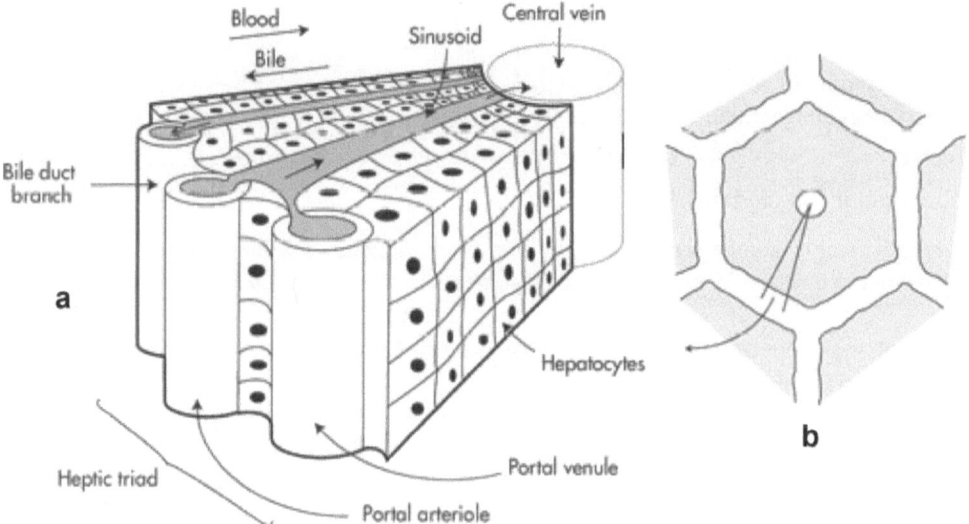

FIGURE 8.17   A liver lobule: (a) The hepatic triad consists of the arteriole, portal venule, and bile duct. Blood from the arteriole and portal venule mixes and flows down the sinusoid towards the central vein. Bile drains the other way towards the branch of the bile duct in the triad. Liver cells (hepatocytes) carry out the liver functions from products recovered from the blood, and they produce the bile. (b) An overall view of the whole liver lobule with the segment (shown in A) identified.

2. Conversion of amino acids from one readily available form to another form which is in short supply.
3. The formation of most blood proteins, such as **albumin**, and the clotting proteins, such as **prothrombin** and **fibrinogen**, the **lipoproteins**, and the protein for transporting iron **transferrin,** and **transcobalamin** for transporting **vitamin B$_{12}$.**
4. Storage of glucose in the form of **glycogen**.
5. Conversion of **fructose** and **galactose** to glucose.
6. Preparation of fats for use as an energy source when glucose, the main energy source, is in short supply.
7. Conversion of fats into a form used for **adipose**, that is, fat storage in the form called **triglycerides**.
8. Usage of fats for lipoproteins and for **phospholipids**; the formed fats are used in cell membranes.
9. Production of bile.
10. Metabolism of drugs in two phases: a **phase I reaction** and a **phase II reaction** called **conjugation**, meaning, joining drugs to other substances, for excretion.
11. Storage of iron; vitamins A, B$_{12}$, and D; and folic acid.

Liver cancer

There are various types of liver cancer:

- **Hepatocellular carcinoma (HCC)**, the commonest form of liver tumour
- **Fibrolamellar carcinoma**, a variant of HCC
- **Cholangiocarcinoma**, an adenocarcinoma
- **Hepatoblastoma**, an embryonic carcinoma
- **Angiosarcoma** of connective tissue origin
- Others (including secondary metastases)

Hepatocellular carcinoma (HCC)

This is a relatively common primary tumour worldwide, although the disease is less common in the Western world and more common in South-East Asia. Some of the causative factors include:

- Infection with **hepatitis B virus (HBV)** (see Figure 4.2c, Chapter 4, p. 61), even if it is mild with no symptoms
- The presence of **cirrhosis**, a disease of the liver where hepatocytes are replaced by fibrosis and abnormal nodule formation, often caused by chronic alcohol abuse
- Metabolic disorders, for example, **haemochromatosis**, a disease where excessive iron is absorbed and stored, damaging several organs
- Some drugs (e.g. chronic alcohol abuse) and toxins (e.g. from smoking)

The commonest features are **hepatomegaly** (enlargement of the liver) and abdominal pain with discomfort, but other symptoms include a loss of appetite (**anorexia**), nausea, fatigue, jaundice, weight loss, and fever. Swelling, pain, and discomfort in the abdomen are an indication of developing **ascites**, a collection of lymphatic fluid within the abdomen. It is a lymphatic oedema (see 'Causes of oedema', Chapter 10, Table 10.1, p. 198) due to obstructive lymphatic drainage within the liver. **Jaundice** is a yellow colour of various tissues, notably the skin, which is also itchy, due to deposits of **bilirubin** in the extracellular (tissue fluid) space; the bilirubin may be either *free* or *conjugated* (Figure 8.18). Many of these symptoms do not occur at first, and a continued worsening of these symptoms is suggestive of a developing tumour.

Bilirubin is normally a bile pigment derived originally from **haemoglobin (Hb)** and excreted through the urine and faeces (Figure 8.16). The normal level of bilirubin in the blood plasma is about 0.5 mg/dl (milligrams per decilitre of blood plasma), and this is mostly *free* bilirubin. In jaundice, it can rise to 40 mg/dl, mostly of the *conjugated* type (Figure 8.18).

The three main causes of jaundice are:

1. **Haemolytic jaundice** – excessive **haemolysis**, that is, breakdown of red blood cells, releasing too much Hb

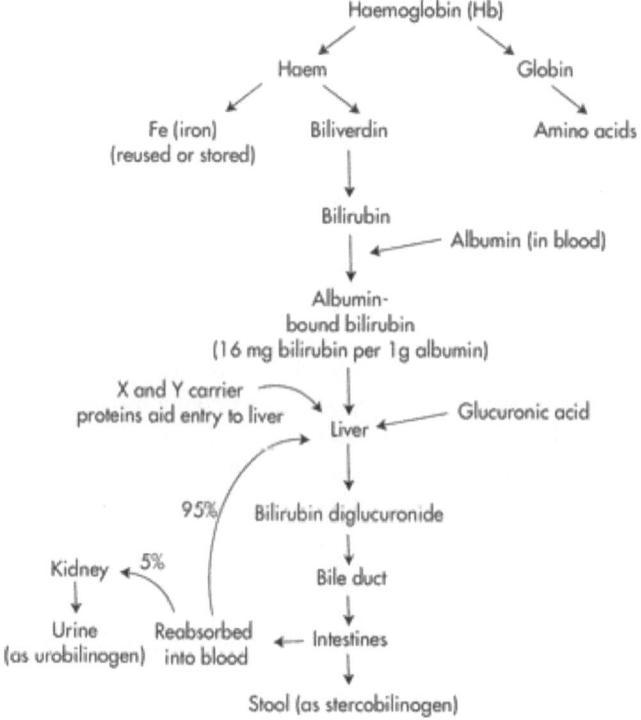

FIGURE 8.18   The natural history of bilirubin. When haemoglobin (Hb) is released from old red cells, Hb splits into the *haem* component and the *globin* component. Globin can be broken down to recover the amino acids. From the haem component, the iron can be recycled, but the biliverdin must be removed. It is first converted to bilirubin and then bound to albumin. This enters the liver with the assistance of carrier proteins X and Y. In the liver, bilirubin is bound to glucuronic acid, that is, it becomes conjugated, and this makes it soluble in water. It enters the bile duct as a component of bile. Bile reaches the intestines and is partly reabsorbed. Most of it goes back to the liver; the rest is excreted in the urine as urobilinogen. What is not absorbed from the bowel is excreted in the stools as stercobilinogen.

2. Liver disease, for example, liver failure due to cirrhosis or cancer of the liver
3. **Obstructive jaundice**, where the bile drainage is blocked, often by bile stones, but can also be by cancer, especially cancer of the head of the pancreas (Figure 8.4, p. 151)

Variations occur in the pathology of hepatocellular carcinoma. It may be a large single mass, or it may be infiltrative or multifocal. It can spread through the branches of the portal vein and hepatic artery, although distal metastases usually occur only late in the course of the disease. Another variation of the histology is **minute carcinoma**, that is, tiny patches of carcinoma, sometimes set against a widespread cirrhosis of the liver. Less common are the **pedunculated tumours**, which protrude from the liver surface.

HCC tumour cells produce a marker which can be a useful diagnostic tool: **alpha (α)–fetoprotein (AFP)**. This is not normally found in circulation after birth, and blood serum levels consistently above 500 μg/L are highly suggestive of liver cancer. However, the minute carcinoma, pedunculated tumours, and fibrolamellar carcinoma are exceptions, since they produce only low levels of AFP.

HCC has a poor prognosis, death being caused by **cachexia** (see 'Kwashiorkor and cachexia', Chapter 18, p. 327), bleeding into the digestive tract, **liver failure** causing hepatic coma, and more rarely, liver rupture. *Liver failure* means failure of the functions of the liver, listed on p. 173. This condition is recognised by the presence of:

- Jaundice.
- Low blood albumin levels (**hypoalbuminaemia**), leading to tissue oedema (see Table 10.1, Chapter 10, p. 198).
- High blood ammonia levels (**hyperammonaemia**) and other metabolic disturbances, leading ultimately to coma.
- The presence of a characteristic musty body odour (called **fetor hepaticus**).
- Impairment of the blood clotting mechanism (a **coagulopathy**), which leads to bleeding, notably into the digestive tract. It is also partly due to the raised back pressure of blood along the portal vein, called **portal hypertension**, from the obstructed liver. Portal hypertension can lead to bleeding from oesophageal varices or the rectum (Figure 8.19).
- Various skin manifestations, such as **spider angiomas**, that is, small spider-like collections of blood vessels seen in the skin, or **palmar erythema**, that is, local vasodilation and redness, both caused by abnormal oestrogen metabolism.
- Failure of other body organs, called **multi-organ failure**, in particular the kidneys.

Other liver and biliary cancers

1. **Fibrolamellar carcinoma (FLC)**, also called **fibrolamellar hepatocellular carcinoma (FLHCC)**, is a type of liver cancer usually seen in teens and adults below 40 years of age who have an otherwise healthy liver. About 65% arise in the left lobe of the liver. It consists of islands of tumour cells with collagen bands running between them. This tumour carries a better prognosis than HCC.
2. **Hepatoblastoma** is an **embryonic carcinoma**, which means the tumour contains cell types normally seen in the developing embryo. It arises in children (mostly boys) up to 2 years of age. Primitive foetal liver cells make up the **epithelioid** type, and in the **mixed** type, primitive stromal cells separate foetal from embryonic liver cells. The children suffer

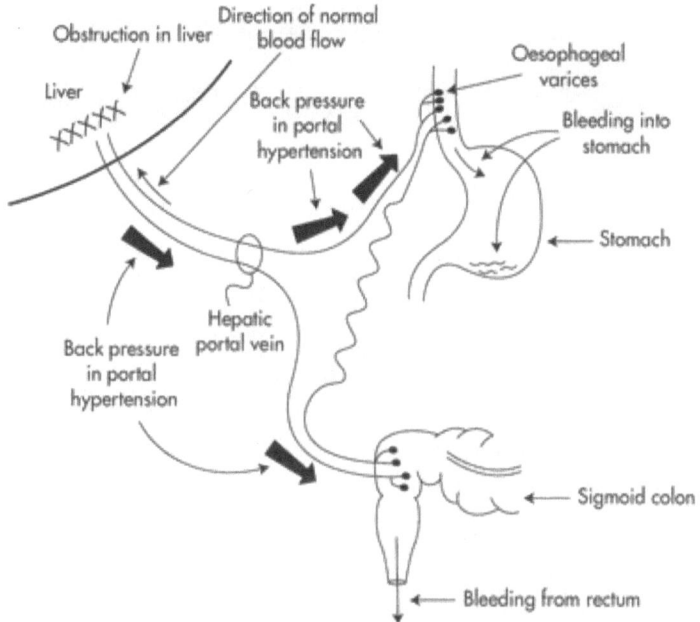

FIGURE 8.19 Hepatic portal hypertension. The passage of portal blood through the liver is obstructed, possibly by a tumour. The pressure of the blood builds up in the portal vein, putting increasing pressure on the vein's capillary bed that spans almost the entire digestive tract, from the lower oesophagus to the rectum. The capillaries swell with blood, especially at the lower oesophagus (varices) and rectum. Bleeding is sometimes a feature at these sites.

anorexia, nausea and vomiting, and abdominal pain. The liver is usually enlarged, and they have a raised serum **alpha-fetoprotein (AFP)** (see 'Hepatocellular carcinoma (HCC)', p. 174).

3. **Angiosarcoma**, also called **haemangiosarcoma**, is a rare tumour of blood vessel origin. This is found mostly in older adult males, often with a background of cirrhosis or history of exposure to industrial chemicals, such as **arsenic** or **vinyl chloride**. The liver is very enlarged, and spread of metastases is usually rapid. The tumour carries a very poor prognosis, with patient survival usually being little more than one year from presentation.

4. **Cholangiocarcinoma** (biliary duct cancer) is a rare **adenocarcinoma** arising from the bile ducts. **Intrahepatic cholangiocarcinoma (ICC)** starts in the bile ducts *inside* the liver. It is the least common but aggressive form, occurring mostly in older people. The more common **extrahepatic cholangiocarcinoma** starts in the bile ducts *outside* the liver. Extrahepatic can be subdivided into **perihilar, gall bladder**, and **distal bile duct cancers** (Figure 8.20). The tumour cells secrete mucin, and the spread to distant organs is more common in this tumour type than for hepatocellular carcinoma (HCC). Symptoms include jaundice, fatigue, loss of appetite, pyrexia, shivers, nausea and vomiting, and abdominal pain, which may be sharp in nature. One symptom which may highlight the possible existence of the cancer is an aching or dragging feeling in the right side of the abdomen. Aggregating factors that may lead to this cancer are being overweight, diabetes, the presence of gallstones, and a **porcelain gall bladder**, a heavily calcified gall bladder, which may be linked to gallstones.

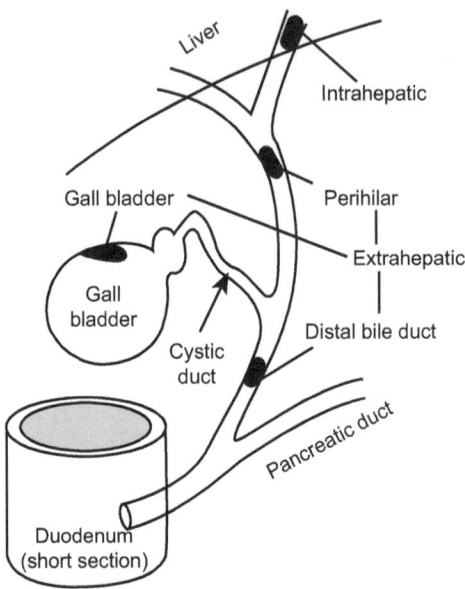

FIGURE 8.20 The sites for biliary tract cancers. Intrahepatic are within the ducts *inside* the liver; extrahepatic are within the ducts *outside* the liver (see also Figure 8.3).

Some gene mutations that are linked to liver cancers are *FOS* (see 'FOS, chromosome 14', Addendum, p. 355), *LAMC2* (see 'LAMC2, chromosome 1', Addendum, p. 343), and *DPP4* (see 'DPP4, chromosome 2', Addendum, p. 344).

Liver secondary tumours

The liver is the site for many metastases, and the majority of liver tumours are caused by metastatic spread from a primary elsewhere. Approximately 40% of cancer patients are likely to have liver metastases. Most of these secondaries will have come from a primary tumour in the stomach, pancreas, gall bladder and bile ducts, large bowel, lung, breast, kidney, or a **malignant melanoma** (see 'Malignant melanoma', Chapter 13, p. 247) (Figure 8.21). The tumours that arise from the metastases develop as nodules mostly on the liver surface, but some occur deeper in the organ. A rise in the serum level of **alkaline phosphatase**, an enzyme involved in phosphate metabolism,[5] is an early warning that liver secondaries are likely to be present. This is followed later by the development of jaundice and other symptoms. Untreated, the prognosis following the discovery of liver metastases is poor. Resection of these tumours should improve the prognosis, with 40% of patients surviving three years or more.

Key points

Oral cancers

- Digestive cancers can seriously impact the patient's nutritional status.
- Smoking and alcohol are often major contributors to oral cancers.
- About 95% of cases of mouth cancers are squamous cell carcinomas.

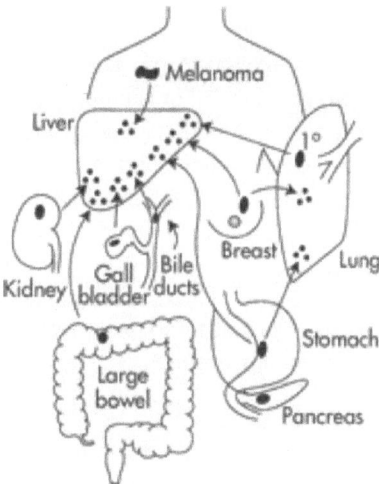

FIGURE 8.21   Liver and lung metastases. The main sites for primary tumours causing liver metastases (black dots) are melanomas of the skin, lung ($1°$ is a primary tumour), kidney, gall bladder, bile ducts, breast, large bowel, pancreas, and stomach.

Oesophageal cancers

- Most oesophageal cancers are squamous cell carcinomas or adenocarcinomas.
- Oesophageal cancers can spread locally into the wall and beyond into the lower respiratory tract, the lung, and the mediastinum.

Gastric carcinoma

- Gastric carcinoma occurs in two forms, the intestinal and the diffuse forms, and two locations, cardia and non-cardia.
- The degree by which the cancer has infiltrated into the stomach wall is an important factor.
- Gastric carcinoma usually begins insidiously and may be asymptomatic at first.
- The earliest symptoms are usually abdominal discomfort and weight loss.
- Gastrectomy can cause pernicious anaemia due to the loss of intrinsic factor in the formation of vitamin B_{12}, and this is corrected by vitamin B_{12} injections.

Intestinal cancers

- About 45% of small bowel cancers are adenocarcinomas, about 30% are carcinoid tumours, a further 10% are small bowel lymphomas, and the rest are sarcomas.

Pancreatic cancer

- Pancreatic cancers are mostly adenocarcinomas.
- The two forms of pancreatic cancer are the ductal and non-ductal types.
- The ductal type accounts for most of the pancreatic tumours, and two-thirds of them arise from the head of the gland.

Colorectal cancers

- Non-malignant (benign) and non-neoplastic (no malignant potential) polyps of the large bowel are growths arising from the mucosal or submucosal lining of the gut wall.
- *Adenomas* are neoplastic tumours (with malignant potential) derived from the glandular epithelial components of the mucous membrane lining of the bowel.
- Adenocarcinoma is the malignant growth of the small or large bowel.

Stomas and surgical complications

- A *colostomy* and an *ileostomy* are openings into the bowel.
- *Paralytic ileus* is a complication of bowel surgery.

The liver

- Liver cells (hepatocytes) are packed in liver lobules.
- The hepatic portal vein conveys blood rich in digestive nutrients from the digestive system to the liver.
- The hepatocytes produce bile, which drains from the liver via the small biliary ducts into the larger common bile duct and on to the duodenum.
- Other functions of the liver relate to protein, glucose, and fat metabolism; the storage of certain nutrients; and the metabolism of drugs.

Liver cancer

- There are various types of liver cancer, the commonest being hepatocellular carcinoma (HCC).
- Common features are hepatomegaly (enlarged liver) and abdominal pain.
- *Jaundice* is a yellow colour of various tissues, notably the skin, due to deposits of bilirubin in the extracellular (tissue fluid) space.
- Liver failure involves bleeding caused by impairment of the blood clotting mechanism (a coagulopathy) and by portal hypertension from the obstructed liver.
- The liver is the site for many metastases, and most of liver tumours are caused by metastatic spread from a primary elsewhere.

Notes

1 The inside lumen of the digestive tract is technically part of the *outside* of the body. That may seem strange, but in order for something to *enter* the body from the digestive system, it must first be absorbed through the gut wall. The *gut wall* is the interface between the outside world and the inside of the body. This makes it easier to understand how microorganisms can exist within the gut lumen whilst the inside of the body remains sterile.
2 Chronic inflammation as a cause of cancer is seen throughout all the bowel cancers.
3 *Enterochromaffin-like cells* are neuroendocrine cells found in gastric mucosal glands and are involved in gastric acid production by releasing histamine. Neuroendocrine cells are similar to neurons because they receive impulse signals from the nervous system and respond by producing hormones.
4 *Dyschesia* is difficulty in passing faeces due to constipation or bowel obstruction.
5 Metabolism, such as the chemistry of glucose, cell membrane phospholipids, DNA, and the calcification of bone.

9

CANCER OF THE RESPIRATORY SYSTEM

- Introduction: oxygen and carbon dioxide
- The airway and gas diffusion
- Laryngeal cancers
- Cancer of the bronchus and the lung
- Symptoms of lung cancer
- Stages and treatment of lung cancer
- Mesothelioma
- Key points

Introduction: oxygen and carbon dioxide

Oxygen (O)[1] is a waste removal system, and as such, it is essential for keeping the cell chemistry going, that is, **metabolism** (Figure 9.1). Without it, the wastes rapidly build up and the cell's chemistry will fail. Given that a large component of metabolism is energy production, failure means all energy production stops and the cell will die if the oxygen supply is not restored.

There are three steps in energy production, and oxygen removes waste from two of them (Figure 9.1). In the **tricarboxylic cycle** (previously known as the **Krebs cycle**), there is a tendency to build up too much carbon waste. So for each carbon atom (C) that needs to be removed, two oxygen atoms ($O + O = O_2$) combine with the carbon to form carbon dioxide ($C + O_2 = CO_2$). The CO_2 is then removed in the blood and eliminated through the lungs. In the final stage of energy production, there is a surplus of hydrogen (H), which, if allowed to accumulate, would cause acidic conditions to develop, known as **metabolic acidosis**. Instead, every time two excess hydrogens (2H) need removal, a single oxygen atom (O) comes in and combines with the hydrogen to form water ($2H + O = H_2O$). Water is removed from the body by the kidneys and, to a lesser extent, through the lungs. Water is also essential in the body since it is a large component of the cells and tissues, but similar to CO_2, it is kept in strict balance.

DOI: 10.4324/9781003389125-9

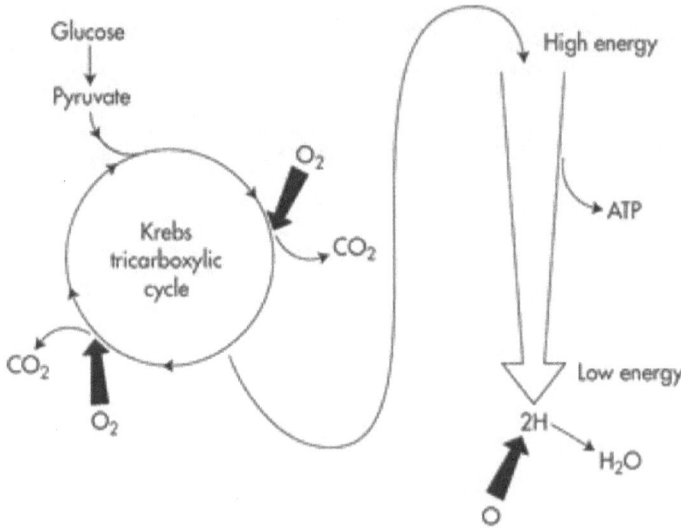

FIGURE 9.1 Oxygen is the waste removal system. In the Krebs/tricarboxylic cycle, oxygen collects unwanted carbon and removes it as carbon dioxide. Oxygen also collects unwanted hydrogen (2H) and removes it as water at the end of ATP production.

The airway and gas diffusion

The airway begins at the nose and mouth and ends at the microscopic air sacs in the lungs, called **alveoli** (Figure 9.2). The tubes that make up this airway have a **smooth muscle** wall (see 'Muscle tissue', Chapter 1, p. 13) with **mucous membrane** (see 'Epithelial tissues', Chapter 1, p. 9) lining the inner surface. The **larynx**, the **trachea**, and the **bronchi** also have cartilage, the purpose of which is to stop the airway from collapsing.

The larynx (Figure 9.3) is a cartilaginous hollow chamber with a mucous membrane lining from which the **vocal cords** are fashioned. The vocal cords are stretched across the **glottis**, the narrowest part of the airway inside the larynx. Above the glottis is a flap, the **epiglottis**, which closes the glottis during swallowing to prevent food and water from entering the respiratory passages.

Below the larynx is the **trachea** (the 'windpipe') (Figure 9.3), which passes down from the larynx into the **thorax**. The trachea is lined with ciliated mucous membrane (see 'Tobacco smoking, mucociliary escalator', Chapter 3, p. 48). The lower end divides into two **primary bronchi** (singular = **bronchus**), one for each lung (Figure 9.2). These also have cartilaginous rings, and they subdivide into **secondary bronchi**. These supply air to the many tiny branches (**bronchiole**) that serve the terminal air sacs, known as **alveoli**. There are 300,000,000 microscopic alveoli, which are held together with **yellow elastic connective tissue** (see 'Elastic connective tissue', Chapter 1, p. 11). Alveoli have very thin walls (only one cell thick) to allow exchange of the gases, oxygen and carbon dioxide, with the blood (Figure 9.4). Oxygen leaves the alveoli and enters the blood by means of **diffusion** down a **concentration gradient**, that is, oxygen moving from a high concentration in the alveoli into a low concentration in the blood. Carbon dioxide moves in the opposing direction, again from a high concentration in the blood to a low concentration in the

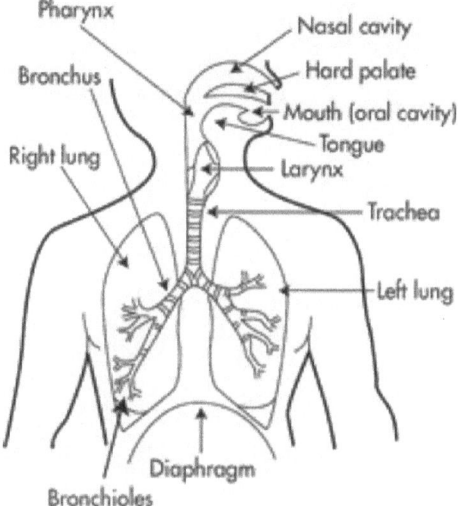

FIGURE 9.2 The respiratory system. The trachea divides into the left and right bronchus.

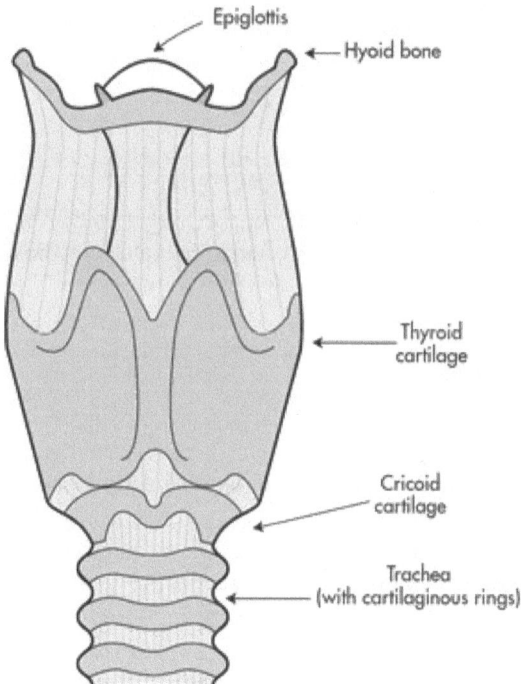

FIGURE 9.3 The larynx and trachea. Cartilage holds the larynx and trachea open for the passage of air.

Source: Redrawn from Martini et al. (2023).

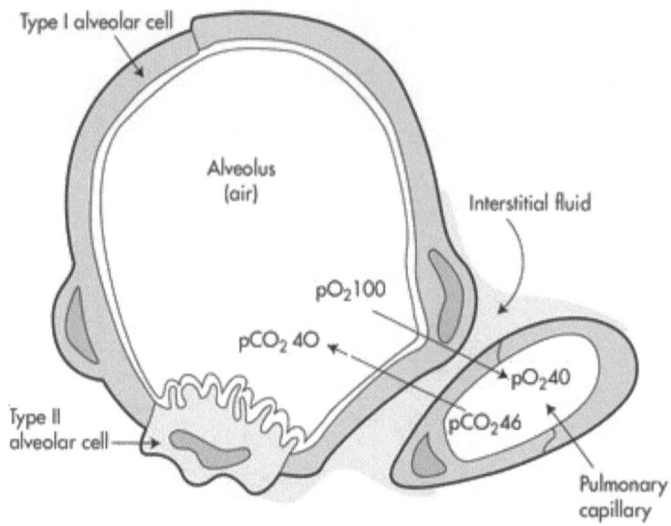

FIGURE 9.4 Microscopic view of the lung. An alveolus, containing air, with walls of type I and type II cells, is next to a pulmonary capillary containing blood. There is interstitial fluid between them. The direction of gas movement and the pressures, in mmHg, for pO_2 and pCO_2 in the blood and air are shown. pO_2 and pCO_2 are partial pressures, that is, that part of the total pressure each gas contributes. Each gas flows down its concentration gradient from high to low pressure (arrowed). In this way, blood gives up carbon dioxide and takes on oxygen simultaneously.

Source: Redrawn from Blows (2024).

alveoli (Figure 9.4) (Blows 2024). Blood is the transport system to deliver oxygen to all parts of the body, mostly attached to **haemoglobin (Hb)**, and to return carbon dioxide back to the lungs, mostly in the plasma.

Laryngeal cancers

Only about 2% of all cancers in men are of the larynx, and only 0.4% in women. This disease occurs most frequently after the age of 40 years. The overwhelming factor in virtually all cases is tobacco smoking. This one factor alone is essentially responsible for this disease, which means that the prevention of laryngeal cancer is clearly available to everyone. Drinking alcohol may play a less-significant role in the cause, but alcohol consumption combined with smoking carries the biggest risk. Most laryngeal cancers (95%) are **squamous cell carcinomas**, with a very small number of **adenocarcinomas** seen. Both are derived from the mucosal lining of the larynx. The commonest site of tumour growth is the vocal cords (Figure 9.4) within the glottis, and these are known as **glottic tumours**, accounting for up to 65% of laryngeal cancers. But cancers may arise from anywhere within the larynx (**intrinsic tumours**) or from outside (**extrinsic tumours**) (Figure 9.5). Intrinsic tumours can develop from above the vocal cords, called **supraglottic**, that is, about 35% of cases, or from below the glottis, called **subglottic**, that is, less than 5% of cases. **Transglottic** tumours extend across the

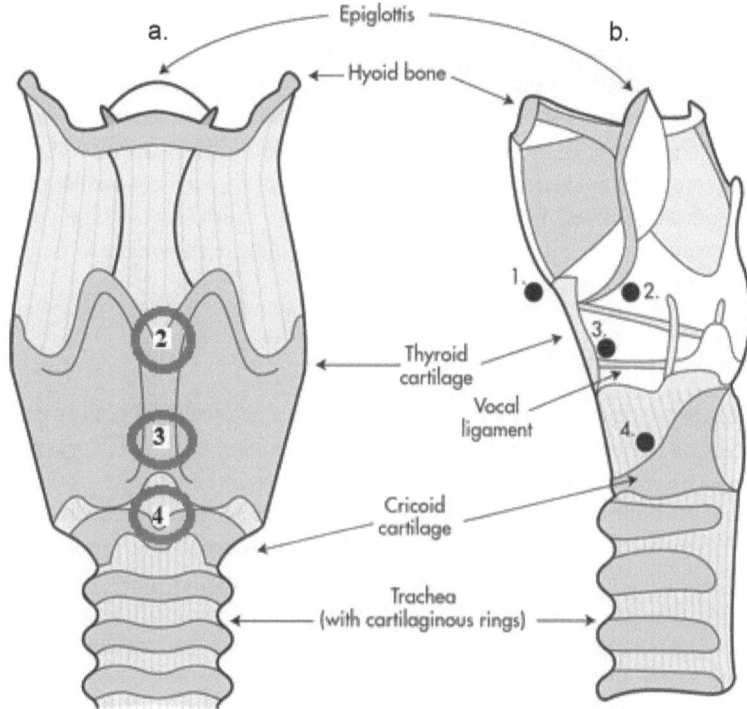

FIGURE 9.5 The laryngeal cancer sites: (a) anterior (front) view; (b) left lateral (side) view of cut section, with cancer sites shown as grey circles or black spots: (1) extrinsic, (2) supraglottic, (3) glottic, (4) subglottic (2, 3, and 4 are all intrinsic).

Source: Redrawn from Martini et al. (2023).

laryngeal ventricle, the space within the larynx. Spread from these locations usually follows these patterns:

1. Glottic tumours remain confined within the larynx for long periods of time, giving the patient a better chance of a long-term prognosis. The reason for this is that the laryngeal cartilaginous wall surrounding the tumour contains the growth, with only a few lymphatic vessels available for spread.
2. Supraglottic tumours can spread into the local spaces within the larynx and to the **cervical** lymph nodes found in the neck area. The prognosis is reasonable, with a 65% five-year survival rate.
3. Subglottic tumours most often involve the vocal cords as well as the structures below, and they frequently spread into the local tissues, especially the thyroid gland, the **cricoid cartilage** (Figure 9.5), and the trachea. The survival rate at five years is about 40%.
4. Transglottic tumours are prone to spread more than the other types to the cervical lymph nodes, and they require extensive excision of all affected tissues. The five-year survival rate is about 50%.

Persistent hoarseness of the voice, beyond that expected from a sore throat, is a primary symptom. This is followed later by pain, **haemoptysis** (coughing of blood), and **dysphagia** (pain or difficulty with swallowing).

The treatment for some of these tumours is surgical removal of the larynx, called a **laryngectomy**. Since the larynx is the 'voice box', surgical removal means that the postoperative patient will no longer be able to speak. Older techniques exist which allow the patient to 'fashion' a voice from air released from the stomach, and this method would have to be taught to the patient. However, modern technology allows for 'synthesised' voices to be generated by a computer, and this speaks for the patient.

Cancer of the bronchus and the lung

Bronchial cancers are one of the commonest causes of cancer deaths in both sexes, and in common with laryngeal and mouth cancer, the main cause is smoking. Other factors play a role in the causation of this disease, such as air pollution in urban areas, where deaths from this disease are twice as common as in rural areas; radiation; genetics; and asbestos, but their effects are small compared with smoking. Air pollution causes 10% of lung cancers in the UK, mostly due to inhaled tiny particulate matter known as PM2.5, that is, air particles measuring less than 2.5 μm (micrometres) in diameter, made from soot, smoke, dust, and minute biological matter, such as bacteria, pollen, and mould spores. The remaining 90% of lung cancer deaths are mainly due to smoking, which has historically meant more men than women being diagnosed. However, more recently, diagnoses have decreased in males by 29% but increased in females by a staggering 102%. As with laryngeal and mouth cancer, individuals have a choice whether to run the risk and smoke or not.

The disease usually starts in the bronchial mucosa close to the tracheal bifurcation, the point where the trachea divides into the two main bronchi (Figure 9.2). From here it will spread into the lung, and metastases will spread to other parts of the body, commonly the cervical lymph nodes, the pleura, the liver, the adrenal glands, the brain, and the bones (Figure 9.6). There are several different types[2] of lung cancer (Table 9.1).

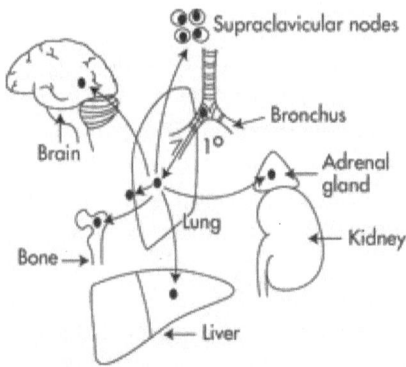

FIGURE 9.6 The spread of lung cancer. The primary site (1°) in this figure is at the division of the trachea into two bronchi. From here it can spread into the lung and pleura, to the bone, brain, liver, adrenal gland, and the supraclavicular lymph nodes.

TABLE 9.1 The types and frequencies of lung cancer

Cancer	Frequency (%)	Variant types
Non-small-cell lung cancers (NSCLC) (about 90% of lung cancers) Adenocarcinoma	30–50% of NSCLC	1. Acinar adenocarcinoma 2. Papillary adenocarcinoma 3. Lepidic predominant adenocarcinoma 4. Solid carcinoma with mucus formation 5. Low-grade adenosquamous carcinoma
Squamous cell carcinoma	25–40% of NSCLC	
Large-cell lung carcinoma (LCLC)	10–20% of NSCLC	1. Large-cell carcinoma 2. Large-cell neuroendocrine carcinoma (LCNEC)
Carcinoid tumour	1–2% of NSCLC	1. 'Typical' 2. 'Atypical'
Bronchial gland carcinomas	Rare	1. Adenoid cystic carcinoma 2. Mucoepidermoid carcinoma
Small-cell lung cancers (SCLC) (about 10% of lung cancers) Small-cell carcinoma		1. Combined oat cell carcinoma 2. Oat cell carcinoma

Non-small-cell lung cancers (NSCLC) (about 90% of all lung can*cers)*[3]

See footnote 2.

Adenocarcinoma

Adenocarcinoma of the lung is the commonest form of NSCLC, and it is closely associated with smoking. The growth arises from mucosal glandular secretory cells. The early stages of the disease tend to be asymptomatic. Adenocarcinomas can be preinvasive, minimally invasive, and invasive. Several subtypes are:

1. **Acinar adenocarcinoma** is a common glandular cancer where cuboidal and columnar cells (see Figure 1.8, Chapter 1, p. 10) form **acinars**, that is, multiple-lobed nodules, similar to raspberries. It has a low five-year survival rate of 16–22%. Mutations of *HRAS* (see 'HRAS, chromosome 11', Addendum, p. 352) and *FES* (see 'FES, chromosome 15', Addendum, p. 355) genes are linked to this form of cancer.
2. **Papillary adenocarcinoma** is characterised by finger-like projections extending into the alveoli. It affects mostly the elderly, and a major risk factor is smoking. The *micropapillary* variant spreads quickly and carries a poor prognosis.
3. **Lepidic predominant adenocarcinoma** is characterised by growth along the inner lining of the alveoli from the lung periphery. It progresses slowly and may be multicentric. Some produce mucus, and those that do are found mostly in smokers.
4. **Solid carcinoma with mucus formation** occurs as a solid growth pattern involving columnar 'goblet' cells (see 'Epithelial tissues', Chapter 1, p. 9) producing mucus. It is linked to distant metastases and a poor prognosis. Mutations of the *KRAS* gene (see 'KRAS, chromosome 12', Addendum, p. 353) are common in this tumour.

5. **Low-grade adenosquamous carcinoma** is a rare variant of adenocarcinoma that affects both squamous and glandular cells. It carries a high risk of spread to lymph nodes and other distal organs. It is strongly linked to smoking and mutations of the *EGFR* gene (see 'EGFR, chromosome 7', Addendum, p. 348).

Squamous cell carcinoma (epidermoid carcinoma)

Squamous cell carcinoma has the strongest link of all with smoking. This type of cancer accounts for an average of 30% of bronchogenic carcinomas, that is, those arising in the bronchus. It starts as a dysplasia (Figure 1.14, Chapter 1, p. 18) of flat squamous cells (Figure 1.8, Chapter 1, p. 10). They metastasise late in the course of the disease, but they are linked with two complications: **pneumonia** (fluid congestion of the lung) and **atelectasis** (lung collapse). Mutations of the *TP53* gene (see 'Chromosome 17', Addendum, p. 356) are seen in 81% of cases.

Large-cell lung carcinoma (LCLC)

Large-cell lung carcinoma consists of large abnormal cells with clear cytoplasm. They can grow quickly and spread in such a manner as to distort the trachea. **Large-cell neuroendocrine carcinoma** (**LCNEC**) is a rare and aggressive subtype of this cancer. It is usually seen in heavy-smoking older males. It is characterised by large cells with a lot of cytoplasm that divide quickly. LCLC and LCNEC are usually diagnosed at post-mortem examination by excluding all other types.

Carcinoid tumour

This is a rare, slow-growing neuroendocrine tumour that can remain asymptomatic for years. Most are diagnosed around the age of 50 years. There are two forms, the **typical** (90% of carcinoid tumours) and the **atypical** (10% of carcinoid tumours). Typical tumours grow slowly, and they tend to stay within the lungs. Atypical tumours grow more quickly and may spread beyond the lungs. Being neuroendocrine, these tumours sometime produce excessive hormones, which can cause symptoms such as skin flushes or wheezing.

Bronchial gland carcinomas

These are tumours occurring in the trachea or the bronchus. There are two subtypes: **adenoid cystic carcinoma** (**ACC**) and **mucoepidermoid carcinoma** (**MEC**). ACC is the second most common tracheal tumour, consisting of nodular growth within the trachea which can extend around the circumference of the tube. This type of growth can narrow the trachea, obstructing the passage of air. MEC affects segments of the bronchi that enter the lung. It is more aggressive than ACC and may produce metastases that affect thoracic lymph nodes. Both forms are locally invasive.

ROS1-positive lung cancer

Any lung cancer can be *ROS1* gene–positive, that is, a fusion between the *ROS1* gene and another gene (see 'ROS1, chromosome 6', Addendum, p. 348). This fusion occurs in about 1–2% of NSCLC, mostly adenocarcinomas, and is found more often in younger women. It causes the tumour to become especially aggressive and to metastasise quickly, spreading secondaries to the brain and bones. By identifying this genetic error in a biopsy of the tumour, patients can be given targeted drug therapy, notably **crizotinib** (see 'Protein kinase inhibitors', Chapter 16, p. 303), which is usually very effective, except in some cases that may become crizotinib-resistant. However, this form of targeted treatment may avoid the need for chemotherapy and radiotherapy.

Small-cell lung cancer (SCLC) (about 10% of all lung cancers)

Small-cell carcinoma is the fastest-growing and most malignant of all the lung cancers and carries the worst prognosis, that is, less than 2% of patients are alive two years after diagnosis. There is a strong link with smoking. On diagnosis, it may be confined to one lung and the lymph nodes associated with that lung (*limited stage*) or may have spread beyond that (*extensive stage*). The cells are tiny, with very little **cytoplasm** (see 'The cell', Chapter 1, p. 1). SCLC can exist combined with any other lung cancer type, and this is called **combined SCLC (C-SCLC)**. It is also sometimes called **oat cell carcinoma** if the cells are compressed into ovoid shapes. Mutations of the *TP53* gene (see 'TP53, chromosome 17', Addendum, p. 356) occur in up to 90% of cases.

Symptoms of lung cancer

The patient with bronchogenic lung cancer is typically middle-aged with a history of smoking. They may have or develop the following symptoms:

- **Persistent cough** caused by the irritation of the tumour within the airway or may be caused by smoking.
- **Sputum** is a lung or bronchial secretion produced by the mucous lining of the respiratory tract and then coughed up. Sputum usually contains microorganisms or cells, and these can be identified in the laboratory and may aid in the diagnosis. Sputum samples may be required from the patient for this purpose.
- **Haemoptysis**, that is, coughing up blood from the respiratory tract, may occur at a later phase of the disease and suggests erosion of blood vessels in the lung.
- **Dyspnoea**, that is, difficulty in breathing causing breathlessness with or without a **wheeze**. During the advanced stages of the disease, the breathless state can become **air hunger**, where the patient is fighting for every breath.
- **Chest pain**, made worse by deep breathing or coughing.
- **Chest infections** that return repeatedly.
- **Fatigue** can be profound and affects more than 90% of patients.
- **Muscle weakness** due to **anorexia** and **malnourishment**, and in time, they will show evidence of body **wasting**, that is, loss of body fat and, eventually, **muscle loss** associated with **weight loss**.
- **Anxiety** and/or **depression**.

Stages and treatment of lung cancer

Lung cancer development has been staged by two different systems: the number system and the TNM systems, which, when used in combination, provide a staging system suitable for all situations.

The numbering system

Stage 1: This stage means the tumour is small, it has only slightly invaded the local tissues, and there are no metastases or spread to lymph nodes.

Stage 2: The tumour is larger, and there may be local lymph nodes involved or wider spread into local tissues.

Stage 3: The tumour has increased in size, and there is spread into local structures and lymph node involvement in areas some distance from the lung.

Stage 4: The tumour is any size and involves wider lymph node involvement and spread of metastases into other organs, for example, the liver.

The TNM system

T: Describes the size of the tumour.

N: Describes if lymph nodes are involved.

M: Describes if metastases have reached other body organs.

Stages 1 to 4 use TNM to describe each stage, creating a complex of substages which cover every possibility (Cancer Research UK 2023).

The treatment is surgery, whenever possible, to remove that part of the lung that contains the primary growth. A **lobectomy** is the removal of one lobe of one lung, whilst the removal of one whole lung is a **pneumonectomy**. Patients in this latter category of treatment must rely on their one remaining lung for the rest of their lives. Whilst this is adequate for sustaining life, it does curtail energetic exercise, where greater oxygenation of the blood is required. Radiotherapy and cytotoxic therapy (chemotherapy) may also be required.

A new test for a protein called **TLR2** in lung tumours is in development. This protein is encoded by the *TLR2* gene (see 'TLR2, chromosome 4', Addendum, p. 346). This gene is a member of the **toll-like receptor family**, and the protein product recognises many aspects of pathogenic microorganisms and activates the innate immune response (see 'Innate (non-specific immunity)' Chapter 5, p. 78). Although the gene is linked to colorectal cancer (see 'Colorectal cancers', Chapter 8, p. 164), the protein is also found in senescent, malignant cells in early-stage lung tumours but is absent from advanced lung cancers. Therefore, testing for the protein TLR2 in lung tumours becomes a useful way to assess the stage of the tumour, and drugs that activate the *TLR2* gene boosts the innate immune response, causing reduction of growth in early-stage tumours.

The drug **sunvozertinib**, currently in clinical trials, targets non-small-cell lung cancers (NSCLC) that have an **EGFR (epidermal growth factor receptor)** tyrosine kinase mutation (see 'EGFR, chromosome 7', Addendum, p. 348). This mutation, found in 2% of lung cancer patients, has shown to be resistant to other treatments, resulting in a poor outcome. Sunvozertinib is an EGFR tyrosine kinase inhibitor that has shown a 61% anti-tumour activity response in early clinical trials.

Mesothelioma

Covering the lungs are two layers which form a single membrane, the **pleura**, which has a fluid-filled cavity between the layers. **Mesothelioma** is a malignant tumour developing usually on the pleura. It tends to spread through the pleural double layers and may involve the pericardium, the covering of the heart. Less often, the primary site may be the peritoneum. The majority of cases are caused by exposure to **asbestos**, that is, the inhalation of extremely fine asbestos fibres (less than 0.5 μm in diameter, 8 μm in length), that is, asbestos dust. *Asbestos* is a naturally occurring mineral and had been used for many years as a building material to act as a fire retardant. This is now no longer the case, but many old buildings will still have asbestos as part of their construction.

The long delay between exposure and the start of the disease, some 20 to 40 years, means that despite the precautions now taken with asbestos and its removal from buildings where possible, the legacy of the past remains, and the disease is still on the increase. Males are affected more than females, possibly because males undertake the building jobs where asbestos is found, and it occurs mostly in the 50–70 years age range.

The tumour grows along the membrane and covers the lung, making surgical removal possible only in a small number of cases where diagnosis is made early. There are *epithelial* and *sarcomatous* types and tumours of mixed types. Spread outside of the pleura, which occurs more often in the sarcomatous type, involves the local lymph nodes, the kidney, the liver, and the brain.

The features of the disease are increasing chest pain, dyspnoea, fatigue, persistent cough, loss of appetite, and loss of weight. These symptoms gradually get worse as the tumour covers the lung and causes considerable incapacitation, with reduced chest wall movements during breathing. **Pleural effusion**, that is, excessive fluid collecting in the pleural space between the two layers, is common, adding to the dyspnoea by putting pressure on the lungs. The prognosis is poor due to the limited ability to treat this condition satisfactorily. An early diagnosis is essential for a good outcome, but this is rarely achieved. The hope for the future is that the precautions taken with asbestos now will result in a decline in the numbers of patients with this tumour.

Key points

Respiratory system

- Oxygen is a waste removal system and is essential for maintaining the cell chemistry.
- The airway begins at the nose and mouth, then the larynx, trachea, and bronchi, leading to the air sacs, called alveoli.
- Oxygen and carbon dioxide move down a concentration gradient from a high concentration to a low concentration, and this moves gases between the alveoli and the blood.

Laryngeal cancer

- The overwhelming causative factor in virtually all cases of laryngeal cancer is tobacco smoking.
- The vast majority of laryngeal cancers (95%) are squamous cell carcinomas; the remainder includes some adenocarcinomas.
- The commonest sites of tumour growth are the vocal cords within the glottis.
- Persistent hoarseness of the voice, beyond that expected from a sore throat, is a primary symptom.
- The treatment for some of these tumours is surgical removal of the larynx, called a laryngectomy.

Bronchial carcinoma

- Bronchial carcinoma usually starts in the bronchial mucosa close to the tracheal bifurcation.
- All lung cancers have a causative link with smoking, but squamous cell carcinoma has the strongest link.
- Lung cancers are divided into two major groups: non-small-cell lung cancers (NSCLC) and small-cell lung cancers (SCLC).
- Spread is into the lung, and metastases will spread to other parts of the body, commonly the cervical lymph nodes and pleura.
- The patient with bronchogenic lung cancer is typically middle-aged with a history of smoking.
- Symptoms include persistent cough (especially productive or excessive sputum or blood), pain on breathing, persistent hoarse voice, dyspnoea, fatigue, malnutrition, and weight loss.
- The treatment is surgery, that is, a lobectomy or a pneumonectomy, followed by chemotherapy and radiotherapy.
- *Mesothelioma* is a cancer of the pleura surrounding the lungs caused by inhalation of asbestos dust.

Notes

1 The chemical symbol for oxygen is O, not O_2, since the chemical symbol for an element is the same as *one atom* of the substance, and the symbol O_2 represents *two* atoms together, that is, a *molecule* of oxygen.
2 Nomenclature and classification of lung cancer vary to some extent according to the country and authority involved. Therefore, names of types and subtypes of certain cancers may vary from those used here.
3 New techniques are allowing researchers to grow NSCLC cells, obtained by biopsy, in the laboratory. These cell colonies, called spheroids, can be studied in 3D to establish their structure and genetic mutations, and they can be treated with drugs to determine the best therapy for each individual patient.

10

CANCER OF THE RENAL SYSTEM

- **Introduction**
- **The renal system**
- **Cancer of the kidney**
- **Bladder cancers**
- **Key points**

Introduction

The renal system is essential both as an excretory pathway for wastes and as a regulatory system for fluid, electrolyte, and pH balances. The respiratory system (Chapter 9) and renal systems are linked by their combined role as excretory organs and by their joint cooperative functions in stabilising the blood chemistry. Stabilisation of the internal body systems and environment is called **homeostasis**, of which the renal system is a major component.

The renal system

The kidneys are a major excretory pathway for the elimination of waste material from the body. The wastes removed through the kidneys are:

- **Urea**, a waste product from protein metabolism
- **Uric acid**, a waste product from the nucleic acids RNA and DNA
- **Creatinine**, waste resulting from muscle breakdown

The kidneys

Both kidneys, left and right, are positioned one on each side of the lumbar spinal column and attached to the back wall of the abdomen. They each have about 1 million **nephrons**. A *nephron* (Figure 10.1) consists of a microscopic tuft of **arterioles**, that is, mini arteries, called the **glomerulus**. This is surrounded by the **Bowman's capsule**, the collecting 'cup' for what is called

DOI: 10.4324/9781003389125-10

filtrate, that is, the fluid product extracted from the blood though the glomerulus. Leading from this are two **convoluted tubules**, the first (*proximal*) and the second (*distal*), and these are separated by the **loop of Henle**. Finally, the nephrons join **straight collecting ducts** that drain urine into the renal pelvis in the centre of the kidney (Figures 10.1 and 10.2).

Inside the cortex is the **medulla**, which consists of the **pyramids**. These are made from numerous straight collecting ducts from one region of the cortex joined together and converged towards a point. Urine from a pyramid first arrives in a cup-like structure called a **calyx**, then into the renal pelvis, the hollow core where urine collects. From here it drains down the ureter to the bladder (Figure 10.2).

The kidneys each have three surface coverings; the innermost **renal capsule**; the middle layer of fat, called the **adipose capsule**, which helps attach the kidney to the posterior abdominal wall; and the outermost **renal fascia**, made of dense fibrous tissue. This last structure is also important for anchorage of the kidney in place.

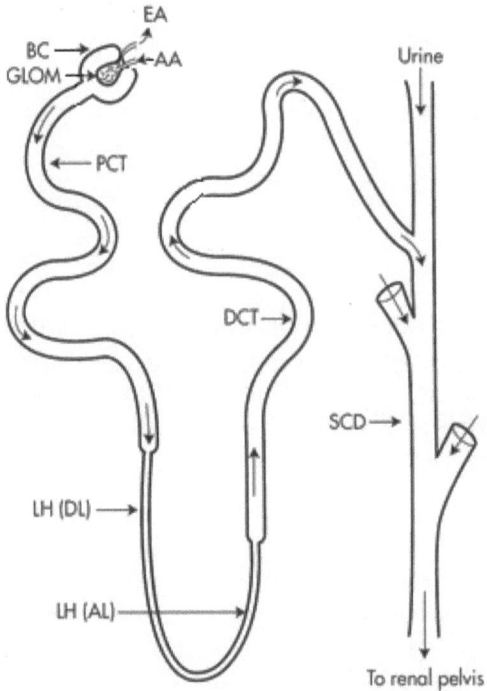

FIGURE 10.1   The renal nephron. Blood enters the glomerulus (GLOM) via the afferent arteriole (AA) and leaves via the efferent arteriole (EA). Filtrate from the blood enters the Bowman's capsule (BC) before draining into the proximal convoluted tubule (PCT). Here, substances that are required by the body are selected to return to the blood. The filtrate continues into the descending limb (DL) of the loop of Henle (LH), followed by the ascending limb (AL), before entering the distal convoluted tubule (DCT), where further products, including a lot of the water, are reabsorbed back into the blood. Finally, the filtrate, which is now urine, drains down the straight collecting duct (SCD) towards the renal pelvis (see 'Urine formation', p. 195) (Redrawn from Blows 2024).

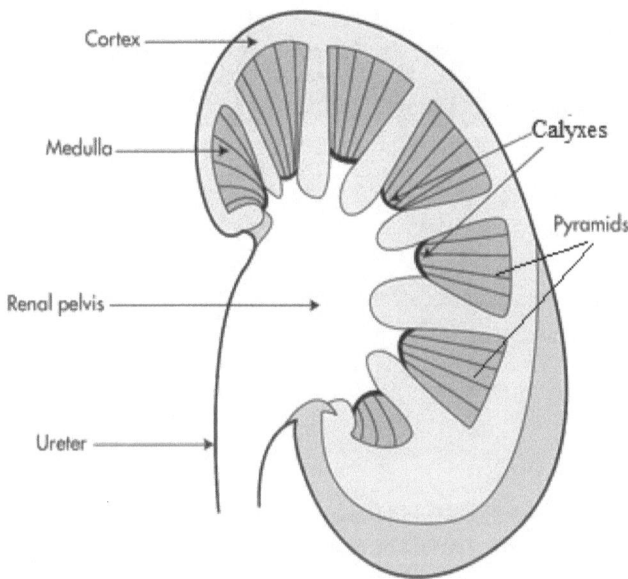

FIGURE 10.2   A section through a kidney. The medulla is made from pyramids, which are collections of straight collecting ducts converging and emptying into the calyxes. From here, urine drains into the renal pelvis and onto the ureters on the way to the bladder.

Urine formation

Urine formation occurs in three main stages:

1. **Filtration** of the blood through the glomerulus. The filtrate enters into the Bowman's capsule.
2. **Re-absorption** of many substances in the filtrate that the body requires. This occurs in the proximal and distal convoluted tubules.
3. **Tubular secretion**, that is, returning some specific substance back into the filtrate. This occurs in the straight collecting ducts.

Filtration from the glomerulus is the result of pressure from the blood in the glomerulus forcing fluid into the Bowman's capsule (Figure 10.3) (Blows 2024). The kidneys work on blood pressure. If the blood pressure falls, kidney filtration becomes less efficient, until the **systolic** blood pressure falls below 50 mmHg, at which point the kidney is likely to stop filtration completely, a condition called **renal failure** and often referred to as **renal shutdown**. The systolic blood pressure is the maximum pressure of blood at the time the heart is contracting. Blood pressure is measured in **mmHg**, that is, **millimetres of mercury**. The blood supply to each of the kidneys is via the **renal arteries** (left and right), and these are branches of the **abdominal aorta**. Anything that interferes with the renal artery supply to the kidneys, for example, tumours, may significantly disturb the kidney's ability to filter the blood and can cause renal shutdown. The blood returns from the kidneys via the **renal veins** to the **inferior vena cava**, the main vein returning blood to the heart from the lower parts of the body.

Once filtrate is produced by the glomerulus and has entered the Bowman's capsule, it flows on into the first (proximal) convoluted tubule, where essential substances, like glucose, are

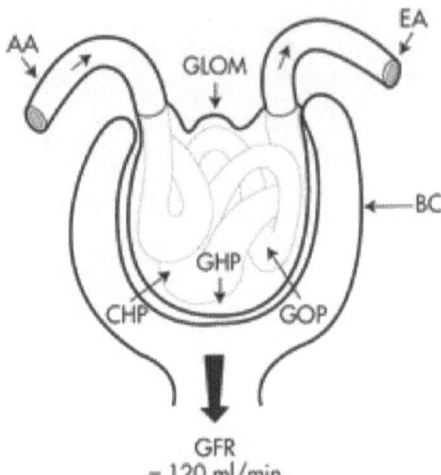

FIGURE 10.3 The glomerulus (GLOM) and Bowman's capsule (BC). Blood enters the glomerulus via the afferent arteriole (AA). The glomerular hydrostatic pressure (GHP) is created by the blood pressure and pushes the filtrate out of the blood. The blood leaves via the efferent arteriole (EA). The forces opposing GHP, that is, the capsular hydrostatic pressure (CHP) and the glomerular osmotic pressure (GOP) caused by blood proteins, return some filtrate back to the blood. The result of these forces is the glomerular filtration rate (GFR) of about 120 ml per minute.

re-absorbed back into the blood. The loop of Henle, distal convoluted tubule, and straight collecting duct all have a role to play in maintaining correct fluid and electrolyte balance. The kidneys carry out the following vital functions:

1. Water balance in the body, excreting surplus water if there is too much or conserving water if there is not enough (see 'Water balance', p. 196)
2. Electrolyte balance in the body, for example, balancing positively charged particles, such as sodium (Na^+), with negatively charged particles, such as chlorine (Cl^-)
3. pH balance, that is, the maintenance of blood pH close to 7.4 by the removal of H ions (H^+)
4. Excretion of wastes
5. The production of some hormones, notably **erythropoietin**, which stimulates erythrocyte production, and other substances, for example, modification of **vitamin D**

Water balance

The volume of water in the body must remain approximately stable. Whilst the water itself is always changing, the overall volume must remain constant. Therefore, water entering the body must be balanced by water leaving the body (Figure 10.4).

Problems start to occur if the loss exceeds the gain (Figure 10.5). The body will be getting dryer, a state called **dehydration**. The reasons for this are shown in Figure 10.5.

The opposite, that is, water retention, leading to **oedema**, is also a possible cause of problems. The causes of oedema are shown in Table 10.1. Both dehydration and oedema are possible complications of cancer.

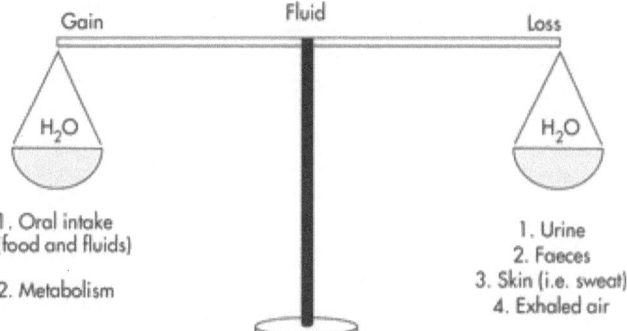

FIGURE 10.4 Normal fluid balance. Oral intake and the much smaller amount of water produced by metabolism must match the output from urine, faeces, and water lost through the skin and lungs.

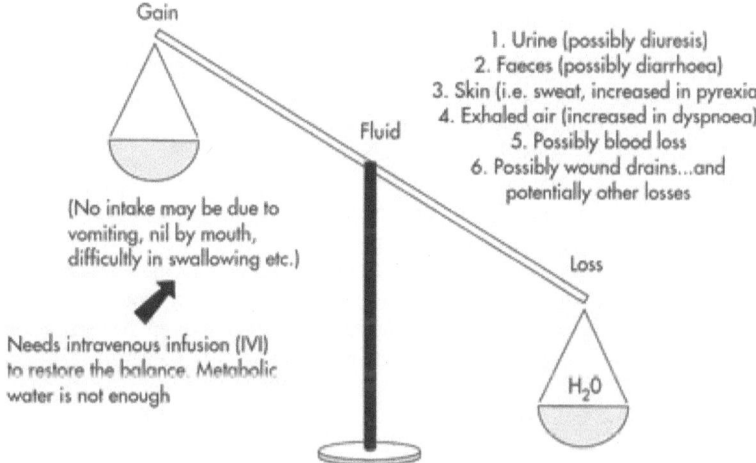

FIGURE 10.5 Abnormal fluid balance. If oral intake is no longer available and the loss of water may be increased (as shown), then a state of dehydration may soon occur. Intravenous infusion of fluids is required to correct the balance and prevent dehydration.

Water imbalance is also linked to electrolyte imbalance (see 'Electrolytes', Figure 18.1, Chapter 18, p. 324). The presence of one imbalance often results in the presence of the other imbalance. This is because electrolytes are usually dissolved in water and are excreted in a water medium. Excessive water loss often causes excessive electrolyte loss, and vice versa. Also, sodium, a major electrolyte in the body, attracts water and therefore has significant influence over water movement in and out the cells and the body (see 'Low plasma sodium level', Table 10.1).

The main electrolytes of the body are sodium (Na^+), calcium (Ca^{2+}), chloride (Cl^-), and potassium (K^+). They often form molecules, for example, NaCl and KCl, which are neutral, that is, no charge, but can disassociate again back to the original electrolytes.

TABLE 10.1 Causes of oedema

Cause of oedema	Physical mechanism	In cancer
Low plasma protein level	Plasma proteins attract water out of the tissues back into blood. Low levels will have the effect of leaving the tissue fluid to accumulate in the tissues.	This can be the result of poor diet, notably low protein, due to prolonged anorexia, weakness, or vomiting.
Low plasma sodium level	Plasma sodium similarly attracts water out of tissues back into the blood, and low levels fail to do this.	This can be the result of prolonged vomiting or diarrhoea coupled with poor dietary sodium intake.
Lymphatic obstruction	A major route for the return of tissue fluid to the blood is via the lymphatic system. Obstruction of this system allows tissue fluid accumulation (called lymphoedema).	Due to lymphatic node obstruction by the cancer cells (i.e. nodal secondaries), or caused by surgical removal of lymph nodes.
Venous blood obstruction or congestion	Tissue fluid normally returns to venous blood plasma. Venous obstruction or congestion prevents the plasma from taking further tissue fluid, and it accumulates in the tissues.	Obstruction of the veins by a tumour pressing on them from outside, or by infiltrating and blocking the veins.
Increased capillary permeability	The capillaries in the tissues are semi-permeable membranes that allow fluid through from the blood at a specific rate. Increasing that permeability causes a rise in the rate of fluid passing through the wall, and this excess fluid can accumulate in the tissues.	This occurs in inflammation and is the cause of the swelling associated with inflamed areas. Some cancers cause inflammation in the tissues surrounding them.

The bladder

Once formed, urine flows down the **ureters** into the **bladder** (Figure 10.6). The *ureter* is a smooth muscle tube connecting the kidney to the bladder below. The bladder is also made from smooth muscle lined with mucous membrane which is made from **transitional epithelium** (see 'Epithelial tissues', Chapter 1, p. 9). Three openings occur in the bladder: the two ureters, left and right, where urine enters from the kidneys, and the one **urethra**, where urine leaves. The patch of bladder floor between the three openings is the lowest part of the bladder and is called the **trigone** (Figure 10.6). There is a ring of smooth muscle, called the **internal sphincter**, which guards the bladder exit into the urethra. Outside this internal sphincter is a second ring, the **external sphincter**, made from **skeletal voluntary muscle** (see 'Muscle tissue', Chapter 1, p. 13). When urine is collecting in the bladder, the sphincter muscles contract, causing the sphincters to tighten up and close the exit. At the same time, the muscles of the bladder wall relax and stretch to allow the organ to fill with urine. At about 300 ml or so of urine, signals are sent via the nervous system to the brain, which then coordinates emptying of the bladder.

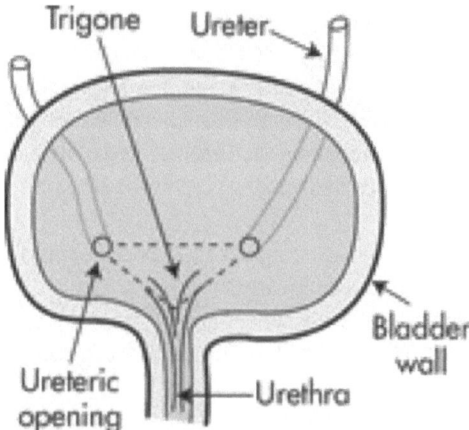

FIGURE 10.6   The urinary bladder in section. The ureters drain urine from the kidneys, and the ure-thra drains urine from the bladder to the outside world. Between the two ureteric open-ings and the urethra is the trigone, shown by a dotted triangle.

During the passage of urine (called **micturition**), both sphincter muscles relax and the sphinc-ters open; the internal sphincter opens automatically, but the external sphincter remains closed until opened voluntarily. This allows urine to pass through the urethra to the outside world. Simultaneously, the bladder wall muscles help push urine out by contracting.

Cancer of the kidney

The *malignant* tumours of the kidney

Malignant tumours of the kidney fall into three categories:

1. **Renal cell carcinoma (RCC)**, that is, those of the kidney substance seen in *adults*
2. **Urothelial carcinoma (transitional cell carcinoma)**, that is, those cells of the kidney, pel-vis, and bladder seen in *adults* (see 'Bladder cancers', this chapter)
3. **Wilms tumour, rhabdoid tumour**, and **clear cell sarcoma**, that is, those of the kidney sub-stance seen in *children*

Renal cell carcinoma (RCC)

Renal cell carcinoma (RCC) (or renal adenocarcinoma) starts in the epithelial cells of the renal tubule. It is the cause of 85–90% of all adult kidney malignancies. The age of onset is usually middle to later life, rising to a peak incidence in the seventh and eighth decades of life. Men over the age of 60 account for twice as many cases as women, and smoking doubles the risk for this disease. Other risk factors include obesity, hypertension, diabetes, and the chronic use of analgesia.

Renal cell carcinoma causes pain and a mass (or lump) in the loin, with haematuria (blood in the urine) as an important sign, seen in 60% of cases. Haematuria will require detection by testing the urine during the early stages of the disease, and if this is not done routinely, the disease could be missed in its early stages. RCC may also cause loss of appetite, weight loss, and tiredness. Invasion of the tumour at a later stage involves spread from the cortex into the medulla, extending into the renal pelvis. There can be spread along the **renal vein**, the vessel that drains blood from the kidney, and along the **inferior vena cava.**

Variations of the tumour cell types include:

- **Clear-cell RCC (ccRCC)** (75%) is an aggressive cancer arising from the epithelium of the proximal convoluted tubule. It is seen mostly in the over 50s.
- **Papillary RCC** (10%) is an aggressive cancer arising from the epithelium of the distal convoluted tubule in the over 50s. It is papillary in nature (see 'Polyps', 'Hyperplastic polyps', Chapter 8, p. 164).
- **Cystic-solid RCC** (1–4%) is similar to clear-cell RCC, but without nodules. It occurs in the 40s–50s and is slow-growing with no metastases, that is, it is indolent.
- **Chromophobe RCC** (5%) is a tumour arising from the distal tubule in the over 50s and having a low mortality rate.

Other variants of RCC, which are very rare, include collecting duct and medullary tumours. **Sarcomatoid renal cell carcinoma** is no longer a separate category since sarcomatoid features can occur in all the RCC subtypes. Sarcomatoid changes display elongated, spindle-shaped cells with excessive numbers of cells (high cellularity) which appear atypical.

The genes involved in ccRCC are:

- *Von Hippel–Lindau* (**VHL**) (see 'Chromosome 3', Addendum, p. 345)
- *PBRM-1* (see 'Chromosome 3', Addendum, p. 345)
- *SETD2* (see 'Chromosome 3', Addendum, p. 345)
- *BAP-1* (see 'Chromosome 3', Addendum, p. 345)
- *KDM5C* (see 'Chromosome X', Addendum, p. 361)
- *MTOR* (see 'Chromosome 1', Addendum, p. 343)

In addition, the loss of the short arm ('p' arm) of chromosome 3, that is, 3p, is found in about 95% of patients with ccRCC. Other chromosomal errors are a gain of additional 5q in 69% of patients, part loss of 14q in 42%, gain of 7q in 20%, 8p deletion in 32%, and loss of 9p in 29%. Rarely, mutations of the *VHL* gene can be passed on to future generations in an *autosomal dominant* manner (von Hippel–Lindau disease) (see 'Gene inheritance', Chapter 2, p. 30), as well as occurring in sporadic cases. The gene encodes for a protein (pVHL) which is a tumour suppressor. It forms a complex with other proteins, notably **elongin B** and **elongin C**, and **cellulin 2** (the VBC complex), and this complex regulates the degradation of other proteins in the cell. pVHL also regulates the level of the proteins HIF1A and HIF2A (hypoxia-inducible factor 1 alpha and 2 alpha), which, in combination, act as transcription factors causing an increase in the production of the growth factors **vascular endothelial growth factor (VEGF)**, **platelet-derived growth factor beta (PDGFB)**, and **transforming growth factors alpha (TGFA)**. These growth factors are key to the growth of a tumour and its blood supply (VEGF). Therefore, mutations of the *VHL* gene result in a loss of control over the HIF1A-2A complex, which then goes on to promote these growth factors and tumour formation (Figure 10.7).

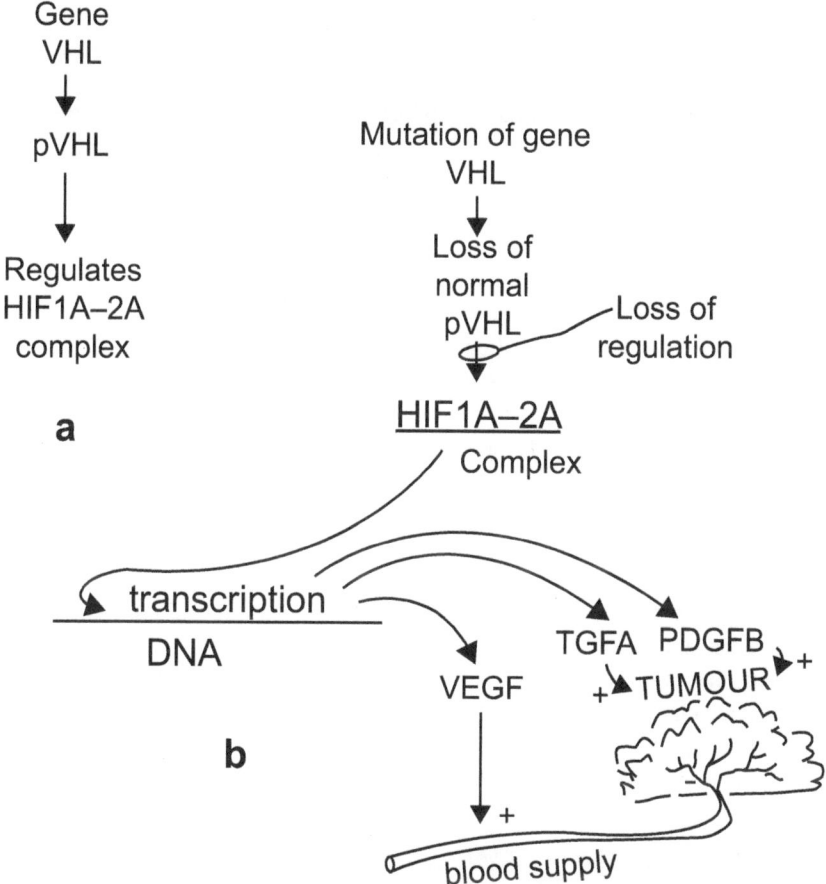

FIGURE 10.7 The *VHL* gene: (a) The normal *VHL* gene product, protein VHL (pVHL), regulates the proteins HIF1A and HIF2A. (b) Mutations of *VHL* gene result in a loss of that regulation, and the increase of the HIF1A–2A complex promotes the genetic transcription of growth factors VEGF, PDGFB, and TGFA. These then promote tumour formation and its blood supply (VEGF).

The staging of RCC is complex (American Cancer Society 2023; Cancer Research UK 2020).

Survival averages out at about 45% for RCC, with poor prognosis (10–15%) for those with metastases, but good prognosis (70%) for those without metastases.

Wilms tumour (nephroblastoma)

Child kidney tumours are rare, but Wilms tumour, also called **nephroblastoma**, is the commonest of these tumours, occurring mostly between the ages of 1 and 4 years of age. It arises from excessive growth of **nephroblasts**, which are immature kidney cells. It may be associated with other medical conditions or appear alone.

Several genes are known to be mutated in many cases of this disease. One of these genes is *WT1* at 11p13 (see 'Chromosome 11', Addendum, p. 352), which appears to result in the loss of this **tumour suppressor gene** (see 'Tumour suppressor genes', Chapter 2, p. 25). Other genes include *AMER1* (*WTX*) (see 'Chromosome X', Addendum, p. 361) and *REST* (see 'Chromosome 4', Addendum, p. 346).

Wilms tumour causes abdominal pain, a palpable abdominal mass and distension, blood in the urine, nausea, vomiting, loss of appetite, dyspnoea, hypertension, and fever.

The staging of Wilms tumour identifies five points:

I   Tumour is confined to the kidney.
II Tumour extends beyond the kidney into local tissues.
III Some tumour remains after surgical removal, lymph node involvement.
IV Distant blood-borne metastases, often spread to the lungs.
V   The tumour is bilateral, that is, present in both kidneys.

Prognosis has much improved with the introduction of surgery in combination with chemotherapy and radiotherapy.

Rhabdoid tumour of the kidney (RTK)

This is a rare, aggressive cancer of early-age onset, usually within the first year of life. It occurs in boys more often than girls. It is highly malignant, and therefore difficult to treat, and has a poor prognosis, that is, only about 25% survival after two years. The abnormal cells resemble immature muscle cells, called rhabdomyoblasts. They are large cells with excessive cytoplasm and eccentric nucleus, that is, positioned up against the inside of the cell membrane. Some genes are involved, the main one being *SMARCB1* (see 'Chromosome 22', Addendum, p. 360).

Clear-cell sarcoma of the kidney (CCSK)

This is a rare but highly malignant renal tumour occurring in children mostly under 3 years of age. It consists of small round cells with clear cytoplasm. A mass forms inside the kidney and soon dominates part or all of the kidney. The tumour spreads via the lymph and blood to many parts of the body, including bone metastases. An important gene mutation involved with this tumour is *BCOR* (see 'Chromosome X', Addendum, p. 360).

The *benign* tumours of the kidney

Oncocytoma is a common benign tumour of the elderly. They have a particular cell type, called an **oncocyte**. These are epithelial cells with abundant fine granular cytoplasm, the granules consisting of numerous abnormally large **mitochondria** (see 'The cell', Chapter 1, p. 1). The nucleus is small and round, with a prominent **nucleolus** (see 'The cell', Chapter 1, p. 1). This tumour is three times more common in men than in women, and it has a benign growth pattern with a good prognosis.

Bladder cancers

Urothelial carcinoma (**transitional cell carcinoma, TCC**) starts in the transitional cells of the bladder or renal pelvis. These cells can stretch to accommodate urine, and they are also found in the tubes (ureters and urethra) and in the bladder, where this cancer is the most common (90%). Of the remaining 10% of bladder cancers, 5% are **squamous carcinomas**, and 5% are a mixture of the two. Bladder cancer affects men three times more than women, usually in middle to late age. The risk factors include smoking; industrial carcinogens, especially those found in the cloth dyeing or rubber industries; drug abuse, especially analgesic drugs; and as a side effect of treatment with the drug **cyclophosphamide**. The mechanism of carcinogenesis is likely to involve the excretion in the urine of toxic carcinogens from smoking, industry, and drugs that are held in the bladder for some hours before voiding.

There are four morphological (= shape) types of transitional cell carcinoma of the bladder (Figure 10.8), where the invasive types are more advanced:

1. **Papillary carcinoma** (Figure 10.8a)
2. **Invasive papillary carcinoma** (Figure 10.8b)
3. **Flat, non-invasive carcinoma** (Figure 10.8c)
4. **Flat, invasive carcinoma** (Figure 10.8d)

(Kumar et al. 2022)

Grading of the tumours is important because, like in other tumours, early staging is conducive to better survival rates at 95% survival, rather than late staging at only 36% survival. Several staging systems are in practice, and the following is a basic I, II, III staging system which can be applied to most TCCs:

I Papillary tumours, non-invasive; tissue remains clearly transitional epithelium with some loss of orientation, and little mitosis is evident.
II Tumours made from tissue that remains clearly transitional epithelium; greater degree of cell mitosis and growth than in grade I, with more variation in the nucleus and greater disorientation of the tissue.
III A carcinoma, with loss of identity as transitional epithelium; loose cells washed off into the urine (**exfoliation**); later invasion of the bladder wall and metastases.

Other grading/staging systems are available (ASCO 2023).

The benign papillomas, which are small nipple-like growths on the inner surface of the bladder wall, may be the original source of any malignancy, so they should be removed when found. They can reoccur after removal, so regular, often annual, checks would be advisable. Checking consists of a **cystoscopy**, where the inner bladder wall is viewed using a **cystoscope** passed up

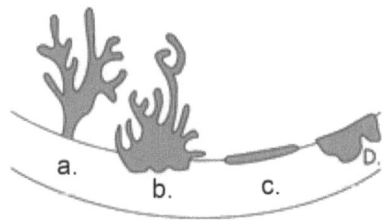

FIGURE 10.8   Bladder cancers: (a) papillary carcinoma, (b) invasive papillary carcinoma, (c) flat non-invasive carcinoma, (d) flat invasive carcinoma.

the urethra under anaesthetic. Cystoscopy is often accompanied by **biopsy** of any lesion found for **histological** examination.

The malignant transitional cell carcinomas may be linked to mutations of the *Tp53* gene (see 'Chromosome 17', Addendum, p. 356). There is a well-established association between the presence of extra chromosomal material, which includes extra DNA, called **aneuploidy** (see 'Chromosomal abnormalities', Chapter 2, p. 32); the depth of the tumour invasion; and the patient's response to various treatments. Also, expression of any mutation of the *RAS* genes (see 'Chromosome 1', 'Chromosome 11', and 'Chromosome 12', Addendum, p. 342, 352, and 353) is often associated with the higher-graded tumours, and therefore a worse prognosis. There are other genetic mutations found in bladder cancers (Table 10.2).

Carcinoma *in situ* (CIS) (see 'The malignant cell', Chapter 1, p. 15) may occur adjacent to papillary lesions in the bladder wall, and 50% of CIS will become invasive carcinomas. These tumours, at first, cause a painless **haematuria** (blood in the urine), frequency and urgency of micturition, or some obstruction to the flow of urine, with or without **dysuria**, that is, difficulty or pain on passing urine.

Urine as a liquid biopsy

Liquid biopsy is the term used when testing body fluids, for example, blood, cerebrospinal fluid (CSF), and urine, to acquire information about a disease for diagnostic purposes or to monitor disease progression. Liquid biopsies can often now replace solid tissue biopsies, which require surgery to obtain. Urine liquid biopsies:

- Are non-invasive, unless a catheter is required
- Are easily repeated at any time required
- Are able to detect disease cells, DNA, and biomarker molecules (see 'Immunotherapy', Table 5.4, Chapter 5, p. 97), especially from cancers of the urinary system, notably the bladder
- Allow for regular monitoring of the disease progression or the results of therapy
- Are able to provide results quickly

TABLE 10.2 The genetic mutations found in bladder cancers

Chromosome	Mutation
2	*MSH2* and *ERCC3* mutations
5	5p (short arm) changes found in 40% of cases
7	Trisomy 7 in some cases
9	Monosomy 9 seen in 50% of cases; 9q (long arm) deletions seen in 67% of advanced bladder cases
11	11p deletions seen in 40% of cases
13	*BRCA2* mutations
17	*TP53* gene mutations found in 63% of cases, or loss of the gene, and even loss of the p arm, found in many invasive bladder cancers; over-expression of this gene associated with poor prognosis
22	*BRCA1* mutations; *CHEK2* mutations

Note: See corresponding genes in Addendum.

For these reasons, urine is sometimes called 'liquid gold' because it becomes a rich source of material derived from the tumour.

Biopsies, either solid or liquid, are generally the future of prescribing cancer treatment. Mini-tumours, grown in the laboratory from cancer cells obtained from biopsies, can be tested to find the best treatment for each cancer before being given to the patient. This targeted approach is much better than traditional medication, which is based on the type of tumour presented. The success rate of targeting treatment in this way is greater, with fewer side effects (Wilson 2024).

Key points

Renal system

- The kidneys provide water balance, electrolyte balance, pH balance, excretion of wastes, and the production of some hormones.
- Blood pressure is the driving force for renal filtration.
- Urine formation occurs in three main stages: filtration, reabsorption, and tubular secretion.

Kidney cancers

- The malignant tumours of the kidney are renal cell carcinoma and transitional cell carcinoma, both seen in *adults*, and Wilms' tumour, rhabdoid tumour, and clear-cell sarcoma, all seen in *children*.
- Renal cell carcinoma, the commonest form of kidney tumour, causes pain and a mass in the loin, with haematuria as an important sign.

Bladder cancers

- The benign papillomas of the bladder may be the source of malignancy, so they should be removed when found.
- The malignant bladder cancers are 90% transitional cell carcinomas, 5% squamous carcinomas, and 5% a mixture of the two.
- Initially, these tumours cause a painless haematuria, frequency, and urgency of micturition, with or without dysuria.

Liquid biopsies

- Urine liquid biopsies allow for quick and easy access to cancer biomarkers for the purpose of diagnostics and monitoring disease or treatment progress.
- Mini-tumours grown from cancer cells obtained from biopsies can be used to test various treatments before prescribing.

11

CANCERS OF THE FEMALE REPRODUCTIVE SYSTEM

- **Introduction: the oestrogens**
- **The breasts**
- **Breast cancer**
- **The ovaries and ovarian cancer**
- **The female reproductive tract**
- **Uterine and cervical cancer**
- **Vaginal and vulval cancer**
- **Key points**

Introduction: the oestrogens

Cancers found specifically in women are often linked by one factor, a hormone group called the **oestrogens**. There are three different oestrogens that are active at various stages of life: **oestrone (E1)**, **oestradiol (E2)**, and **oestriol (E3)**. They are produced originally from **cholesterol** (see Figure 4.8, Chapter 4, p. 68) and are, therefore, fat-based (or lipid-based) hormones known as **steroids**.[1] Another female hormone, called **progesterone**, is also produced in the same sequence from cholesterol. In women, the oestrogens are produced mostly in the **ovaries**, with smaller quantities being produced by the **adrenal cortex**. Oestradiol (E2) is the most potent of the oestrogens, and the one that has the greatest physiological effects, especially during the reproductive years. The potency of E2 is 12 times that of oestrone and 80 times that of oestriol. This hormone promotes the development of the female reproductive tract during the embryonic stages, and breast development during puberty. It continues to have an important influence throughout life, promoting cell division and growth and maintaining health of the reproductive tissues. Oestrogen binds to **oestrogen receptors (ER)** within the cell (see footnote 1). Cells that have oestrogen receptors are said to be **ER-positive (ER+)**. On binding to the receptor, E2 forms a complex with the receptor, and this complex then binds to a **gene promoter** region on the DNA (see Figure 4.10, Chapter 4, p. 69). The binding of a second oestradiol–receptor complex to the same promoter site, that is, two E2 + ER complexes together, is called a **dimer**. This initiates

DOI: 10.4324/9781003389125-11

gene promotion, that is, it sets into motion the activation of the gene so that protein synthesis will commence (also known as **gene expression**). The genes that are switched on in this way are, first, the genes that replace the original ER; otherwise, the cell would use up all the ERs and become ER-negative (ER−), that is, no longer able to respond to E2. Other genes are also activated, including those that code for **PgR** (the **progesterone receptor**) and various growth hormones.

E1 (oestrone) is held in the body mostly in an inactive form, bound to the protein **albumin** in the blood. It also stimulates breast cell growth, but to a lesser extent than E2. It becomes a more important oestrogen in women after the menopause, when levels of E2 drop.

E3 (oestriol) is the weakest[2] of the oestrogens. E3 may have a beneficial effect on the prevention of breast cancer by occupying ER instead of E2. E3 is the form in which much of the oestrogen is excreted from the body.

The breasts

The breasts (Figure 11.1) are modified sweat glands.[3] They are constructed in the form of **lobes**. There are between 15 and 20 lobes set in a circular fashion, like spokes of a wheel, around a central point, the **nipple** (also called the **mammary papilla**). Each lobe is sectioned off from the neighbouring lobes by a wall of connective tissue. Lobes contain a root-like system of ducts called a **lobule**, that is, the milk-producing, or secretary, portion of the breasts (Marieb and Hoehn 2022). A *lobule* consists of one central duct with multiple branching ducts, each ending

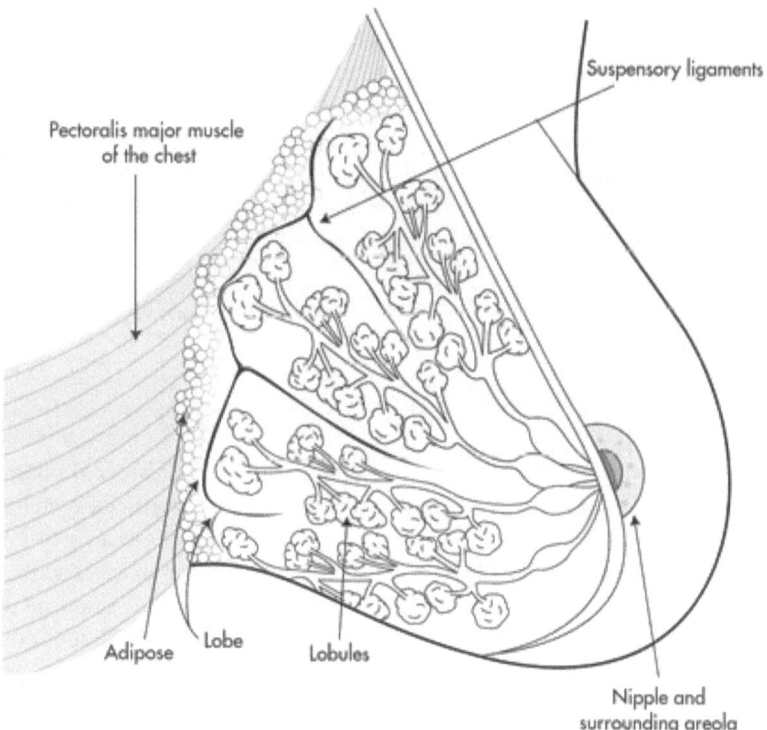

FIGURE 11.1   Internal structure of the breast.

Source: Redrawn from Martini et al. (2023).

in a dilated segment (called **acini**). The walls of the acini form terminal sac-like structures called **alveoli**, that is, the same name as the sac-like structures of the lungs. The cells of the alveoli walls produce breast milk, when required, under hormonal control (called **lactation**). Outside the alveoli, **myoepithelial cells** have long thin extensions forming a network around the alveoli. Under hormonal control, these cell extensions contract, similar to miniature muscles, and squeeze milk from the alveoli into the central duct. The central duct of the lobule drains the milk towards the nipple (Figure 11.1).

The nipple has a covering of pigmented and folded **epidermis** which is rich in **sebaceous glands** producing **sebum**, an oily fluid that protects the skin surface during breastfeeding. Inside the nipple is **dense collagen** connective tissue with many elastic fibres. These fibres continue beneath the **areola**, a pigmented area of epidermis around the nipple, which is also rich in sebaceous glands.

The breast is packed with a fibrous connective tissue called **stroma**, and this includes a number of supportive structures. The **adipose** tissue, that is, fat, is present in variable amounts, and the volume of fat present determines the size of the breasts. Fat has nothing to do with milk production. There are loose connections between the breasts and the **deep pectoral fascia**, a connective tissue layer covering two main chest muscles, the **pectoralis major** and the **serratus anterior**. These muscles are sometime involved in advanced breast cancer.

Blood supply to the breast comes from branches of the **axillary artery** and the **internal thoracic artery**, plus some **intercostal arteries**. Venous drainage is via a **venous plexus** beneath the areola, then the **internal thoracic** and **intercostal veins**. The **lymphatic** drainage is important for the understanding of how breast cancers spread. Over 85% of lymph drains from the breast into the **axillary lymph nodes**, that is, those of the armpit. There are 20 to 30 large lymph nodes, plus a number of smaller ones, clustered in the axilla, and these are grouped into five sets, the **anterior**, **posterior**, **lateral**, **central**, and **apical** (or **infraclavicular**) sets. The anterior sets are several large nodes with contacts within the tail of the breast that extend beneath the axilla (called the **tail of Spence**).

Two sets of lymphatic vessels drain the breast of lymph:

1. The **cutaneous lymphatic** plexus, which is within the skin, except the nipple and areola, and drains the skin surface
2. The **subareola plexus** (or **plexus of Sappey**), which drains lymph from the secretory tissues, that is, the ductal system of the lobules, and the areola

The remaining 15% of the lymph drainage passes either into the **parasternal nodes** along the edge of the **sternum** (the breastbone) or crosses the midline via superficial lymphatic vessels from one breast to the other. Crossing between the breasts allows the cancer to involve both breasts by this means. There are lymphatic connections between the breasts and the pectoralis major muscle, allowing for spread to the chest wall and some lymphatic drainage through the diaphragm, giving the potential for spread to the abdomen. The cells and tissues present in the breasts are listed in Table 11.1.

Breast cancer

Breast cancer is a very important subject for two reasons: (1) it is still the cause of many needless deaths in women, and (2) because of the uncertainty surrounding the role of hormones, that is, the contraceptive pill and hormone replacement therapy, in the course of this disease.

TABLE 11.1 The cells and tissues of the breast

Tissue type	Examples in the breast	Notes
Epithelial	Alveolar	Milk-producing cells; cuboidal in non-lactating phase, becoming columnar when lactating; ER+
Epithelial	Duct lining	Cuboid or columnar; ER+
Epithelial	Myoepithelial	Long branching processes containing two contractile proteins, actin and myosin; responds to the hormone oxytocin by contracting and squeezing the alveoli, pushing milk towards the nipple; ER+
Connective	Stroma	Connective tissue fibres containing fibroblasts, adipocytes, neutrophils, macrophages, lymphocytes

TABLE 11.2 Abbreviations and terms used in breast cancer classification

Abbreviation	Full name	Explanation
ER	Oestrogen receptor	Binds the hormone oestrogen. May be present (positive) or absent (negative).
PR	Progesterone receptor	Binds the hormone progesterone. May be present (positive) or absent (negative).
HER2	Human epidermal growth factor receptor 2 (see 'MABs known as ADCs', Chapter 5, p. 105)	One of a group of epidermal growth factor receptors that are essential for cell proliferation and differentiation.
Ki-67	Antigen Kiel 67	A nuclear protein involved in cell proliferation and acts as a proliferation marker in cancers.
CK	Cytokeratins	Keratin proteins found in the cellular framework (cytoskeleton) of epithelial cells.
BRCA1	Breast (BR) cancer (CA) gene 1	Gene linked to breast cancer at 17q21.31 (see 'Chromosome 17', Addendum, p. 356).
BRCA2	Breast (BR) cancer (CA) gene 2	Gene linked to breast cancer at 13q13.1 (see 'Chromosome 13', Addendum, p. 354).

The pathological types of breast cancer

The types of breast cancer can be classified into two groups, **non-invasive** and **invasive**, and are located as either **ductal**, that is, arising from, or located within, the ducts, or **lobular**, arising from the lobes (Table 11.2) (Kumar et al. 2022).

Luminal A carcinoma

These are slow-growing, low-grade tumours that are ER-positive and/or PR-positive, but they lack the HER2 growth factor. They also have less than 20% of Ki-67 (Table 11.2). Prognosis is good, with low frequency of relapse and longer life expectancy.

Luminal B carcinoma

These are faster-growing and higher-grade than luminal A tumours. They have a lower expression of ER-positive and may be PR-negative, but most have the HER2 growth factor. They have greater than 20% of Ki-67 and raised levels of cell cycle genes. They have a high rate of visceral and bone metastases, with a prognosis worse than luminal A.

HER2-positive

The HER2 status of breast cancer tissue cells falls into several main groups (Table 11.2):

- HER2 1+ is negative.
- HER2 2+ is negative.
- HER2 1+ and 2+ mix of cells is called 'low'.
- HER2 3+ is positive.

HER2 3+ positive cancer cells are classified as having high levels of HERS, that is, *HERS* gene is over-expressed, with both ER and PR negative. Growth is faster and more aggressive than in luminal group cancers, and it carries a worse prognosis. Metastases, especially in the brain and bones, occur frequently, but the tumour responds well when treated early with chemotherapy combined with targeted therapy (see 'Monoclonal antibodies (MABs) known as antibody–drug conjugates (ADCs)' Chapter 5, p. 105).

Triple-negative breast cancer (TNBC)

These tumours are negative for ER, PR, and HER2. There are a number of subtypes, each with their own genetic variability and clinical outcomes. Two of these subtypes are basal and non-basal TNBC. Basal TNBC expresses the cytokeratins 5/6 (Table 11.2), but non-basal TNBCs do not express cytokeratins. Overall, they are aggressive; consist of high-grade, highly proliferative cells; and often first present at an advanced stage. They also relapse early in the course of the disease. Included in this group are most (80%) of the breast cancers linked to *BRCA1* and *BRCA2* gene mutations. Other mutations in DNA repair genes are also common in this type of tumour. **Adenoid cystic carcinoma (ACC)** is a subtype of TNBC. It is an important cause of salivary gland cancers, but it also accounts for about 0.1–0.2% of breast carcinomas. While ACCs of the breast have a triple-negative ER, PR, and HER2 profile, they are usually low-grade with indolent behaviour. The tumour is a mix of two cells, luminal and basaloid cells. It presents as a painful lump, about 1 to 5 cm in size, close to the areola, usually in older women. It has few metastases, and there is a good prognosis following treatment (see 'Salivary gland cancer', Chapter 8, p. 155).

Clinical types of breast cancer

The most common clinical types of breast cancer, based on location and spread, are:

- Ductal carcinoma in situ (DCIS)
- Invasive ductal carcinoma (IDC)
- Lobular carcinoma in situ (LCIS)
- Invasive lobular carcinoma (ILC)

Ductal carcinoma in situ (DCIS)

DCIS causes 20% of all breast carcinomas, with malignant cells occupying the ducts but remaining within the basement membrane. It is regarded as early, or pre-invasive, cancer, and the

TABLE 11.3 Nipple disorders in breast cancer

Nipple disease	Description
Paget's disease	Paget cells are large with abundant pale cytoplasm and large nuclei with a prominent nucleolus. They occur in the surface epithelium of the nipple (i.e. epidermis) and are probably derived from glandular cells, that is, ductal cells; therefore, they are a type of adenocarcinoma. They originally cause simple reddening of the nipple and areola with pruritis. This leads on to scaling, that is, eczema-like changes, and eventually to erosion of the skin (ulceration). Often, there is a painless palpable mass in the underlying breast tissue in about 50% of cases. Up to 95% of patients have underlying carcinoma, frequently intraductal carcinoma, although it is not always palpable. Paget's disease of the nipple is generally unilateral but can be bilateral.
Nipple duct carcinoma (NDC)	This can be mistaken for Paget's disease. It is usually unilateral. Nipple discharge is commonly reported in about 60–70% of cases. Then enlargement follows, and induration of the nipple with ulceration. There is also pain, itching, or burning. The margins of the lesion are well-delineated. Cystic dilation can occur in the underlying ducts. The pathology begins with a small number of ductules clustered around a major duct. The advanced lesion replaces part or all of the nipple stroma, causing enlargement and expansion of the nipple and erosion of the surface epithelium (ulceration).

prognosis is excellent. DCIS may be **comedo**, that is, poorly differentiated with central necrosis (dead cancer cells), or **non-comedo**, that is, differentiated with no central necrosis. Comedo can reach a large size; 50% are over 2 cm across. DCIS with **Paget's disease** is seen mostly in older women (Table 11.3). If the nipple is affected, the symptoms are similar to eczema, that is, ulcerated, fissured, and oozing fluid.

Invasive ductal carcinoma (IDC)

This is the most common form of breast cancer (70–85% of patients). It usually appears as a very hard nodule, making it easily detected by palpation. It is composed of dense fibrous stromal cells mixed with tumour cells, where the surface of the tumour often infiltrates the surrounding tissues, including blood vessels. Variations of this type are seen, with different tumour cell types and abnormal tissue structures. Generally, hard tumours cause inflammation at the interface between the tumour and surrounding tissues, and this results in **fibrosis**, involving cells called **fibrocytes**. This is not the case with soft tumours. **Apocrine carcinoma** is a type of IDC forming a solid mass, about 2 cm in diameter. Apocrine cells are normal milk-producing exocrine glandular cells that release their product into the ductal system. **Apocrine metaplasia** is a pre-malignant change in these cells sometimes seen in otherwise-normal breasts in women over 20 years of age. It consists of pink cells present during fibrocystic changes, increasing the risk of malignancy.

Lobular carcinoma in situ (LCIS)

This is a distinct form of the disease that is found by tissue biopsy and examination. It can be multifocal (many sites within the breast, accounting for 70% of patients) or bilateral (involving both breasts, about 30–40% of patients). Small uniform cells occur within the smaller ducts or acini, and these become distended with central necrosis. Later invasion of surrounding tissues can occur in about 30% of patients.

Invasive lobular carcinoma (ILC)

This accounts for about 5–10% of all invasive breast tumours. One-fifth of these are bilateral (in both breasts), and they tend to become multifocal. The cells are smaller and more uniform than in ductal carcinoma, causing a poorly circumscribed mass, that is, the edges are not easily defined.

Rare types of breast cancer

Medullary carcinoma is rare and accounts for about 3% of all breast cancers. It forms a mass, from 2 cm up to 10 cm in diameter, which is soft in nature, with a well-defined edge. Growth causes the tumour to 'push' into the surrounding tissues rather than infiltrate. The large cells of the tumour grow in sheets with no stroma between them.

Colloid (mucinous) carcinoma accounts for about 1–2% of breast cancers. Most are seen in women after menopause, and they have a good prognosis, owing to very few nodal metastases. The tumour is a jelly-like bulky mass with a well-defined edge. It is largely **mucin** produced by the islands of tumour cells scattered throughout.

Tubular carcinoma accounts for about 2% of invasive carcinomas. It is slow-growing and has a good prognosis. It consists of a small tumour, about 1 cm in diameter, with a poorly defined edge. The cells have a tubular shape, which can be oval or elongated and arranged randomly. It may develop from DICS (see 'Ductal carcinoma in situ (DCIS)', p. 210). It is usually seen in women above 50 years of age, and there is a family history of the disease in about 40% of patients.

Invasive papillary carcinoma accounts for only about 1.5–2.5% of breast cancers. The highest incidence of this disease occurs in post-menopausal and non-Caucasian women. It is an intraductal palpable tumour with finger-like projections known as papules. The invasive form grows inside the ducts before infiltrating local breast tissues and lymph nodes. It should not get confused with **intraductal papilloma**, which is a benign (non-malignant) growth of the milk duct cells.

The risk factors linked to breast cancer

The disease increases with **age**, doubling the risk every ten years until menopause, then the risk increase slows down. Also, **menarche**, the age at first period, before 11 years, and late **menopause**, that is, after 54 years, have higher risk, twice the risk of those women with later menarche and menopause at about 45 years. The reasons are not clear but perhaps could be to do with the length of time the breasts are exposed to the oestrogens. Oestrogens are highest between menarche and menopause, and the more years this involves, the greater the risk. Oestrogen causes chromosomes to fuse, break, and make additional copies of cancer-causing DNA. This disruption to DNA is called **translocation-bridge amplification** and probably triggers and supports cancer development.

First pregnancy after the age of 30 years doubles the risk compared with those whose first pregnancy is before 20 years. **Breastfeeding** for a long term is protective against the disease. **The contraceptive pill** and **hormone replacement therapy (HRT)** as risk factors are inconclusive.

Family history of the disease increases the risk by three or more times that of the general population in all the female members of that family. Increased risk is seen in women who have a **first-degree relative**, that is, mother, sister, or daughter, with bilateral breast cancer or unilateral breast cancer under 40 years of age or have combined breast and ovary cancer. Also at higher risk are women who have two **first-** or **second-degree relatives**, that is, granddaughter, grand-mother, aunt, or niece, with breast cancer diagnosed between 40 and 60 years of age, or three first- or second-degree relatives with breast and ovarian cancer on the same side of the family. Four or more family members with breast cancer, with or without ovarian cancer, within three generations put the other women in that family at a very high risk. Identifying who is at risk is important because these high-risk women should then be screened at very regular intervals, as well as performing self-checks at home (Figures 11.2 and 11.3), and they may be tested for the presence of specific genes.

Previous history of benign breast disease is important. Women with severe atypical epithe-lial hyperplasia have four to five times greater risk of breast cancer. Women with benign breast changes like this and with a family history of breast cancer carry nine times higher risk.

Lifestyle factors, such as **diet, alcohol, smoking**, and **night work** affect the risk. Smoking and alcohol are risk factors women have control over, and they can choose not to take that risk. Smoking particularly involves the inhalation of many cancer-causing chemicals (see Table 3.1, Chapter 3, p. 44). Smoking 20 cigarettes per day increases the risk by four times.

The risk is doubled with post-menopausal **obesity**, and eating high levels of meat and dairy products increases the risk. This is thought to be due to the consumption of higher levels of **IGF-1 (insulin-like growth factor-1**; see Table 4.1, Chapter 4, p. 66) associated with these foods. Post-menopausal women with higher-than-normal IGF-1 intake have three times the av-erage risk of breast cancer. In women below the age of 50 years, the risk is higher, that is, up to seven times the average.

Women who work **night shifts** have been shown to increase their risk by 1.5 times. The reason is not clear but may be due to working in artificial light conditions and with **melatonin** production. *Melatonin* is a hormone produced by the **pineal gland** in the brain, and whilst its

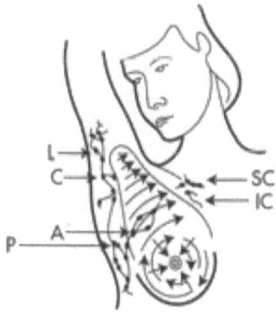

FIGURE 11.2   Self breast examination. The breast is examined by palpation with the three middle fingers. It can be examined in different directions, either circular, or from the outside towards the nipple, as shown by the arrows. It is important to feel the entire surface and to examine the tail of Spence under the arm. Also check visually in a mirror, comparing right and left breasts, looking for any symptoms mentioned in *the symptoms of breast cancer* (p. 214). The lymph nodes are also shown. *A* = anterior; *C* = central; *L* = lateral; *P* = posterior; *IC* = inferior clavicular; *SC* = superior clavicular.

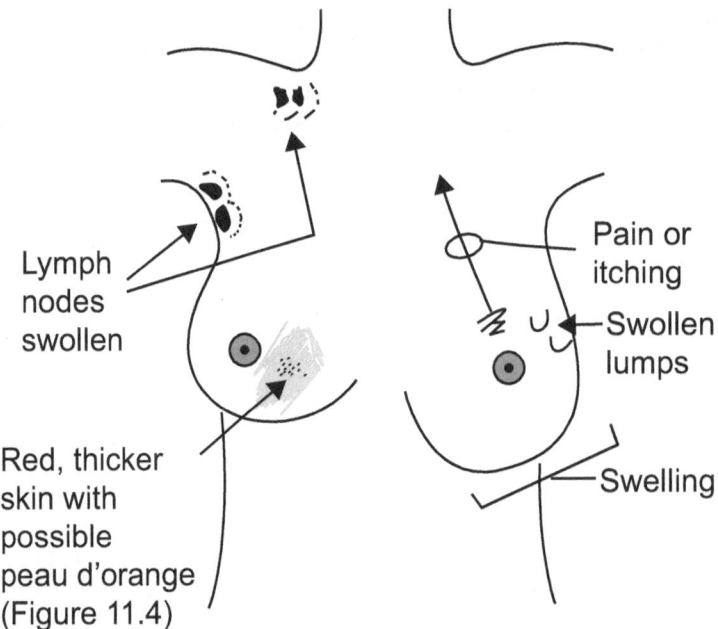

Lymph nodes swollen

Pain or itching

Swollen lumps

Red, thicker skin with possible peau d'orange (Figure 11.4)

Swelling

FIGURE 11.3 Signs of breast cancer. When viewed in a mirror, the breasts may appear asymmetrical, with one breast swollen. There may be palpable lumps, redness, and thicker skin, with possible peau d'orange (Figure 11.4), pain or itching of the breast or nipple, and possible lymph node involvement.

functions are not fully understood, it is thought that this hormone has some influence over the sleep–wake cycle. The link between night duty and breast cancer is best explained by the following theory. Melatonin is produced mainly at night in dark conditions, but artificial light on night duty would suppress this natural cycle. Melatonin is also thought to suppress oestrogen levels, so oestrogen would be naturally lower at night. It is possible that women on regular night work have constantly low melatonin levels, which results in maintaining a high oestrogen level day and night. A persistently high level of oestrogen would promote breast cell replication and may therefore contribute towards breast cancer. Taking this theory further, blind women, because they never see any light and therefore are likely to have raised melatonin levels and correspondingly lower oestrogen, have been shown to have 50% *less* risk of breast cancers.

Radiation increases the risk of breast cancer. The greatest risk is exposure to radiation at an early age, particularly between 10 and 14 years of age, when breast tissue is undergoing rapid development. Radiation-induced breast cancer comes on later in life, with a gap of at least 10 to 15 years after the exposure before symptoms arise. The effects of the radiation have been shown to last for 35 years, maybe longer.

The symptoms of breast cancer

The symptoms of breast cancer may be the presence of a solitary painless lump in the breast, often found by the patient at self-examination (Figures 11.2 and 11.3). Lumps in the breast are *not* always cancer; most lumps have benign causes, like **fibrocystic** changes, that is, non-malignant

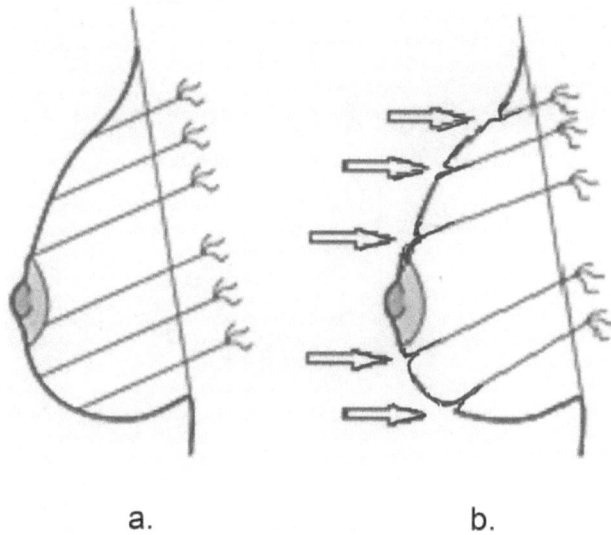

a.   b.

FIGURE 11.4   Side views of a breast showing the cause of the peau d'orange effect: (a) The normal breast showing suspensory ligaments. (b) The breast is swollen, and the suspensory ligaments are holding parts of the breast skin back, causing a dimpling effect (arrowed).

lesions of epithelial origin that come and go in relation to the ovarian cycle (Figure 11.5). The involvement of swollen axillary lymph nodes in combination with breast lumps is a sign of advancement of the disease. The removal of the lump (often called a **'lumpectomy'**) is a first step, and subsequent treatment depends on the histopathological result of the removed tissue.

Mammography, an X-ray procedure of the breast, can show shadows of dense tissue or **calcification** in the breast, although benign lesions can also calcify and show up on mammography. A valuable use of this examination is as an annual screening test for those women who carry a higher risk of the disease.

Breast pain is not commonly an early symptom but may be a feature in advanced disease, that is, 60–70% of patients with *advanced* breast cancer complain of pain. Breast pain generally may be *cyclic,* that is, occurring at specific points in relation to the menstrual cycle, or *non-cyclic,* that is, unrelated to the menstrual cycle. Cyclic breast pain (**cyclic mastalgia**) is due to hormonal changes and is not often caused by breast cancer. Non-cyclic pain is far less common and feels very different from cyclic pain. It does not vary over the menstrual cycle; it is often of unknown cause and usually in one spot or area, that is, a '**trigger zone pain'**, suggesting it is anatomical rather than hormonal in origin. Breast pain may sometimes be caused by trauma to the breast. In some cancers, there may be discharge of fluid from the nipple, an asymmetry in size or shape of one breast, and inflammatory redness or ulceration of the skin.

The spread of **metastases** from tumours is suggested by:

1. The tumour size being larger than 5 cm.
2. The formation of **oedema** (see Table 10.1, Chapter 10, p. 198) of the skin around the tumour. Swelling causes dimpling of the skin where the ligaments attaching the breast tissue to the skin pull the skin in, called **peau d'orange**, or orange peel appearance (Figure 11.4).
3. Ulceration of the skin over the tumour.

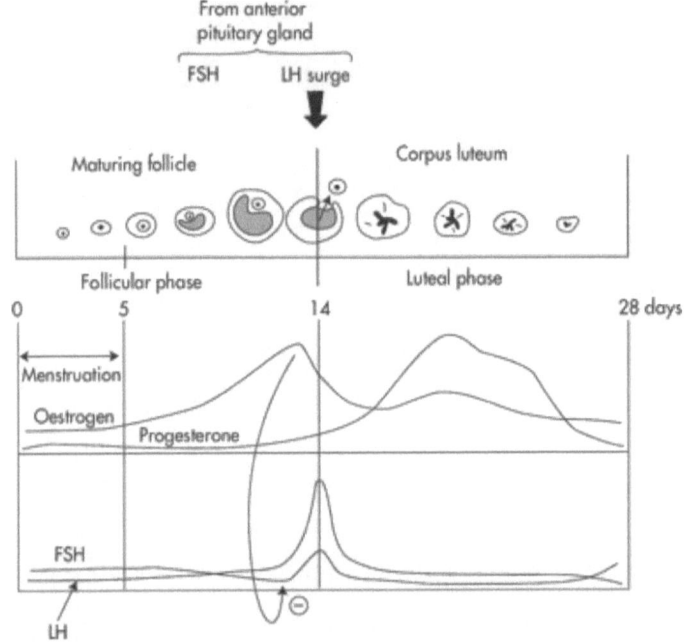

FIGURE 11.5   The ovarian cycle. The cycle is shown here over an average of 28 days, although a variety of different time spans is seen. The first 14 days is the follicular phase, the second 14 days the luteal phase, with ovulation occurring about day 14 due to a surge in LH (luteinising hormone). The maturing follicle in the first half releases more oestrogen as it gets bigger. This rise in oestrogen has negative feedback [Θ] on FSH (follicle-stimulating hormone), which then falls. Progesterone is released from the corpus luteum in the second half and rises to a peak before falling again as the corpus luteum disappears. Progesterone sustains the endometrium of the uterus, and due to the decline in progesterone towards the end of the cycle, this lining is then shed over days 1 to 5 of the next cycle, a process called menstruation.

4. Adhesion of the breast on the chest wall muscles, preventing movement of the breast.
5. **Superclavicular**, that is, above the collarbone, lymph nodes can be felt by palpation.
6. Large lymph nodes (e.g. walnut size) are found in the axilla.
7. The skin around the tumour mass is inflamed.

The genetics of breast cancer

About 5% of breast cancers are caused by a **dominant** gene (see 'Gene inheritance', Chapter 2, p. 30). This means that about 1 in 200 women in the Western world will develop a genetic predisposition for breast cancer.

The **TP53 gene** at 17p13.1 (see 'Chromosome 17', Addendum, p. 356) is an important **tumour suppressor gene** and a factor in this disease. **Li–Fraumeni syndrome** is a rare **autosomal dominant** inherited disorder (see 'Gene inheritance', Chapter 2, p. 30) involving the *TP53* gene, which causes the development of multiple cancers, including multifocal breast cancer early in life.

Other genes involved in breast cancer include the following:

- *MLH1* (see 'Chromosome 3', p. 344) and *MSH2* (see 'Chromosome 2', Addendum, p. 344) are DNA repair genes, that is, they code for proteins which repair mismatched bases on DNA. They cause breast cancer in those families with **hereditary non-polyposis colorectal cancer (Lynch syndrome type II)** (see Table 8.4, Chapter 8, p. 163).
- *BRCA1* (**br**east **ca**ncer 1) gene is implicated as a causative factor in all hereditary breast cancers with ovarian cancers. It is a large gene (18 million bases long) at 17q21 (see 'Chromosome 17', Addendum, p. 356). The normal gene product may be involved in the suppression of oestrogen-dependent breast cell proliferation, possibly by inhibiting ER production (see p. 209), and appears to have some control over the cell cycle by interacting with the protein products of the genes *Tp53* (Chapter 2, p. 30) and *RB1* (Chapter 2, p. 30) (Passarge 2017). Women with mutations of the *BRCA1* gene lose this function and therefore have a 56–85% increased chance of developing the disease (estimates of the importance of this gene vary). Five different mutations have been found for this gene, and during screening, the entire gene must be examined for errors. With a gene this large, screening is a huge undertaking.
- *BRCA2* (**br**east **ca**ncer 2) at 13q12.3 (see 'Chromosome 13', Addendum, p. 354) is found in about one-third of all familial breast cancer patients. It appears to have a similar role in controlling the cell cycle as *BRCA1* (Passarge 2017). The inheritance of *BRCA1* and *BRCA2* is *autosomal dominant* (see 'Gene inheritance', Chapter 2, p. 30).
- Less is known about the *BRCA3* (**br**east **ca**ncer 3) gene than *BRCA1* or *BRCA2*. There appears to be a link between this gene and breast cancer similar to *BRCA2*.
- *PALB2* (see 'Chromosome 16', Addendum, p. 356).
- *BRIP1* (see 'Chromosome 17', Addendum, p. 356).
- *ERB-B2* (see 'Chromosome 17', Addendum, p. 357).

Important prognostic markers are:

1. **Lymph node metastasis,** that is, the more nodes involved, the worse the prognosis.
2. **Tumour size,** that is, the larger the tumour, the worse the prognosis. Generally, tumours less than 1 cm have an excellent prognosis.
3. **Histological grade**, using cellular differentiation, nuclear pleomorphism, and the number of mitotic figures present in the tumour.

    - **Cellular differentiation.** *Well-differentiated* means that the cells look normal, the same as the tissue of origin; *poorly differentiated* means that cells appear grossly abnormal.
    - **Nuclear pleomorphism** concerns how abnormal the nucleus looks (*pleo* = more; *pleomorphism* = more or multiple-shaped nucleus).
    - **Mitotic figures**, that is, the number of cells in mitosis within the tissue. The more cells in mitosis, the more aggressive the tumour.

4. **Histological type**, that is, what the abnormal cells are like; for example, **tubular** are cells that appear like tubes, **medullary** are cells which have the colour of the brain (medulla), **mucinous** are tumour cells that produce mucus, and **papillary** are cells that stick out in little finger-like projections called **papules**.

5. **Hormone–receptor status** of the cells (also known as *biological markers*):

   - **Oestrogen receptor positive (ER+)** or **negative (ER−)** (see Table 11.2, p. 209). ER+ tumours allow for treatment with anti-oestrogen drugs. About 60% of breast tumours are ER+.
   - **Progesterone receptor positive (PgR+)** or **negative (PgR−)** (see Table 11.2, p. 209). PgR+ tumour cells exist mostly in relation with ER+, since the presence of PgR is dependent on an intact ER pathway. PgR+ role in causing breast cancer is not clear, and anti-progesterone therapy may only ease symptoms in advanced disease.

6. **Ploidy** is the measurement of the amount of DNA in the cell, that is, **diploid** is the normal chromosome count (46) and carries a better prognosis if found in tumour cells than **aneuploid**, that is, any abnormal chromosome count.

7. **Genetics**, the presence of mutations of the genes, such as ***ERB-B2*** (see 'Chromosome 17', Addendum, p. 357) or ***Tp53*** (see 'Chromosome 17', Addendum, p. 356).

Advanced breast disease is divided into local and metastatic. Locally advanced disease is characterised by the features of skin and chest wall infiltration, with or without axillary node involvement. *Skin features* include ulceration and the presence of satellite nodes, dermal infiltration, peau d'orange (Figure 11.4), and erythema (redness) over the tumour site. *Chest wall features* include fixation of the tumour to the ribs, the intercostal muscles, or the serratus anterior muscle. *Axillary node* features are where the nodes are fixed to each other or to other structures, that is, they become matted together. **Lymphoedema** is the collection of fluid in the tissues due to obstruction of the lymphatic drainage. In cancer, this is due either to blocking of lymph nodes with malignant cells, as in lymph metastases, or from treatment, for example, surgical removal or irradiation of the lymph nodes (see 'The causes of oedema', Table 10.1, Chapter 10, p. 198). Upper-limb lymphoedema is often caused by local recurrence of the disease within nodes of the axillary and supraclavicular regions. It is a cause of pain, discomfort, and distress.

    Metastatic disease may involve any site, but more often bone, lymph, and chest wall (better prognosis), or lung, liver, or brain (poorest prognosis).

    Hypercalcaemia (high blood calcium) can be caused by bone disease releasing calcium into the blood. The loss of calcium from the diseased bones makes them weaker and at risk of **pathological fractures**. Breathlessness can be caused by pulmonary (lung) disease, and **raised intercranial pressure (RICP)** may be caused by cerebral (brain) disease.

    Advanced breast cancer is known to gain energy for continued growth from the extracellular matrix (ECM) that surrounds the cells (see 'Extracellular matrix (ECM)', Chapter 6, p. 124). This is because, sometimes, as the tumour gets bigger, the blood supply can become restricted. This reduces oxygen and nutrition to the rapidly growing tumour cells, yet they continue to grow. Breast tumour cells are 'scavenging' from the ECM, mostly collagen, then breaking it down in the lysosomes with enzymes that break down substances. The amino acids tyrosine and phenylalanine are important in this process. New treatments could target the use of these amino acids and therefore prevent breast cancer cells from further development when blood restriction occurs. This may also have implications for other cancers.

The ovaries

The two ovaries are situated low in the pelvis, one on each side of the uterus. They have a close association with the **uterine (or fallopian) tubes**, which carry the **ova** that have been discharged from both ovaries into the uterus. The function of the ovary is to produce the ovum and the hormone **oestradiol**.

The ovarian cycle

The ovarian cycle is based on the standard 28 days, although there is considerable variation in the timing of the cycle in different women (Figure 11.5).

The **ovarian cycle** (Figure 11.5) is controlled by two hormones from the **anterior pituitary gland** at the base of the brain: (1) **follicle-stimulating hormone (FSH)** and (2) **luteinising hormone (LH)**. These are together called the **gonadotropic[4] hormones**. In women, ova develop up to the **antrum stage** (Figure 11.6) without FSH, but FSH is required to stimulate the development of ova from the antrum stage onto full maturity (**follicular maturation**). At first, several ova develop, but then only one goes on to full maturity. They are maturing inside a tiny ball of cells in the ovary called a **follicle**. This occurs during the first 14 days of the cycle, and this period is therefore called the **follicular phase** (days 0 to 14). The maturing follicle produces increasing amounts of oestradiol, so the level of this hormone increases in the blood over the follicular phase. At or about day 14 (mid-cycle), the high oestradiol level causes a surge in the release of LH from the pituitary gland, which, in turn, causes the mature follicle to rupture and release the ovum. The ovum is captured by the **fallopian tube** to begin its journey to the uterus, and it may or may not become fertilised in this tube.

The remains of the follicle in the ovary condense down to form a **corpus luteum**, so the second half of the cycle, after ovulation, is known as the **luteal phase**. During this phase, the condensing corpus luteum produces the hormone **progesterone** that sustains the uterine lining until the fertilised ovum (if it is fertilised) can become embedded in this lining. The decline in progesterone towards day 28, the end of the cycle, due to the gradual disappearance of the corpus luteum, causes shedding of the uterine lining, called **menstruation**, or a **menstrual 'period'**, over the first five days of the *next* cycle (days 1 to 5) in those cycles where fertilisation did *not* occur. If fertilisation does occur, the ovum, which has now developed into a cluster of cells, becomes embedded in the uterine lining and establishes a connection with the maternal blood circulation through the developing **placenta**. Part of the embedding cell cluster (called a **blastocyst**) produces a hormone called **human chorionic gonadotropin (HCG)**, which enters the mother's blood and causes retention of the luteal phase. Keeping the corpus luteum means

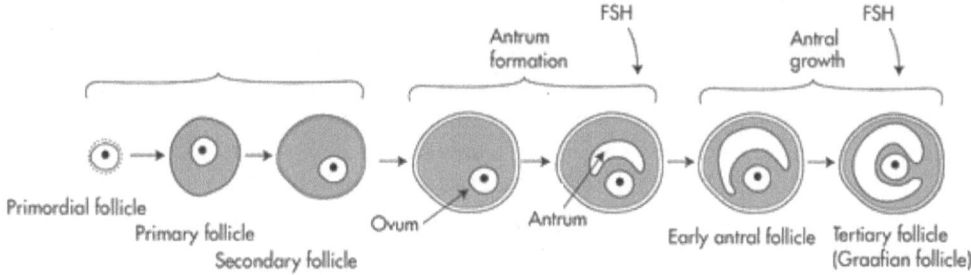

FIGURE 11.6   The developing follicle and ovum (days 1 to 14 of the ovarian cycle). The stimulus for development during the early stages is not known, but from antrum (or cavity) formation onwards, the stimulus is FSH (follicle-stimulating hormone).

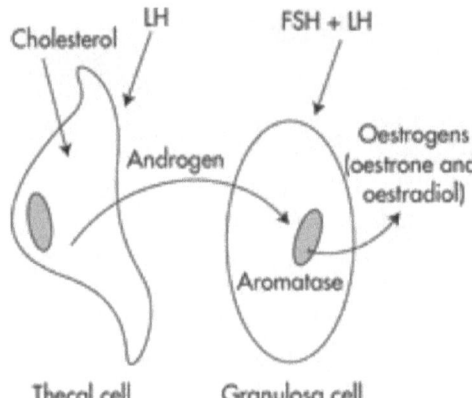

FIGURE 11.7   Two cell types in the ovary. The first, the thecal cell, converts cholesterol to androgens (male hormones), and the second, the granulosa cell, converts the androgen to oestrogen using the enzyme aromatase. The thecal cell responds to LH (luteinising hormone), and the granulosa cell responds to LH and FSH (follicle-stimulating hormone).

that the progesterone production does not diminish, thus preventing the loss of the uterine lining and retaining the pregnancy, so that the menstrual period will be missed because the next cycle will not start. HCG levels rise over the first two months of pregnancy, then fall to a low level by the fourth month, and remain at this lower level for the remainder of the pregnancy (Marieb and Hoehn 2022). Excretion of HCG in the urine forms the basis of pregnancy tests since it can only be present as a product of a blastocyst, that is, a pregnancy.

Two particular cell types are important in the ovary: the **theca** cells and the **granulosa** cells (Figure 11.7). The theca cells are stimulated by LH, and they produce **androgens** (mostly **androstenedione**) from **cholesterol**. The granulosa cells are stimulated mostly by FSH (but also some LH), and they produce oestradiol from the androgen. One effect of oestradiol is to suppress the release of FSH (as a negative feedback system). As the follicle reaches full maturity, the oestradiol reaches the greatest output. This peak of oestradiol blocks FSH release (since FSH will no longer be required for follicular maturation), and the oestradiol also triggers the LH surge that causes ovulation. Oestradiol is therefore a major hormone in the control of the ovarian cycle.

Ovarian cancer

The highest risk of cancer of the ovary seems to be related to a Western lifestyle, with higher risks seen in women who have never had children or have never been pregnant, or those who are smokers or exposed to asbestos. Three categories of malignant potential occur in these tumours, *benign, borderline* (*low malignant potential*), and *overtly malignant*. Many are associated with **cysts**, which are fluid-filled cavities within the tissues. Neoplasms of the ovary are a wide assortment of diseases which can be broadly placed into the following two main groups (according to the cell of origin) (Kumar et al. 2022):

1. Tumours of **surface epithelial** origin make up the largest proportion of ovarian cancers seen. The malignant forms of the disease account for about 90% of all malignant ovarian cancers. The group includes benign and malignant, and there are different types (Table 11.4).

TABLE 11.4 The types of *surface epithelial* ovarian tumours

Tumour type	Notes
Serous (cystadenomas, cystadenocarcinomas)	Most frequent type, presents at 30–40 years of age. Solid tumour often with cysts; 60% are benign, 15% borderline, and 25% malignant.
Mucinous	Very similar to serous, derived from mucin-secreting epithelium. Less likely to be malignant than serous (only 20% are borderline or malignant).
Endometrioid	Usually malignant form derived from the walls of cysts. They take on a microscopic appearance similar to endometrial cells; 30% are bilateral, and 15–30% are associated with endometrial cancer (see 'Endometrial carcinomas', p. 223).
Clear-cell (mesonephroid)	A spongy, partly cystic tumour of cells with clear cytoplasm. Most are malignant.
Brenner	Rare, mostly benign, solid tumour of transitional epithelium set in stromal cells.
Cystadenofibroma	Similar to serous cystadenoma, malignancy is rare.

TABLE 11.5 The types of *germ cell* ovarian tumours

Tumour type	Notes
Teratoma	About 15–20% of all ovarian tumours. They appear at an early age. *Mature* and *immature* forms occur. Mature are rarely malignant (99% are benign), but immature have a greater tendency to become malignant (see 'Non-seminomas', Chapter 12, p. 237).
Dysgerminoma	These appear around 20–30 years of age. They are solid malignant tumours; about one-third spread to other sites.
Endodermal sinus tumour (yolk sac tumour)	Appears in the young (average age is 19 years). It is highly malignant. The tumour secretes a protein called α-fetoprotein (AFP), which can be monitored to assess the progress of the disease.
Choriocarcinoma	Appear in those under 30 years of age. They are malignant and metastasise early. They often have areas of necrosis and haemorrhage.
Sex cord tumours	*Sex cords* are primitive germ cells that migrate into the ovary during embryonic development. They retain the ability to differentiate into the adult ovarian follicles and can give rise to tumours. This category includes granulosa theca cell tumours, which account for about 1.5% of all ovarian tumours and which may produce oestrogens; thecomas (benign thecal cell tumour seen in post-menopausal women); and Sertoli–Leydig tumours, which are very rare (0.2% of ovarian cancers).

2. Tumours of **germ cell** origin account for about 3–5% of all malignant ovarian tumours. Germ cells are the ova and its surrounding follicular tissues. Like surface epithelial tumours, there are several different types (Table 11.5).

Ovarian cancers are often asymptomatic at first, which gives the tumour time to spread, unless found on routine examination. When symptoms do occur, they are often pain in the abdomen, swelling of the abdomen, and sometimes **ascites**, that is, oedema collecting in the abdomen. In advanced disease, the patient can suffer from nausea and vomiting, bowel changes, and vaginal bleeding from local spread into the vagina.

Staging for ovarian cancer uses four major grades, **1** to **4**, with divisions **A**, **B**, and **C**.

Stage 1: Cancer contained within the ovary

1A: One ovary involved, capsule intact, no ascites
1B: Both ovaries involved, capsules intact, no ascites
1C: Capsule involved, and malignant cells present in peritoneal fluid

Stage 2: Cancer growing outside the ovary into the pelvic cavity

2A: Extension of the cancer into the fallopian tubes or uterus
2B: Extension of the cancer into other pelvic organs, for example, the bladder

Stage 3: Cancer growing outside the pelvic cavity into the abdomen

3A: Cancer has spread to the lymph nodes at the back of the abdomen
3B: Cancer growths 2 cm or smaller on the peritoneum
3C: Cancer growths larger than 2 cm on the peritoneum

Stage 4: Cancer now growing in organs outside the abdomen, for example, the lungs

Usually, **oophorectomy**, the surgical removal of an ovary, is the first option for treatment, followed by other treatments, depending on the stage of the disease.

The female reproductive tract

The **uterus** (Figure 11.8) is the main organ low in the female pelvis, where development of, first, the embryo and, later, the foetus takes place. It is a hollow organ with a smooth muscle wall (the **myometrium**) lined internally by a layer of glandular cells set in stromal connective tissue

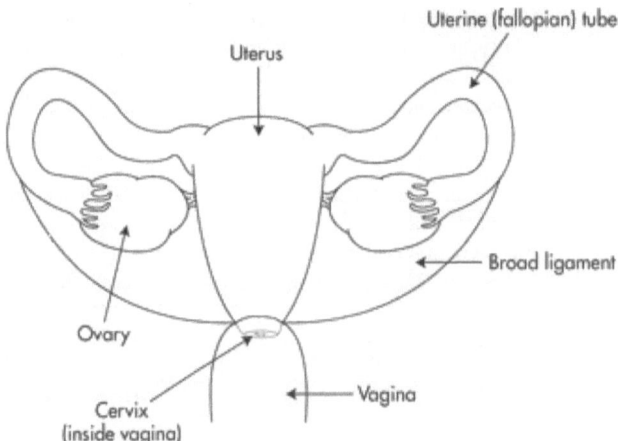

FIGURE 11.8   The female reproductive tract. The ovaries are suspended on the broad ligament. Ova shed from the ovaries are captured by the fimbriae (finger-like projections from the fallopian tubes). The cervix is the opening of the uterus into the vagina.

Source: Redrawn from Martini et al. (2023).

(the **endometrium**). This inner layer has a rich blood supply and is shed regularly as part of the **uterine cycle**. This cycle is linked to the ovarian cycle (Figure 11.5).

Over the first five days of the ovarian cycle, some of the endometrial lining is lost through the vagina in a flow known as **menstruation**. It then begins to thicken over the remaining follicular phase up to day 14 but becomes thicker still under the influence of progesterone during the luteal phase (day 15 onwards). Towards the end of the 28-day cycle, the progesterone production from the corpus luteum that had sustained the endometrium declines, and the endometrium can no longer survive. By day 1 of the next cycle, the endometrium is shed and a new menstruation starts (Figure 11.5).

Linking the uterus to the ovaries are the **fallopian** (or **ovarian**) **tubes**, one each side, and these capture and pass the released ova from the follicle of the ovary to the uterine body (Marieb and Hoehn 2022). If fertilisation has taken place in the fallopian tube, which is the commonest site for fertilisation of the ova by the sperm, then the developing cells of the **blastocyst** will attach to the endometrium and become buried in it (called **implantation**). The lower portion of the uterus is the **cervix** (meaning *neck-like*), with a narrow opening into the **vagina**. The *vagina* is a collapsible tube extending from the cervix to the outside world and is the organ of **coitus** (sexual intercourse). It is also the *birth canal*, that is, the route for the natural birth of a foetus, and the route for menstrual flow. It is made of smooth muscle with a mucous membrane lining.

The **external genitalia** in females, that is, the **vulva**, consists of the (1) **mons veneris**, the skin-covered pad of fat over the symphysis pubis bearing pubic hair; (2) **labia majora**, the folds of skin-covered fat on each side of a space called the **vestibule**; (3) **labia minora**, the smaller folds inside the labia majora; (4) **clitoris**, an erectile organ, the tip of which is positioned at the anterior union of the two labia minora; (5) **urethral opening**, for the passage of urine, just anterior to the **vaginal opening**, both openings in the vestibule; and (6) **Bartholin's glands** and **Skene's glands**, which secrete lubricating fluid and mucus, respectively, into the vestibule.

Uterine and cervical cancer

Endometrial carcinomas

The tumours of the uterus are usually **endometrial carcinomas**. They are quite rare under 40 years of age but are more often seen in women aged 55 to 65 years. Risks factors of the disease are the presence of obesity, diabetes, hypertension, and infertility, and some of these, like obesity, are linked to raised levels of oestrogen in circulation. The origin of the disease often lies in the occurrence of **endometrial hyperplasia**, that is, excessive overgrowth of the endometrium, and post-menopausal women who develop endometrial hyperplasia whilst on **hormone replacement therapy (HRT)** are at particular risk. This disease is often associated with breast cancer. Uterine cancers erode into the muscle wall of the uterus and fill the uterine cavity. They are mostly **adenocarcinomas**, derived from, and looking like, the glandular cells of the endometrium. Some may also contain well-differentiated squamous-like cells, and then the tumour is called an **adenocarcinoma with squamous metaplasia**. Squamous cells that become overtly malignant within an adenocarcinoma produce a tumour called an **adenosquamous carcinoma**.

Types and grades

There are two types of this cancer:

1. Type 1 are mostly endometrial adenocarcinomas linked to high levels of oestrogen. They are the most common type, slow-growing with low potential for spreading.
2. Type 2 are faster-growing, with greater potential for spreading. They are not linked to oestrogen levels and include various subtypes, such as clear-cell carcinoma and uterine serous carcinoma.

Three grades are identified:

Grade 1: The cells are well-differentiated and appear normal. They tend to be slow-growing and are less likely to spread than higher-grade cancer.

Grade 2: The cells are moderately differentiated and appear more abnormal. They are more likely to spread than grade 1.

Grade 3: The cells are poorly differentiated and appear very abnormal. They grow quickly and have high potential to spread, usually to the pelvis, abdomen, lungs, liver, and bones.

An early sign of an endometrial carcinoma is irregular vaginal bleeding, which, in a post-menopausal woman, is indicative that something is wrong. Bleeding is from erosion of the endometrial surface. In time, the uterus may become enlarged and palpable. Spread beyond the uterus can cause fixation of the uterus against surrounding structures.

The genes involved in endometrial cancers are shown in Table 11.6.

Myometrium cancers

The smooth muscle layer of the uterine wall is the site of origin for the **leiomyosarcoma**, a moderately rare neoplasm affecting older, post-menopausal women aged 50 years old or more. The prognosis is not good, with about 20–30% surviving for five years. A poorer prognosis is associated with the onset in a younger, pre-menopausal woman. Spread can be into the pelvic organs and the lungs.

Cancer of the cervix

Cancer of the cervix is, worldwide, the second most common female malignancy after breast cancer. The link between cervical cancer and the woman's sexual history relates to the age

TABLE 11.6 Genes linked to endometrial cancer

Gene	Locus	Further information
JAZF1	7p15.2–p15.1	See 'Chromosome 7', Addendum, p. 349.
PHF1	6p21.32	See 'Chromosome 6', Addendum, p. 348.
EPC1	10p11.22	See 'Chromosome 10', Addendum, p. 352.
MEAF6	1p34.3	See 'Chromosome 1', Addendum, p. 343.
YWHAE	17p13.3	See 'Chromosome 17', Addendum, p. 357.

at first intercourse, that is, before 18 years of age increases the risk by 2.5 times, and the number of sexual partners, that is, the more the partners, the greater the risk. This suggests a viral agent may be a major causative factor, and the **human papillomavirus (HPV)** (see Figure 4.2b, Chapter 4, p. 61) is a common cause. There are over 50 different varieties of HPV, and HPV types 16 and 18 are oncogenic. HPV is sexually transmitted, and it appears to infect the cells of the cervix, which then produce proteins that interfere with the function of the *RB1* gene (see 'Chromosome 13', Addendum, p. 354). Another causative factor is smoking. Both **nicotine** and its breakdown product, called **cotinine**, are found in the cervical cells of smokers.

A pre-malignant phase occurs where the squamous epithelial cells of the cervical mucosa show increasing degrees of abnormal change, for example, dysplasia (see Figure 1.14, Chapter 1, p. 18). Identifying these pre-malignant changes is the goal of **cervical cytology**, where screening by cervical smears can allow early intervention to save lives and improve the prognosis. **Cervical intraepithelial neoplasia (CIN)** is the termed used to describe the degree of these dysplastic changes:

- **CIN I** means one-third or less of the cells show dysplasia, that is, mild.
- **CIN II** means that one- to two-thirds of the cells show dysplasia, that is, moderate.
- **CIN III** means that more than two-thirds of the cells show dysplasia, that is, severe, or *carcinoma in situ*.

Evidence for the inclusion of HPV is strong for CIN I and II, but rarer for CIN III, where full integration of the HPV genome into the host cell makes the virus invisible.

About 70% of invasive cancers of the cervix are **squamous carcinomas** (Kumar et al. 2022). Spread from the site of origin can occur directly to the uterus above, to the vagina below, or into the bladder or rectum. Lymph node involvement and blood-borne metastases also occur, leading to secondaries in the lungs, liver, and bone at a later stage. Survival rates at five years stand overall at about 55%.

The removal of the uterus is a **hysterectomy**, although not all cancers are treated by total removal of the organ. Cervical cancers, especially in the early stages of the disease, may be treated by the removal of the affected tissues only, resulting in various degrees of cervical **resection**.

Vaginal and vulval cancer

Vaginal cancer

Most vaginal cancers are those spread from the cervix. Malignancies primarily occurring in the vagina are rare, about 1% of all cancers of the female reproductive tract. Most are **invasive squamous carcinomas** occurring in the upper parts of the vagina in elderly women, but some **adenocarcinomas** occur. Spread is into the bladder, the rectum, and the local lymph nodes, and in the later stages, secondaries in the lungs and bone can be seen. Several variations of adenocarcinoma of the vagina occur, and one of these, called **clear-cell adenocarcinoma**, is a rare but important disease as it causes cancer in *young* women of about 17 years of age. It is very rare in girls before the age of 12 years, and in women after the age of 30 years. It therefore affects women, in most cases, *before* child-bearing has occurred.

The staging of vaginal cancer is:

1. Tumour is limited to the vaginal wall. It has a very good prognosis, with 80% of patients surviving for at least five years.

   1A The cancer is 2 cm or less and has not spread to local lymph nodes.
   1B The cancer is larger than 2 cm and has not spread to local lymph nodes.

2. The cancer involves local tissues, but not the pelvic wall.

   2A The cancer is 2 cm or less but has spread outside of the vagina, but it has not reached the pelvic wall or local lymph nodes.
   2B The cancer is larger than 2 cm and has spread outside of the vagina, but it has not reached the pelvic wall or local lymph nodes.

3. The cancer has reached the pelvic wall. There may be local lymph nodes affected. The survival rate is poor.
4. The cancer has grown outside the pelvis. The survival rate is poor.

   4A The cancer has reached the bladder or rectum.
   4B The cancer has reached organs outside the pelvis, notably the lungs and bones.

The grading types for vaginal cancer are:

1. Grade 1: Normal-looking cells that are well-differentiated and slow-growing. There is a low risk of the tumour spreading.
2. Grade 2: Moderately differentiated abnormal-looking cells with a higher risk of spread to other areas.
3. Grade 3: Very abnormal-looking, poorly differentiated cells that grow quickly, with high risk of spread.

Visual examination of the vagina and the cervix (called **colposcopy**) is done using an instrument called a **colposcope**. Surgery on the vagina may be required as a first step in the management of this disease. Reconstruction surgery to create a new vaginal opening, known as a **vaginoplasty** or **colpoplasty**, is available in most cases and is essential in menstruating women.

Vulval cancer

Neoplasms of the **vulva** fall into two categories: **Paget's disease** of the vulva and **invasive carcinoma** of the vulva. Paget's disease is the presence of Paget cells (Table 11.3, p. 211). These cells invade the epidermis of the vulva in about 70% of patients or invade the local glands in about 30% of patients. Invasive carcinomas are mostly squamous in origin in about 90% of cases. It affects mostly women in their 60s with a history of smoking and sexually transmitted diseases. It affects the **labia majora** in most patients, with the **clitoris** being the second commonest site. Itching or irritation of the vulva (**pruritis vulvae**) is a common sign, with the formation of a mass or ulceration of the tissues, bleeding, and local discharge. Spread into the lymph nodes on both sides of the vulva can happen, and surgical removal of the tumour usually involves dissection of lymph nodes on both sides.

Staging consists of:

1. Confined to vulva, tumour is 2 cm or less.
2. Nearby structures involved, for example, urethra, vagina, or anus.
3. Tumour extends to include lymph nodes.
4. Spread to other organs, such as the liver, lungs, or bones.

Patients with early-stage disease have a good prognosis, up to 90% with five-year survival rates. Only 25% survival rates occur in women with pelvic node involvement.

Surgical removal of the vulva (a **vulvectomy**) is a radical means of eliminating the tumour and can involve removing the labia, the clitoris, much of the surrounding skin and subcutaneous tissues, and the regional lymph nodes.

Key points

Hormones

- Three oestrogens are found in women: oestradiol (E2), oestrone (E1), and oestriol (E3).
- In women, the oestrogens are produced mostly in the ovaries.
- Oestrogen binds to oestrogen receptors (ER) within the cell, and cells that have these receptors are said to be ER-positive (ER+).
- Oestradiol (E2) is the most potent of the oestrogens.
- Another female hormone, called progesterone, is produced by the corpus luteum in the ovaries.

The breasts

- Epithelial cells make up the alveolar (milk-producing), ductal, and myoepithelial cells.
- The breast is packed with a fibrous connective tissue called stroma.
- The adipose (fat) tissue is present in variable amounts.
- Over 85% of lymph drains from the breast into the axillary (armpit) lymph nodes.
- Breast cancers can be classified into non-invasive and invasive and are located as either ductal or lobular.
- Invasive ductal carcinoma is the most common form of breast cancer.

The ovaries

- The two ovaries produce mature ova and the hormones oestrogen and progesterone.
- The control of the ovarian cycle is by the pituitary hormones: follicle-stimulating hormone (FSH) and luteinising hormone (LH).
- The ovarian cycle is linked to the uterine cycle.
- Tumours of surface epithelial origin make up the largest proportion of ovarian cancers.
- Ovarian cancers are often symptom-free at first.

The uterus

- The uterus has a smooth muscle wall (the myometrium) lined by a layer of glandular cells in stroma (the endometrium).

- The tumours of the uterus are usually endometrial carcinomas.
- An early sign of an endometrial carcinoma is irregular vaginal bleeding.

The cervix

- Cancer of the cervix is the second most common female malignancy after breast cancer.
- The human papillomavirus (HPV) is a potential cause of this disease.
- About 70% of invasive cancers of the cervix are squamous carcinomas.
- A pre-malignant phase occurs where the epithelial cells of the cervical mucosa show abnormal changes, and this is the reason screening by cervical smears is so important.

The vagina

- The majority of vaginal cancers are those spread from the cervix.
- Most are invasive squamous carcinomas.
- Clear-cell adenocarcinoma occurs in women of around 17 years of age, that is, *before* child-bearing has occurred in most cases.

The vulva

- Neoplasms of the vulva are either Paget's disease or invasive carcinoma.
- Itching or irritation of the vulva is a common sign, with ulceration of the tissues, bleeding, and local discharge.

Notes

1 Being fat-based, steroids, such as oestrogen, can pass through cell membranes and bind to receptors inside the cell. This is contrary to protein-based hormones, which must bind to receptors mounted on the cell surface (see Figure 4.9, Chapter 4, p. 69).
2 As a comparison, E2 has a thousand times greater effect on breast tissue than E3.
3 This *does not* mean that breast milk is modified sweat! In this case, a gland has been modified in order to generate a completely different product.
4 *Tropic* means 'to influence', that is, they influence the **gonads**, a collective term for the ovaries and testes.

12

CANCERS OF THE MALE REPRODUCTIVE SYSTEM

- **Introduction: the androgens**
- **The male reproductive system**
- **Prostate cancer**
- **Testicular cancer**
- **Penile cancer**
- **Key points**

Introduction: the androgens

The male hormones are three **androgens**:

1. **Testosterone**, the naturally secreted product of the Leydig cells of the testes, but it is converted to **dihydrotestosterone (DHT)** in the prostate gland and testes, and in this form, it is the most potent hormone of the androgen group, being responsible for sexual differentiation during embryo development and male body development during puberty.
2. **Dehydroepiandrosterone (DHEA)** the naturally secreted product of the adrenal gland. It has a wide range of functions and acts as precursor of the oestrogens in females.
3. **Androstenedione** is a naturally secreted product of the adrenal gland and gonads. It has weak androgen hormonal effects. It is the precursor in the production of oestrone and **testosterone**.

The **adrenal gland** cortex is the site of production of these hormones in small quantities in both sexes, but the main source in males is the **testes**. Androgens have masculinisation effects on several types of tissues. For example, they build muscle and bone by inducing cell and tissue growth and are known as **anabolic steroids**. These effects are seen during male puberty, when testosterone levels rise and growth accelerates. It is this cellular growth effect that becomes a problem in a number of male tumours that respond to androgens. Testosterone and the other hormones bind to **androgen receptors (AR)** in cells that are androgen receptor positive, that is, AR+, similar to ER+ in women. Any male tumour that is AR+ will grow faster with androgen stimulation.

DOI: 10.4324/9781003389125-12

The male reproductive system

The organs of the male reproductive system are the testes and its associated ducts, the prostate gland, and the penis (Figure 12.1). The distal urethra is important as the common duct conveying both urine and sperm to the outside world.

Testes

The testes (singular = *testis*) (Figure 12.2) are the organs that produce both sperm (a process called **spermatogenesis**) and the hormone testosterone. They begin by developing within the abdomen and must descend through a canal in the groin region (the **inguinal canal**) to a position within the **scrotum**, the sac of skin behind the penis, prior to birth. The core temperature of 37°C within the abdomen is too high for the testis to function correctly. Babies born with undescended testes (called **cryptorchidism**) must have the problem corrected or risk infertility and testicular cancer later in life.

Internally, the testis is divided into sections (called **lobules**) by **septa** (singular = *septum*, a wall or partition) (Figure 12.2). Each lobule contains a convoluted and twisted tube called the **seminiferous tubule**, where spermatogenesis takes place (*seminiferous* means 'sperm-carrying'). The septa are internal extensions of the outer coat of the testis, called the **tunica albuginea**. Outside this layer is the double membrane of the **tunica vaginalis**, with a fluid-filled cavity between the membranes. The seminiferous tubules from the lobules unite in a network of tubes

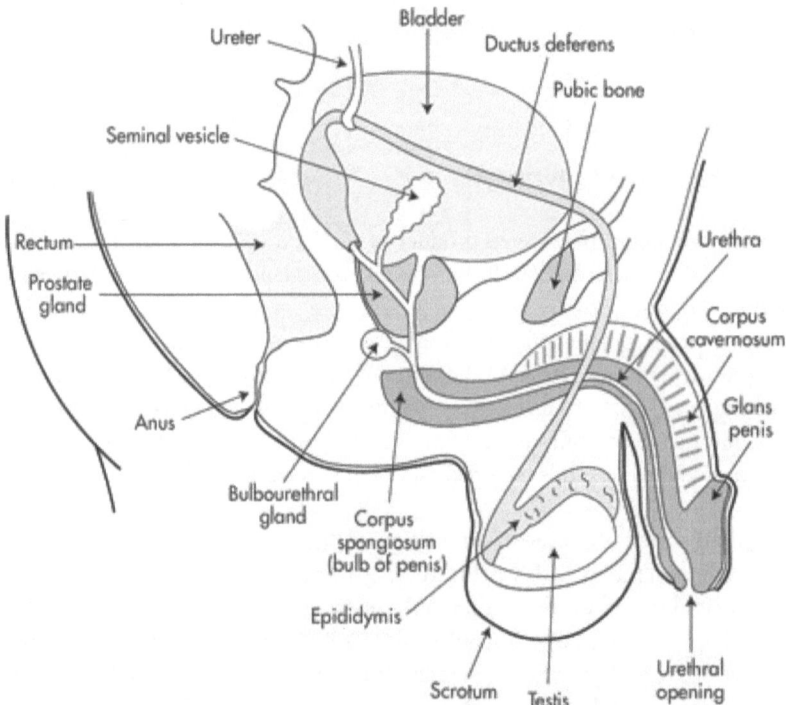

FIGURE 12.1   Section through the male reproductive system.

Source: Marieb and Hoehn (2022).

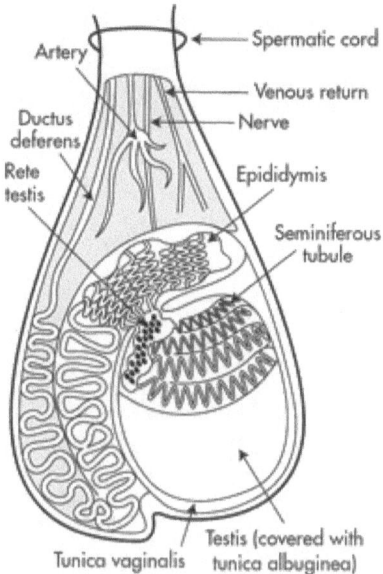

FIGURE 12.2   Section through the scrotum and testis showing the spermatic cord.

Source: Marieb and Hoehn (2022).

called the **rete testis**, and this, in turn, opens into the head of the **epididymis**. This structure is positioned close to the outside of the testis and has a head end (connected to the rete testis) and a tail end. It contains a single tightly coiled tube which, when uncoiled, would be 6 m (20 ft) in length. It takes about 20 days for sperm to move through this duct, and it is the site for the storage of sperm for up to several weeks.

During ejaculation, sperm are pushed by smooth muscle contractions from the tail of the epididymis into the next duct, the **ductus deferens**, or **vas deferens**. This is a much straighter tube that doubles back on itself and enters the **spermatic cord**. The testis is suspended on the spermatic cord, a sheath forming a tube through which the following pass: the ductus deferens, the arterial blood supply, and venous drainage from the testis, and the nerve supply to the testis (Figure 12.2).

Both ductus deferens, one from each testis, extend into the abdomen, over the urinary bladder, and down the posterior wall of the bladder, where they join the duct from the **seminal vesicles** on each side (Figure 12.1). The seminal vesicles produce a fluid which makes up about 60% of the **semen**, the fluid containing sperm that is ejaculated. This alkaline fluid contains sugar and vitamin C for nutrition of the sperm. The ductus deferens and the duct from the seminal vesicles join to form a single duct, the **ejaculatory duct**, on each side. The left and right ejaculatory ducts extend into the **prostate gland** on both sides and both join with the **urethra** inside the prostate.

The prostate gland

This gland lies immediately below the urinary bladder, at the 'neck' of the bladder, and is made up of three main compartments (or zones) (Figures 12.1 and 12.3). The **central zone** surrounds the ejaculatory duct as far as its junction with the urethra. The **transitional zone**, the smallest region, encompasses the *proximal* (upper) portion of the urethra, that is, *before* its junction with

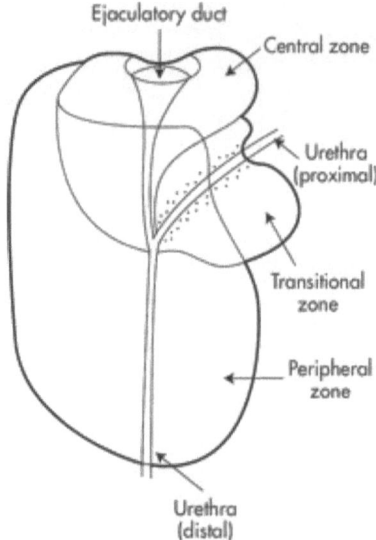

Ejaculatory duct

Central zone

Urethra
(proximal)

Transitional
zone

Peripheral
zone

Urethra
(distal)

FIGURE 12.3   The prostate gland showing three zones and the junction of the ejaculatory duct with the urethra.

Source: Kumar et al. (2022).

the ejaculatory ducts. The largest region, the **peripheral zone**, surrounds the previous two zones on most sides and encompasses the *distal* (lower) portion of the urethra, that is, *after* its junction with the ejaculatory duct (Kumar et al. 2022).

The function of the prostate gland is to produce fluid (about 30% of the fluid component of semen) and to produce other nutrients for sperm (Marieb and Hoehn 2022). The 'gland' is in fact about 25 smaller glands set in a connective tissue called **stroma** (see Table 11.1, Chapter 11, p. 209) surrounded by a fibrous outer cover.

The urethra and the penis

The distal urethra leaves the prostate and extends through the **penis** and opens on the tip of the **glans penis** (Figure 12.1). This portion of the urethra acts as both a duct for urine and for sperm. The body of the organ contains two types of cavity filled with spongy tissue: the **corpora cavernosa** and the **corpus spongiosum** (*corpus* = body). These extend along the full length of the penis. The corpora cavernosa is a pair of cavities touching along the midline and positioned within the dorsal (upper) region of the penis. The single corpus spongiosum is positioned more ventrally, that is, below the corpora cavernosa, and it contains the urethra. It is this cavity that expands at the end of the penis to form the **glans penis**, which is covered by a fold of skin, the **prepuce**. Erection of the penis can occur as a result of filling these cavities with blood, and emptying of blood restores the flaccid state.

Spermatogenesis

Sperm are produced in the seminiferous tubules from **germ cells** called **spermatogonia**. In the healthy adult male, sperm are produced at the rate of *200 to 400 million per day*.[1]

Sperm production requires testosterone, and specialised cells in the testis, called **Leydig cells**, produce testosterone (Figure 12.4). Leydig cells are under the control of the male version of **luteinising hormone**, called **interstitial cell–stimulating hormone (ICSH)**, from the **anterior pituitary gland** (Figure 12.4). Other specialised cells, called **Sertoli cells**, within the lining of the seminiferous tubules are under **follicle-stimulating hormone (FSH)** control from the anterior pituitary gland (Figures 12.4 and 12.5). FSH and testosterone between them stimulate sperm production. The Sertoli cells regulate the process of spermatogenesis and provide nutrition to the germ cells. They also form a barrier, the **blood–testis barrier**, between the outer surface of the tubule (the **basal compartment**) and the inner lumen of the seminiferous tubule (the **adluminal compartment**) (Figure 12.5). The fluid derived from blood in the basal compartment is different from the adluminal compartment fluid, which has the correct constituents needed for developing sperm. The purpose of the blood–testis barrier is to maintain this difference. The Sertoli cells also produce the hormone **inhibin** and a protein called the **androgen-binding protein** (Figure 12.4). The hormone inhibin provides a negative feedback mechanism to the anterior pituitary, regulating the release of FSH, because increasing levels of inhibin will switch off FSH release. The androgen-binding protein binds testosterone, and this ensures the correct concentration of testosterone needed for sperm production (Figure 12.4).

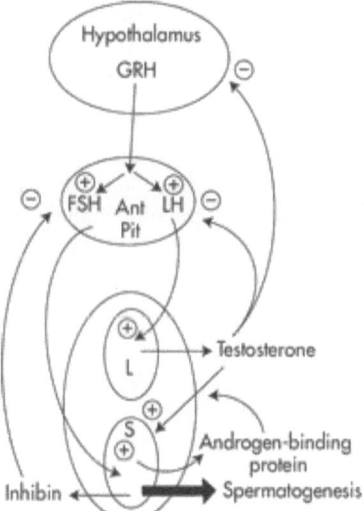

FIGURE 12.4   Control of the testis by the hypothalamus. Gonadotropin-releasing hormone (GRH) causes release of follicle-stimulating hormone (FSH) and luteinising hormone (LH) from the anterior pituitary (Ant Pit) gland. FSH acts on Sertoli cells (S) to promote spermatogenesis and the release of two substances, androgen-binding protein and inhibin. Androgen-binding protein binds testosterone and ensures its concentration needed for sperm production in the Sertoli cells. Inhibin provides a negative feedback system to the anterior pituitary gland, reducing FSH release. LH acts on the Leydig cells (L), promoting the release of testosterone. Testosterone has a double-negative feedback on the anterior pituitary (reducing LH release) and on the hypothalamus (reducing GRH production).

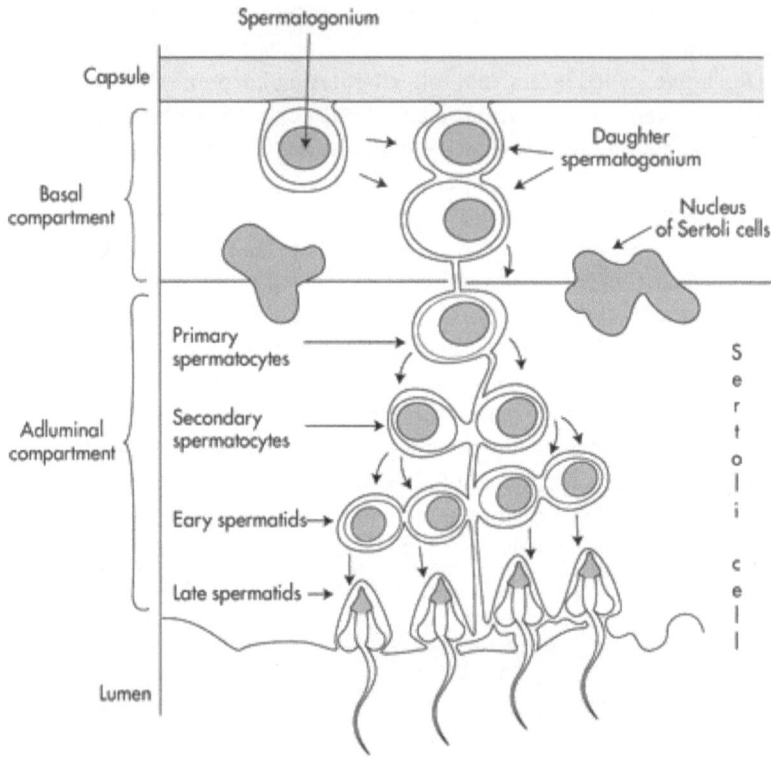

FIGURE 12.5 Sertoli cells nurture sperm production in the seminiferous tubules of the testis. Spermatogonia in the basal compartment divide to form daughter cells. One goes on into the adluminal compartment to further divide into four early spermatids. These will become sperm, which break free in the lumen of the tubule.

Source: Marieb and Hoehn (2022).

Benign prostatic hyperplasia (BPH)

This is a problem experienced by a relatively large number of men in their late middle age or old age. Approximately 50% of males show evidence of the problem by 50 years of age, and 75% of men by 80+ years. BPH is an increase in the size of the prostate gland due to an overgrowth of the cells forming nodules in the periurethral transitional zone (Figure 12.3). This overgrowth encroaches on the urethra and interrupts urine flow. It is generally benign, but some cases may go on to malignancy. The hyperplasia is due to the conversion of testosterone to another hormone, called **dihydrotestosterone (DHT)**, by the enzyme **5α-reductase** (Figure 12.6). Dihydrotestosterone binds to androgen receptors in cells within the transitional zone of the prostate and promotes cell growth there. The symptoms of urinary obstruction are:

- **Hesitancy**, a delay between trying to start urination and the actual flow of urine, which can be a considerable time delay
- **Retention of urine**, that is, incomplete emptying of the bladder
- **Urgency**, the need to pass urine urgently

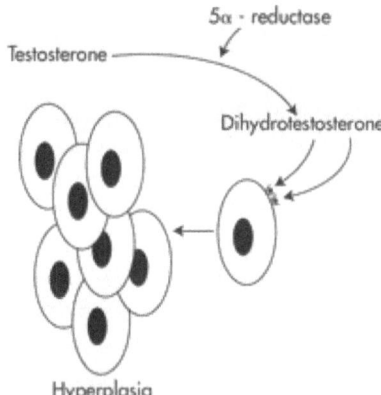

FIGURE 12.6   The conversion of testosterone to dihydrotestosterone by the enzyme 5α-reductase is a factor in prostate gland cells going into hyperplasia.

- **Frequency**, passing urine more than seven times per day
- **Nocturia**, passing urine at regular intervals throughout the night and disturbing sleep

There is a need to exclude prostatic cancer first as the possible cause of the symptoms, even though most men with BPH do not develop malignancy. Treatment options include medication to improve urine flow (**alpha-adrenoceptor blockers**) and medication to block the enzyme that converts testosterone to DHT to shrink the prostate (**5α reductase inhibitors**). Surgical removal of the gland (a **prostatectomy**) or re-establishment of the urethral passage through the prostate is a treatment option for those men where the condition has become urgent (acute urinary retention) or that medication does not help.

Prostate cancer

Cancer of the prostate ranks high in the list of cancer deaths in males over 50 years of age. About 12% of males develop prostate cancer. Most tumours (about 70%) develop from the peripheral zone of the gland (Figure 12.3), with only 25% within the transitional zone, and 5% within the central zone. Peripheral zone tumours cause less urinary obstruction symptoms than hyperplasia, and they are more susceptible to palpation via rectal examination of the prostate. Symptoms of prostate cancer are similar to those of BPH (see 'Benign prostatic hyperplasia (BPH)', p. 234), and this is a good reason to have any symptoms investigated. In addition to the urinary symptoms identified under BPH, the following may also be present:

- Blood in the urine or semen
- Erectile dysfunction
- Unexplained back pain
- Unexplained loss of weight, anorexia, fatigue, and swelling of the feet
- Pain in the hips that may be caused by metastases in advanced prostate cancer

Diagnosis is likely to involved prostate examination, various scans, and specific blood tests to identify markers for the disease in the blood. Tumour marker blood tests are:

1. **Prostate-specific antigen (PSA)** is a glycoprotein normally found in the **endoplasmic reticulum (ER)** (see Figure 1.1, Chapter 1, p. 3) of prostatic cells but released into the blood serum in increased quantities in disease of the gland. The normal PSA in serum is 4 ng/ml (nanograms per millilitre) but can be raised up to 60% in patients with prostate cancers and up to 40% of those with benign hyperplasia. If the PSA test is positive, it may be followed up with a PCA3 urine test. The *PCA3* gene (see 'PCA3, chromosome 9', Addendum, p. 351) is present in prostate cells, and these normally produce only trace quantities of a non-coding RNA molecule. Prostate cancer cells produce between 60% and 100% more of this RNA molecule. The PCA3 test therefore acts as a biomarker for prostate cancer and is more specific than the PSA test.
2. **Prostate screening EpiSwitch** (PSE) is a new blood test still in development which appears to raise the diagnostic accuracy to 94% when used in combination with the PSA test. PSE detects abnormal, cancer-specific chromosome conformations in circulation.
3. **Prostate-specific acid phosphatase** is another marker found in the lysosomes of prostate cells and released into the blood in disease of the gland. It may be raised in 60% of patients with cancer, and 80% of those with bone metastases show raised levels of prostate-specific acid phosphatase.

Prostate cancers are mostly **adenocarcinomas**, that is, derived from glandular tissue that produces the prostatic fluid. They fall into a wide range of behaviour patterns, from those that show no signs of their presence and may only be found at post-mortem to those that are very aggressive and spread widely, often causing the death of the patient. The prognosis in each case can be assessed from the grading of the tumour (Cancer Research UK 2022a). Those that are graded as poorly differentiated tumours tend to grow and spread quickly, whilst those that are well-differentiated tumours progress more slowly.

Other forms of prostate cancer are derived from:

- **Transitional cells** than line the urinary tract through the prostate gland and mostly start in the bladder before invading the prostate.
- **Squamous cells** that cover the prostate. These grow quickly and spread.
- **Small cells** which are a type of neuroendocrine cell (see footnote 3, Chapter 8, p. 180).

Staging of these tumours uses the **tumour, node, metastasis (TNM)** system (Cancer Research UK 2022b).

Testicular cancer

Germ cell neoplasia in situ (GCNIS) describes abnormal cells present on the inner lining of the seminiferous tubules. About 50% of these will go on to develop invasive carcinoma. More than 90% of all testicular cancers arise from the **germ cells** (see 'Spermatogenesis', p. 232). Apart from leukaemia and lymphoma, testicular cancers are the commonest malignant disease in men aged between 15 and 34 years, the time of highest testosterone levels, and most of these cancers have the potential to cause metastases if not found early. Self-examination of the testes is an important step forward in the early detection of cancer (Figure 12.7).

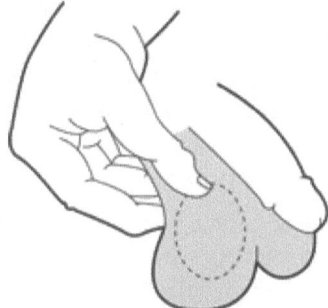

FIGURE 12.7   Self-examination of the testis. The testis should be felt by rolling the fingers over its entire surface to check for enlargement or lumps. Comparison with the other side will help establish what is normal or not. If in doubt, seek advice from a doctor.

Tumours of the testes are not easy to classify because of the variations of tissue types and cell mixtures that occur. They fall broadly into three main categories based on the cell they originate from: (a) germ cell tumours (about 90% of all testicular cancers), divided into seminomas and non-seminomas; (b) sex cord–stromal tumours (about 2% of all testicular cancers); and (c) others, including secondaries, that is, metastases from primary tumours at other sites.

Germ cell tumours

Male germ cells, known as **spermatogonia** (see 'Spermatogenesis', p. 232), are the cells from which the sperm originate within the seminiferous tubules. Tumours can develop from these cells since they are naturally rapidly reproducing cells and they are vulnerable to the effects of radiation. These tumours can be divided into those derived from GCNIS, that is, seminomas, and those of non-GCNIS origin, that is, non-seminomas, and others, for example, malignant lymphoma and adenomatoid tumour.

- **Seminomas** (or **germinomatous, seminomatous,** or **germinomas**), about 50–60% of all germ cell tumours, are the male equivalent of the female ovarian dysgerminomas (see Table 11.5, Chapter 11, p. 221). They are referred to as **classical** (or **typical**), accounting for more than 90% of seminomas, and arise mostly in men between the ages of 30 and 50 years. They consist of sheets of primitive-looking germ cells forming a well-defined mass.
- **Non-seminomas** (**non-germinomatous** or **non-seminomatous**), about 10% of all germ cell tumours, are *not* derived from GCNIS.

  1. **Teratomas** are composed of multiple different cell types. They are caused by abnormal pluripotent, germ cell, and embryonic cell development. They occur most frequently in testes of young men (pre-puberty) and in female ovaries (see Table 11.5, Chapter 11, p. 221). The risk of teratoma of the testes is higher in men with a history of undescended testes. They are not as aggressive as post-puberty tumours, with less chance of spread and with good prognosis. Teratomas often produce markers, such as **alpha-fetoprotein**

or **human chorionic gonadotropin**, which can be monitored to assess the extent of the tumour and progress of the treatment.
2. **Spermatocytic** account for about 5% of seminomas and arise in men around 55 years of age or older. Spermatocytic seminomas are large lesions containing sheets of cells of mixed sizes. They are less aggressive than other tumours, with low risk of spread.

Germ cell tumours usually begin as a painless swelling of one testis (rarely both). The spread of germ cell tumours is first into the retroperitoneal lymph nodes, that is, behind the peritoneum, around the abdominal aorta and iliac regions, then to the supradiaphragmatic lymph nodes, that is, those above the diaphragm, in an **ipsilateral** manner, that is, on the same side as the tumour. Spread can then be into the blood to the liver, bone, and lung.

Sex cord–stromal tumours

These tumours are rare, only 2% of all testicular cancers, and although they can occur at any age, about 40% are found in children. **Sex cords** are the original embryonic cords of cells that, in the adult, form the tissues that house the ova and sperm cells; in females, these are the follicles, and in males, they are the seminiferous tubules. These tumours are a mix of sex cord cells with stromal (connective tissue) cells. The tumour can cause **gynaecomastia**, that is, male breast development, in children below puberty or in men over 50 years of age, and 40% of these tumours can be aggressively malignant. **Leydig** and **Sertoli cell tumours** are types of sex cord cancer. The mass is composed of Leydig or Sertoli cells (see 'Spermatogenesis', and Figure 12.4, p. 233) in sheets or mesh form. They often do not spread and may be treated by surgery.

Others

Malignant lymphoma is the commonest testicular cancer in men over 55 years of age. They are mostly non-Hodgkin lymphomas (see 'Non-Hodgkin lymphoma', Chapter 7, p. 144). There is testicular enlargement, about 60% in one testis, 40% in both. The tumour will infiltrate into the testis. **Adenomatoid tumours** occur mostly in the epididymis of men aged 30–40 years. The first sign is a small lump of 1–2 cm just above the testis. They tend to be benign. The **gonadoblastoma** is a mix of germ cell tumour elements with sex cord cancer components within separate compartments of the tumour. It occurs mostly in men below the age of 20 years who may also have a mix of other male developmental and gender problems.

Surgical removal of the diseased testis (**orchidectomy**) is an important first step in the treatment, particularly since the testes are, in surgical terms, relatively easy to get to. Chemotherapy as a follow-up treatment for any spread of the disease is the usual course.

The staging used for testicular cancers is usually as follows:

0 Germ cell neoplasia in situ (GCNIS), that is, abnormal cells confined to seminiferous tubules. Not actual cancer, but sometimes it may develop into invasive cancer.
1 First stage of cancer, which is not found outside the testis.
2 Cancer spread to lymph nodes in the pelvis or abdomen.
3 Cancer has spread to other organs.

Penile cancer

Squamous carcinomas account for most invasive penile tumours, which are rare in the Western world but more common in parts of Asia, Africa, and Latin America. The disease is closely associated with uncircumcised males; circumcision reduces the risk dramatically, especially if circumcision is carried out at an early age. **Phimosis**, the inability to retract the foreskin, increases the risk further. It is also associated with sexually transmitted **human papillomavirus (HVP)** infection (see 'The virion', Chapter 4, p. 59). The tumour may develop as a mass extending from the **glans penis** or the **prepuce** (Figure 12.1) or as an ulcerating lesion infiltrating into the penis. Excision of the lesion means the loss of part, or all, of the penis.

Key points

Hormones

- The male hormones are androgens: testosterone (the most potent), dehydroepiandrosterone (DHEA), and androstenedione.
- Testosterone binds to androgen receptors (AR) in AR-positive cells.
- Any male tumour that is AR+ will grow faster with androgen stimulation.

The reproductive system

- The testes produce both sperm (spermatogenesis) and testosterone.
- The testis is divided into lobules, each lobule containing a seminiferous tubule where spermatogenesis happens.
- Testes must descend through the inguinal canal to a position within the scrotum prior to birth.
- Undescended testes increase the risk of testicular cancer in later life.
- The prostate lies immediately below the urinary bladder and is made up of the central zone, the transitional zone, and the peripheral zone.
- Sperm are produced in the seminiferous tubules from germ cells called spermatogonia.
- Leydig cells produce testosterone. They are controlled from the anterior pituitary gland by luteinising hormone, also called interstitial cell–stimulating hormone (ICSH) in males.
- Sertoli cells line the seminiferous tubules and are under follicle-stimulating hormone (FSH) control from the anterior pituitary gland.
- The Sertoli cells regulate spermatogenesis and provide nutrition to the germ cells. They also form the blood–testis barrier.
- The Sertoli cells produce inhibin, which provides a negative feedback mechanism to the anterior pituitary, regulating the release of FSH.
- Sertoli cells also produce androgen-binding protein that binds testosterone, essential for spermatogenesis.

Prostatic hyperplasia

- Benign nodular prostatic hyperplasia occurs in late middle or old age in men.
- This is an enlargement of the prostate due to excess cells forming nodules in the periurethral transitional zone, which then encroaches on the urethra.
- This can cause urinary retention.
- Symptoms include frequency and urgency in micturition and nocturia.

Prostatic cancer

- Prostate cancers are mostly adenocarcinomas.
- About 70% of cancers develop in the peripheral zone of the gland.

- Two tumour markers are useful diagnostic tools, prostate-specific antigen (PSA) and prostate-specific acid phosphatase.
- The normal PSA in serum is 4 ng/ml but can be raised in up to 60% of patients with prostate cancers and up to 40% of those with benign nodular hyperplasia.

Testicular cancer

- More than 90% of all testicular cancers arise from the germ cells.
- Testicular cancers are the commonest malignant disease in men aged 15–34 years.
- Self-examination of the testes is an important step forward in the early detection of this cancer.
- Orchidectomy is usually the first-line treatment.

Penile cancers

- Squamous carcinomas account for the majority of invasive tumours of the penis.
- The uncircumcised penis, and particularly phimosis, carries a higher risk of penile cancer.
- A higher risk occurs with a human papillomavirus (HVP) infection.

Note

1 Compare this with the production of ova in women at the rate of one from each ovary per month.

13

SKIN CANCER

- **Introduction: anatomy and functions of the skin**
- **Neoplastic diseases of the skin**
- **Malignant melanoma**
- **Malignant non-melanomas**
- **Vascular tumours**
- **Lipoma and liposarcoma**
- **Key points**

Introduction: anatomy and function of the skin

The skin, also known as the **integumentary system**, is the largest organ of the body. It accounts for 16% of the body weight, is between 1.5 and 2 m² in area, and averages between 2 mm and 3 mm in thickness. In some specific places, such as the soles of the feet, it is often thicker.

Structure and function of the skin

There are two major divisions of the skin, the outer **epidermis** and the deeper **dermis**.

The epidermis has five layers of cells, which are the same cells that begin in the deepest layers and migrate slowly towards the surface. The five layers, starting with the deepest layer, are (Figure 13.1):

1. **Stratum germinativum**, the deepest layer, rests directly on top of the dermis. The basal cells, next to the dermis, are constantly dividing by **mitosis**, that is, standard cell division. From here, cells migrate upwards away from the dermis.
2. **Stratum spinosum** ('spiny layer'), where the cells from the stratum germinativum undergo some cytoplasmic shrinking and many continue to divide.
3. **Stratum granulosum** ('grainy layer'), where cells from the stratum spinosum no longer divide. They produce a fibrous protein called **keratin** (called **keratinisation**). The cell membranes get thicker, and movement of substances across these membranes becomes difficult

DOI: 10.4324/9781003389125-13

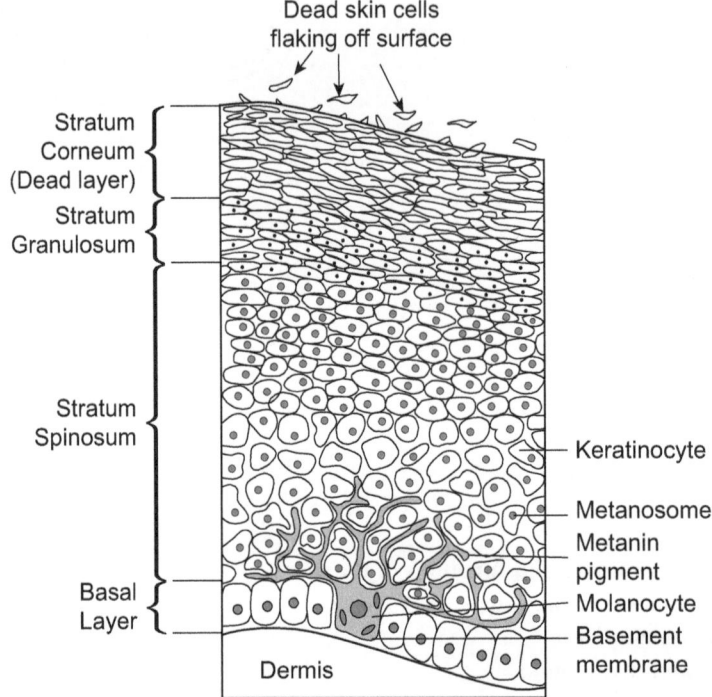

FIGURE 13.1 Section through the epidermis. Melanocytes occur in the deepest layers. They produce a pigment called melanin that is packaged in melanosomes. These melanosomes infiltrate into the keratinocytes and help protect them from sunlight during the early stages of their migration towards the surface. During this migration, the cells flatten and die and fill with keratin.

Source: From Blows (2024).

and gradually declines. Finally, the nucleus and organelles of the cells disintegrate, and the cells die, their cytoplasm filled with keratin. They are then called **keratinocytes**. Towards the upper limits of the layer, the cells begin to flatten out and pack closer together as they dehydrate. This is now effectively a layer of dry keratin.

4. **Stratum lucidum** is a glassy layer of densely packed keratinised cells derived from the stratum granulosum and only found in thick skin areas, for example, the sole of the foot.
5. **Stratum corneum** is the outermost layer, the surface of the skin. These keratinised dead cells, derived either directly from stratum granulosum or via stratum lucidum, form a protective layer for the deeper parts of the skin. Flakes of dead keratin are being shed from the surface all the time, that is, about 30,000 flakes shed per minute. This outer layer is therefore dead tissue.

The epidermis is basically a cell 'escalator', with newly evolved cells in the stratum germinativum moving up through the layers and becoming flat, dead, keratinised cell remnants in the stratum corneum. The epidermis is constantly being replaced with new cells from below. It takes anything from 15 to 30 days for cells to move through the epidermis, and they remain as dead cells on the surface for a further two weeks before being shed into the environment.

Other important cells exist at specific layers of the epidermis:

- **Melanocytes** in the stratum germinativum (Figure 13.1) are pigmentation cells producing the dark-brown pigment **melanin** from the dietary amino acid **tyrosine**. Melanin is packed inside vesicles called **melanosomes**, which are transported into keratinocytes. This protects vital cell structures, for example, the nucleus, against harmful exposure to ultraviolet (UV) light in sunlight as the keratinocytes migrate towards the surface. Eventually, the melanosomes are destroyed as the keratinocyte nucleus degrades and the cells die. The differences between light and dark skin are simply that dark skin has larger melanosomes and the melanin levels are higher and persist for longer than in light skin. The concentration of melanocytes in the epidermis is about 1,000 per mm^2, but this doubles in more heavily pigmented areas of the body, such as the nipples, labia, and scrotum.
- **Langerhans cells** in the stratum spinosum are immune cells able to kill microorganisms from the environment that have penetrated into the epidermis. The skin surface has its own ecosystem of microorganisms consisting of bacteria, yeasts, and viral agents. Each square inch (6.5 cm^2) has approximately 50 million bacteria, a figure that rises to 500 million in areas of skin subjected to rich, oily secretions. On the surface, they are harmless to the skin because they are incapable of causing harm to the dead, keratinised outer layer. But should they penetrate deeper, they may cause infection. Langerhans cells are an important part of our protection against these deeper organisms.

Epidermal growth, that is, the growth of new cells in the stratum germinativum, is promoted by a protein hormone called **epidermal growth factor (EGF)**. EGF is found in some glands of the body, for example, submandibular and parotid salivary glands, and in most body secretions, for example, blood plasma, tears, saliva, urine, and breast milk. It has a range of functions throughout the body, notably within the mucosal lining of the digestive system. In the skin, it promotes growth and cellular differentiation by increasing cell division and keratin production and is an important factor in wound healing. The layer beneath the epidermis is the **dermis**, which is subdivided into two main layers (Figure 12.2).

The outer layer of the dermis is called the **stratum papillare** and is made from **areolar connective tissue** (see 'Connective tissues', Chapter 1, p. 11). Areolar connective tissue contains random collagen fibres, elastic fibres (called **elastin**), and reticular fibres, with small blood vessels, nerve endings, and some open spaces. The junction between the epidermis and the dermis is folded into **dermal papillae**, that is, extensions of the stratum papillare that push upwards into the basal area of the stratum germinativum (Figure 12.2). Dermal papillae contain blood vessels that mark the closest extension of the blood supply to the skin surface.[1] Dilation and constriction of the blood vessels within the papillae, being so close to the skin surface, affect heat loss (dilation) or heat conservation (constriction), part of the body's temperature control system. Some dermal papillae contain **Meissner's corpuscles**, which are sensory nerve endings for the purpose of touch (Table 13.1).

The inner layer of the dermis, the **stratum reticulare**, contains **collagen** fibres in bundles for strength, and **elastin**. **Fibroblasts** are embedded in this matrix, that is, cells for the production of protein fibres, and **macrophages**, that is, specialised cells of the immune system. There are also patches of **adipocytes**, that is, fat cells.

There are additional embedded structures within the dermis (Figure 13.2). These are:

1. **Sweat glands**, which produce sweat from blood plasma. Sweat is released onto the skin surface and contains water, salts, and some urea.
2. **Hair follicles** containing hairs, which grow and protect various body areas. They have **sebaceous glands** attached which secrete **sebum**, an oily fluid that lubricates the hair shaft.
3. **Nails**, which are made from the same dead keratin protein as epidermal keratinocytes but are more densely packed for strength.
4. Nerve endings, making the skin a vital sensory organ (Table 13.1).

Beneath the dermis is the **subcutaneous** tissue, also called the **hypodermis**. It is made from some **areolar** connective tissue with a variable amount of **adipose** (fat) tissue made from **adipocytes**. The dense adipose areas act as an energy store, provide insulation against heat loss, and have a protective role against skin impacts, that is, as a shock absorber. Within the outermost section of the hypodermis, immediately below the dermis, there is a network of larger arteries and veins, the **cutaneous plexus**, that supplies blood to the dermis above.

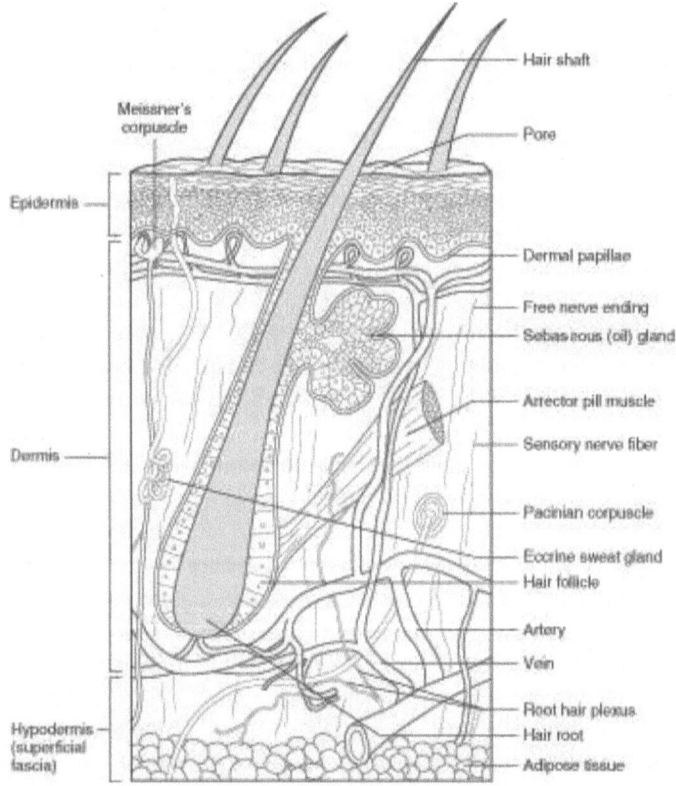

FIGURE 13.2 Section through the skin showing the epidermis, dermis, and hypodermis. Sweat glands, hair roots, and sebaceous glands are shown originating in the dermis. Nerve endings are listed and described in Table 12.1.

Source: From Blows (2024).

TABLE 13.1 Sensory nerve endings in the dermis and their functions

Nerve ending in dermis	Notes
Free dendritic nerve endings	Sensitive to pain, heat, cold, and pressure. Found in most body tissues, including the dermis and lower layers of epidermis.
Root hair plexus	Sensitive to hair movement. Found around hair roots.
Merkel cells with tactile discs	Sensitive to touch and light pressure. Found across the dermis–epidermis border.
Meissner's corpuscles	Sensitive to touch, light pressure, and low-frequency vibrations. Found in the dermal papillae, especially over sensitive areas, such as the nipples, external genitalia, fingertips, and eyelids.
Krause's end bulb	A modified Meissner's corpuscle. Found in mucous membrane and some skin areas.
Pacinian corpuscles	Sensitive to deep pressure, stretching, and high-frequency vibrations. Found in the subcutaneous tissues of the skin, especially on the fingers, feet, external genitalia, and nipples, and also some deeper tissues.
Ruffini's corpuscles	Sensitive to deep pressure and stretching. Found in the dermis and subcutaneous tissues and joint capsules.

The functions of the skin

The skin functions are as follows:

1. It is a barrier against microorganisms, a major part of our **non-specific** immune system (see 'Innate (non-specific) immunity', Chapter 5, p. 78). It is non-specific because it does not distinguish between one type of organism or another. Almost all organisms from the environment, that is, bacteria, most viruses, and fungi, are incapable of penetrating intact skin.
2. The skin is the body's vital touch sensory organ. The rich supply of nerve endings in the skin provides a wide range of sensations, including touch, pain, temperature, and pressure (Figure 13.2 and Table 13.1).
3. The skin is an important excretory organ, allowing the controlled loss of salts, water, and organic wastes, for example, **urea**, through sweat glands.
4. The skin is part of the temperature regulation mechanism since heat is lost through the skin. The deeper layers of the skin often have fat present, and this provides some insulation against the cold.
5. The skin stores some nutrients, for example, lipids in fat cells.
6. It carries out synthesis of vitamin D_3 (**cholecalciferol**) (Figure 13.3). Vitamin D deficiency has been shown to cause several disorders, notably disruption of bone development, **rickets** in children, and **osteomalacia** in adults. But now, vitamin D deficiency has been shown to increase the risk of skin cancers of all types (Kanasuo et al. 2022). Taking daily vitamin D supplements by mouth during long periods of little sun, for example, winter, is an important habit to keep.
7. Skin provides physical protection to underlying structures.
8. It is also a water resistance barrier, but it is *not* waterproof. There is a difference. Rain will drip off the skin (water resistance), but long-term soaking in water will cause the skin to become waterlogged (lack of waterproof).

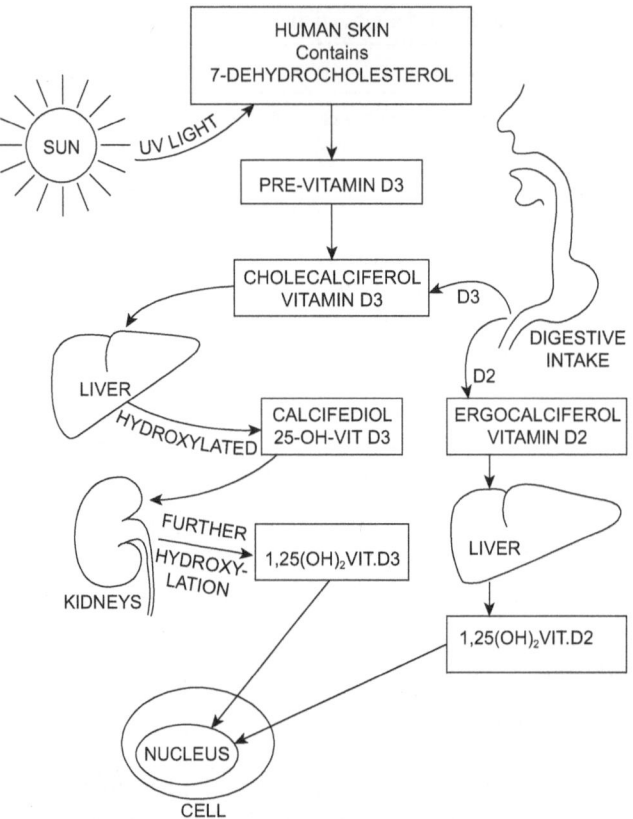

FIGURE 13.3 The production of vitamin D from diet and the skin exposed to sunlight.

Neoplastic disorders of the skin

New growths of various kinds occur on the skin throughout life, but the great majority of them are benign and harmless (Table 13.2). Skin cancers are divided into **melanomas** and **non-melanomas**. Some start off as benign but may turn malignant later in life. Less often, some may begin as malignant. The link between sun exposure and skin cancers is well known (see 'Background radiation', Chapter 3, p. 54), and every effort should be taken to protect the skin, when possible, to keep sun exposure and other ultraviolet (UV) sources to a minimum. Just one sunburn event every two years can triple the risk of skin cancer. UV light is composed of UVA, UVB, and UVC. It is only carcinogenic for the skin since it does not penetrate any deeper than the skin, but it does affect three skin cell types: melanocytes, squamous cells, and basal cells. UVA penetrates deeper than UVB, that is, UVA affects the skin as deep as the dermis, whilst UVB affects cells of the epidermis. UVC rarely reaches the ground since it is filtered out by the ozone layer (Figure 13.4) (Pecorino 2021).

Cells damaged by UV light usually resort to apoptosis, that is, cell death, and this is seen as skin peeling after a sunburn. The gene *Tp53* regulates apoptosis, and mutations of *Tp53* that prevent apoptosis as an option occur mostly in non-melanomas. These cells then proliferate into a tumour. Excessive exposure to ultraviolet (UV) sunlight, especially UVA, mostly affects those

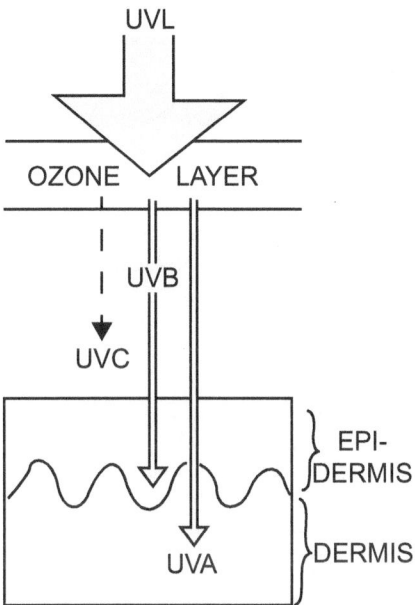

FIGURE 13.4   UV light penetration of the skin. The depth of penetration of UV light (UVL) into the skin is dependent on the wavelength. Long wavelength penetrates further than short wavelength. UVL contains UVA, UVB, and UVC. Most of the UVC (100–290 nm) is absorbed by the ozone layer. UVA (320–400 nm) reaches the dermis, whilst UVB (290–320 nm) penetrates the epidermis.

having fair or red hair and pale skin. They have a higher risk of developing the disease than darker-skinned people (McCance and Heuther 2019).

Malignant melanoma

This is a cancer of the pigment-producing cells, the melanocytes (see 'Melanocytes', p. 243), mostly within the skin. In people aged 25–39, melanoma is the third most common cancer. Most of these cases could be prevented by taking more precautions in sunlight (see 'Background radiation', Chapter 3, p. 54).

An aggregation of melanocytes in the skin is called a **nevus** (or **mole**) (Table 13.3). Most nevi are no problem, but occasionally, one may change to become malignant. The average white person is said to have about 12 pigmented naevi, any of which could become malignant.

More than half of melanomas develop from a pre-existing skin lesion, like a **nevus**. Any changes in a nevus, for example, changes in size, colour, or shape, should be reported to a doctor as soon as possible (Tables 13.3).

There are two ways in which melanomas grow: (1) *radially*, called **radial growth phase (RGP)**, that is, growth is outwards in all directions from the central point, and (2) *vertically*, called **vertical growth phase (VGP)**, that is, growth extends deep into the lower half of the dermis. These two distinctions in growth are accompanied by differences in the type and behaviour of the malignant cells.

TABLE 13.2 Skin lesions

Skin lesion	Description
Bulla (blister)	Similar to vesicle (this table), but larger, that is, greater than 5 mm diameter, and fluid-filled.
Cyst	An encapsulated cavity lined with epithelium within the skin, containing semi-solid material or fluid.
Macule	Localised patch of different skin colour, either darker or lighter than the surrounding skin. Some are normal, for example, freckles, but others indicate skin changes. Usually less than 1 cm in diameter.
Mole (nevus)	A lesion formed from melanocytes accumulating at the basal epidermal layer, forming a macule. Migration into the dermis causes the area to become nodular and palpable (Table 13.3).
Nodule	Larger than a papule, that is, larger than 5 mm in diameter. They can be solid or a fluid-filled raised lump within any skin layer.
Papule	Small solid raised lump less than 5 mm in diameter, for example, a wart.
Plaque	A palpable, slightly raised, flat-topped patch of skin more than 1 cm in diameter but usually below 5 mm in height.
Pustule	A visible collection of pus within a blister formation on the skin surface.
Scale	A thick layer of keratin loosely attached to the skin that can detach easily.
Ulcer	An open cavity, or erosion, that is, a circumscribed area of skin loss, extending into the dermis or deeper.
Vesicle	A small blister, less than 5 mm in diameter, filled with clear fluid occurring within or below the skin.
Wheal	A patch of dermal erythema, slightly raised with local oedema, seen in urticaria.

TABLE 13.3 The ABCDE of nevi (mole) changes that require medical attention

A	Asymmetrical in shape
B	Border irregularity
C	Colour variation
D	Diameter larger than 6 mm
E	Elevation

The types of melanomas are:

- **Superficial spreading melanoma (SSM)** is the most common melanoma (about 67% of cases) and is mostly diagnosed in middle age. Initially, it spreads across the skin surface, that is, RGP is present, and it only becomes a risk of spreading to other organs when it invades the deeper skin layers. Genes have also been linked to this form of melanoma (Table 13.4). The *BRAF* gene (see 'Chromosome 7', Addendum, p. 348) is found in about 50% of all melanomas.
- **Nodular melanoma (NM)** grows quickly and penetrates deeper skin layers at an early stage. RGP is absent; it is only VGP. It appears as a very dark, raised lesion in skin areas most often exposed to sunlight.
- **Lentigo maligna melanoma (LMM)** grows slowly along surface skin layers, that is, RGP is present, from flat patches of brown skin called **lentigo maligna**, or **Hutchinson's melanotic freckle**. Gradually, it may change shape and get larger, forming nodules in deeper

TABLE 13.4 Genes linked to melanomas

Gene	Locus	SSM	NM	LMM	ALM	AM	Page
BRAF	7q34	√		√	√	√	348
NRAS	1p13.2	√		√	√		342
CDKN2A	9p21.3	√	√		√		350
NK1	4p16.3	√					346
CDK4	12q14.1	√	√				353
KIT	4q12			√			346
MC1R	16q24.3		√			√	356
MITF	3p13		√			√	345
TYR	11q14.3					√	352
TERT	5p15.33		√				347
ACD	16q22.1		√				356
BAP1	3p21.1		√				345
TP53	17p13.1			√			356
POT1	7q31.33		√				349
TERF2IP	16q23.1		√				356
NF1	17q11.2				√		356
CCND1	11q13.3				√		352
FGF19	11q13.3				√		353

skin layers. It is mostly seen in the elderly in areas most often exposed to sunlight, such as the face. The most important genes linked to LMM are shown in Table 13.4.

- **Acral lentiginous melanoma (ALM)** is a rare (about 4% of cases) skin cancer seen mostly in the palm of hands and soles of the feet in dark-skinned individuals. It has flat margins that slowly grow by RGP and increase in size.
- **Amelanotic melanoma (AM)** is a rare, colourless cancer and often overlooked because it is mistaken for other benign lesions.

Mutations of the *BRAF* gene are found in 66% of melanomas. This and other genes linked to these melanomas are shown in Table 13.4.

Malignant non-melanomas

Basal cell carcinoma (BCC) (also known as **rodent ulcer**) often appears as an ulcer which does not heal. It has few symptoms and is very slow-growing, having a very low risk of spread to other organs. The most important genes linked to BCC are listed in Table 13.5.

Squamous cell carcinoma (SCC) (also known as **epidermoid carcinoma**) is an aggressive cancer that appears initially as a skin sore that does not heal or a lump in the skin that grows quickly. It usually grows from skin areas damaged by sun exposure or areas associated with a skin would or ulcer. Spread to lymph nodes will occur quickly if not treated. The most important genes associated with SCC are shown in Table 13.5.

Merkel cell carcinoma (MCC) is a rare but aggressive, and often dangerous, cancer of the skin, usually of the head, face, or neck, that begins in the Merkel cells at the base of the epidermis (Figure 13.1, Table 13.1). It appears as a rapidly growing, painless nodule, mostly in people over 50 years of age. It is sometimes caused by the virus **Merkel cell polyomavirus (MCPyV)**, 1 of

TABLE 13.5 Genes linked to BCC and SCC

Gene	Locus	BCC	SCC	Page number
PTCH1	9q22.32	√	√	351
PTCH2	1p34.1	√	√	342
MMP1	11q22.2		√	353
MMP10	11q22.2		√	353
GATA3	10p14		√	351
POU2F3	11q23.3		√	353
BAP1	3p21.1	√		345
MC1R	16q24.3	√		356
TP53	17p13.1	√	√	356

14 species of polyomavirus that can infect humans. Treatment is with the drug *avelumab* (see Table 5.5, Chapter 5, p. 103), which is started at the earliest possible stage.

Vascular tumours

Haemangioma is a mass of tiny blood vessels that occurs as a red or purple tumour on the skin. It can occur anywhere on the body, developing from endothelial cells in the walls of local blood vessels. The most common sites are the head, neck, and face, especially in children, for example, infantile haemangioma. They may be present at birth, when they are called *birthmarks*. Adults can develop them, especially in the over 75 years of age. There are two types:

- **Capillary type**, which includes **infantile haemangiomas**, or **strawberry haemangiomas**, which occur within the first year of life in about 12% of babies. They tend to reach a maximum size of 2 in (5 cm) in diameter, then fade away by the age of 10 years. A second capillary type are the **cherry haemangiomas**, which are tiny raised red spots found mostly on the chest and back in older adults.
- **Cavernous type** develops in the dermis, especially around the eye. They appear as red or blue patches and can cause problems of the eye, such as glaucoma or cataracts.

Kaposi's sarcoma is a rare vascular cancer of the skin and other tissues and is caused by the **human herpes virus 8** (**HHV8**) (see 'The virion, *HHV8*', Chapter 4, p. 60). It affects mostly those with a weak immune system, such as people with the **human immunodeficiency virus** (**HIV**) (see 'The virion, HIV', Chapter 4, p. 61). It occurs as raised or smooth patches which are red, brown, or purple. They form anywhere on the skin, on mucous membrane, or on internal organs. It can cause complications depending on what body systems get involved, such as lymphoedema when the lymph drainage gets blocked, dyspnoea if the lungs are involved, and constipation, passing blood in the stools, or vomiting of the digestive system is involved. Kaposi's sarcoma can cause anaemia from the bleeding, and also, it can cause spread through metastases to the lymphatic system, causing a lymphoma.

There are four types of Kaposi's sarcoma:

- **Classic** form, also called **Mediterranean sarcoma**, because it is mostly seen in men of Mediterranean or Middle Eastern descent aged over 60 years of age. The skin lesions are usually slow-growing, with internal organ metastases.

- **Endemic** form, also called **African sarcoma**, affecting people of equatorial Africa. The disease is similar to the classic form but is mostly diagnosed at a young age.
- **Acquired** form, a very rare sarcoma of the skin seen in those taking immunosuppressive drugs.
- **Epidemic** form, an AIDS-related sarcoma, is a very rare sarcoma seen in the USA in people with HIV infection or acquired immunodeficiency syndrome (AIDS).

Skin cancer stages

Stage 0: Cancer cells in top layer of skin, that is, carcinoma in situ (Chapter 1, Figure 1.14, p. 18).
Stage 1: Although the tumour has grown, it remains small, and there is no spread to lymph nodes.
Stage 2: Tumour has penetrated to deeper layers or widened without spread to lymph nodes.
Stage 3: Local lymph nodes involved.
Stage 4: Distant lymph nodes and/or other organs involved.

Grades of skin cancers

Grade 1 (lowest grade): The cells look close to normal and are well-differentiated.
Grade 2: The cells are becoming obviously abnormal and less well-differentiated.
Grades 3 and 4 (highest grade): Grossly abnormal cells that are poorly differentiated.

New forms of treatment

- With the advancement of drugs known as **monoclonal antibodies** (**MABs**) (see 'Monoclonal antibodies (MABs)', Chapter 5, p. 102), there is a new drug suitable for treating melanomas, especially in the advanced stage. **Pembrolizumab** is a type of MAB called an **immune checkpoint inhibitor** (**ICI**) (see 'Monoclonal antibodies (MABs) known as immune checkpoint inhibitors (ICIs)' and Table 5.5, Chapter 5, p. 103). It blocks (or inhibits) PD-1, a cancer cell surface protein called a checkpoint that deactivates immune T cells. These T cells would attack and kill the cancer cell, but PD-1 prevents this. By blocking PD-1, this drug allows T cells to continue their activity in killing the cancer cell (Figure 5.19, Chapter 5, p. 105).
- A new vaccine is in development based on a modified form of the anthrax toxin (Bachran and Leppla 2016).

Lipoma and liposarcoma

Lipoma is a benign tumour of fat tissue, that is, adipose, usually positioned between the skin and the underlying muscle (see 'Hypodermis', Figure 13.2, p. 244). About 1% of the population have lipomas. They form a soft, painless swelling which may become noticeable to other people if it is on the face or scalp. Lipomas can last a lifetime. It may gradually increase in size, but it is harmless, unless it gets too big, then it may interfere with activities such as dressing or become unsightly. Surgical removal, if necessary, is usually quick and easy. Any lipoma which grows quickly or becomes red, painful, or hard should be seen by a doctor.

Liposarcoma is a rare malignant tumour of the adipose tissue beneath the skin (see 'Hypodermis', Figure 13.2, p. 244). It starts in the adipoblasts, the primitive precursor cells of the mature fat cells, called adipocytes. It occurs mostly in older people, usually within the abdomen or limbs. The four types of liposarcoma are:

- Well-differentiated liposarcoma (WDLS) accounts for 50% of cases.
- Dedifferentiated liposarcoma (DDLS) is the next stage of development from WDLS.
- Myxoid liposarcoma is mostly found in the limbs.
- Pleomorphic liposarcoma is a fast-growing, very rare tumour.

Symptoms include a painful lump under the skin which is growing. Sometimes they can arise from adipose tissue in the abdomen, behind the peritoneum (retroperitoneal), and are likely to cause abdominal swelling, pain, and symptoms of digestive disturbance, for example, nausea, constipation.

Key points

Structure and function of skin

- Skin has an outer epidermis and a deeper dermis.
- Epidermal cells migrate slowly towards the surface.
- *Melanocytes* are pigmentation cells in the epidermis.
- The dermis contains areolar connective tissue and patches of adipose fat tissue.
- The dermis has hair follicles, sweat glands, nerve endings, and blood vessels.
- Skin functions include part of the temperature control system, a sensory organ, barrier against infection, an excretory organ, and vitamin D production.
- Taking vitamin D supplements during the winter months is important and may reduce your risk of skin cancer.

Skin neoplasms

- The two types of skin cancer are melanomas and non-melanomas.
- Malignant melanoma is a cancer of the epidermal melanocytes.
- Exposure to excessive ultraviolet light A (UVA) is a key risk factor.
- Non-melanomas are squamous cell carcinoma and basal cell carcinoma.
- Genetic mutations have a role in the cause of skin cancers.
- *Haemangioma* is a mass of tiny blood vessels that occurs as a red or purple tumour on the skin.
- *Lipoma* is a benign tumour of fat tissue.

Note

1 The epidermis is mostly blood-free, except the basal stratum germinativum, a good reason that epidermal cells are largely dead – they migrate away from their blood supply.

14

CANCERS OF THE SKELETAL AND NERVOUS SYSTEMS

- The skeleton
- Cancer of the bones
- Bone secondary tumours (metastases)
- The brain
- Primary tumours of the central nervous system (CNS)
- Primary tumours of the peripheral nervous system (PNS)
- Brain secondary tumours
- The meninges
- Symptomology: the symptoms of intracranial tumours
- Brain tumour vaccine
- Cancer neuroscience . . . the *safe harbour hypothesis*
- Key points

The skeleton

Chapter 1 discussed bone tissue (see 'Bone tissue', Chapter 1, p. 12) and identified the various types and constituents of bone.

There are 206 bones in the skeleton, counting those in the ears, that is, three ossicles in each ear. The skeleton is usually divided into:

- The axial skeleton, that is, 80 bones, including:

  - The skull, 22 in total, made from bones of the face (14) and the cranium (8).
  - The throat has 1 bone, the hyoid.
  - The vertebrae, 24 in all, divided into 7 cervical (neck), 12 thoracic (back), 5 lumbar, 1 sacrum, and 1 coccyx.
  - The ribs, 24 in all (12 pairs).
  - The sternum (1).

DOI: 10.4324/9781003389125-14

- The sacrum consists of five vertebrae fused into a single bone, the coccyx consists of four small vertebrae fused into a single bone, and the sternum consists of three bones fused into a single bone.
- The appendicular skeleton, that is, the arms and legs, have 126 bones, including:

  - Phalanges of manus (finger bones), 28, that is, 14 for each hand
  - Phalanges of pes (toe bones), 28, that is, 14 for each foot
  - Metacarpals (hand bones), 10, that is, 5 for each hand
  - Metatarsals (foot bones), 10, that is, 5 for each foot
  - Carpal bones (wrist), 16, that is, 8 for each wrist
  - Tarsal bones (ankle), 14, that is, 7 for each ankle
  - Arm bones, 6, that is, 3 for each arm
  - Leg bones, 8, that is, 4 for each leg, including 2 patellas (kneecaps)
  - Pelvis, 6, including 3 fused bones on each side, that is, left and right pubis, ischium, and ilium

Bones are covered by a membrane called **periosteum**, and this is essential for bone growth and healing.

The functions of the skeleton are as follows:

1. Protects vital organs, for example, the skull protecting the brain and the ribs protecting the lungs
2. Provides a system of joints for the purpose of movement
3. Provides an internal framework for the purpose of weight-bearing
4. Provides for the attachment of muscles
5. Provides a mineral store for the body, mostly calcium
6. Provides a 'home' for bone marrow, which serves to produce blood cells of all kinds (see 'Blood cell formation', Chapter 7, p. 130)

Bone cancer

The skeleton is often subject to bone cancers. Primary bone cancers begin in the bone itself, but the bone is more often the site for secondary metastases derived from soft tissue tumours elsewhere. Secondary bone cancers are more common than primary in adults. The bone has a rich blood supply and a community of active cells, so circulating metastases will be delivered to the bone frequently.

Symptoms of bone cancer include:

- Often no symptoms, that is, asymptomatic, at least during the early stages of the disease.
- Bone pain.
- Swelling of the soft tissue around the tumour. This may be the tumour itself or caused by inflammation.
- Tenderness of the affected area, mostly due to inflammation.
- Weight loss and fatigue.
- Fractures, called **pathological fractures**, which can occur even when very little stress is put on the bone. Both primary and secondary bone tumours can cause the bone to become weak and often break.

Primary bone tumours fall into the following groups:

1. **Osteosarcomas**
2. **Chondrosarcomas**
3. **Ewing sarcoma**

Osteosarcomas (osteogenic sarcomas)

These are the commonest form of malignant bone tumour, particularly in teenagers, with an average age for diagnosis being 15 years of age. Most cases (75%) occur in people less than 25 years of age. The most frequent site for osteosarcoma is around the knee, that is, the lower **femur** and upper **tibia**, but other sites include the upper part of the **humerus** and the **ilium** (Figure 14.1). Males develop this disease more often than females. Some gene mutations play an important role in the cause of this disease, notably *TP53* (see 'Chromosome 17', Addendum, p. 356) and *RB1* (see 'Chromosome 13', Addendum, p. 354).

Osteosarcoma usually begins with a pathological fracture at the site, and on physical and X-ray examination, the bone is enlarged by a mass. The tumour destroys the **cortex** (the outer layer of the bone) and extends both outward into surrounding soft tissues and inwards into the intramedullary canal. Tumours tend to metastasise via the blood early in the course of the disease, with most secondary tumours occurring in the lungs.

Patients over 40 years of age are likely to have developed osteosarcoma as a complication of **Paget's disease** of the bone. Sir James Paget described several diseases in the 1800s that now carry his name (see 'Paget's disease', Table 11.3, Chapter 11, p. 211). Paget's disease of the bone is a disorder of bone reabsorption and formation and is not, in itself, a neoplastic disorder, but an osteosarcoma is sometimes seen as a complication of this disease.

Osteosarcomas are classified as:

- High-grade, fast-growing, with rapid cell division. Cells look abnormal and immature. Mostly seen during teenage and in children. There are several subtypes, including osteoblastic, fibroblastic, and chondroblastic.
- Intermediate-grade, with mixed features of high- and low-grade.
- Low-grade, slow-growing, with normal-looking osteoblastic cells embedded in bone matrix, called osteoid. It often occurs in the femur and tibia and can produce metastases in the lungs and other bones.

Chondrosarcomas

This is a group of diseases that are relatively uncommon. The tumour forms a cartilaginous matrix with embedded abnormal, disorganised chondrocyte cells. This grows on the surface of the bone and forms lesions that infiltrate into the bone. It causes a painful mass, often in the pelvis and upper thigh area, with bone and periosteal destruction. It occurs mostly in middle to late life.

Two forms are:

- **Clear-cell chondrosarcoma** (<2%) is a malignant, immature, and low-grade cartilaginous tumour. It is derived from chondrogenic[1] tissue, mostly of the epiphysis[2] of bones. *Clear-cell* means the chondrocytes have abundant vacuolated[3] cytoplasm.

- **Mesenchymal chondrosarcoma**, an excessive and aggressive growth of cartilage with associated small round densely packed 'blue cells' showing biphasic growth, that is, growth in two phases.

Chondrosarcoma involves mutations of genes *IDH1* (see 'Chromosome 2', Addendum, p. 344) and *IDH2* (see 'Chromosome 15', Addendum, p. 355) in approximately 50% of cases.

Ewing sarcoma

This tumour accounts for 14% of all primary bone sarcomas and 5–10% of all bone tumours. It most often affects teenagers and young adults. The pelvis, femur, and tibia are the bones most often affected (Figure 14.1). It can also affect soft tissues, especially those tissues surrounding

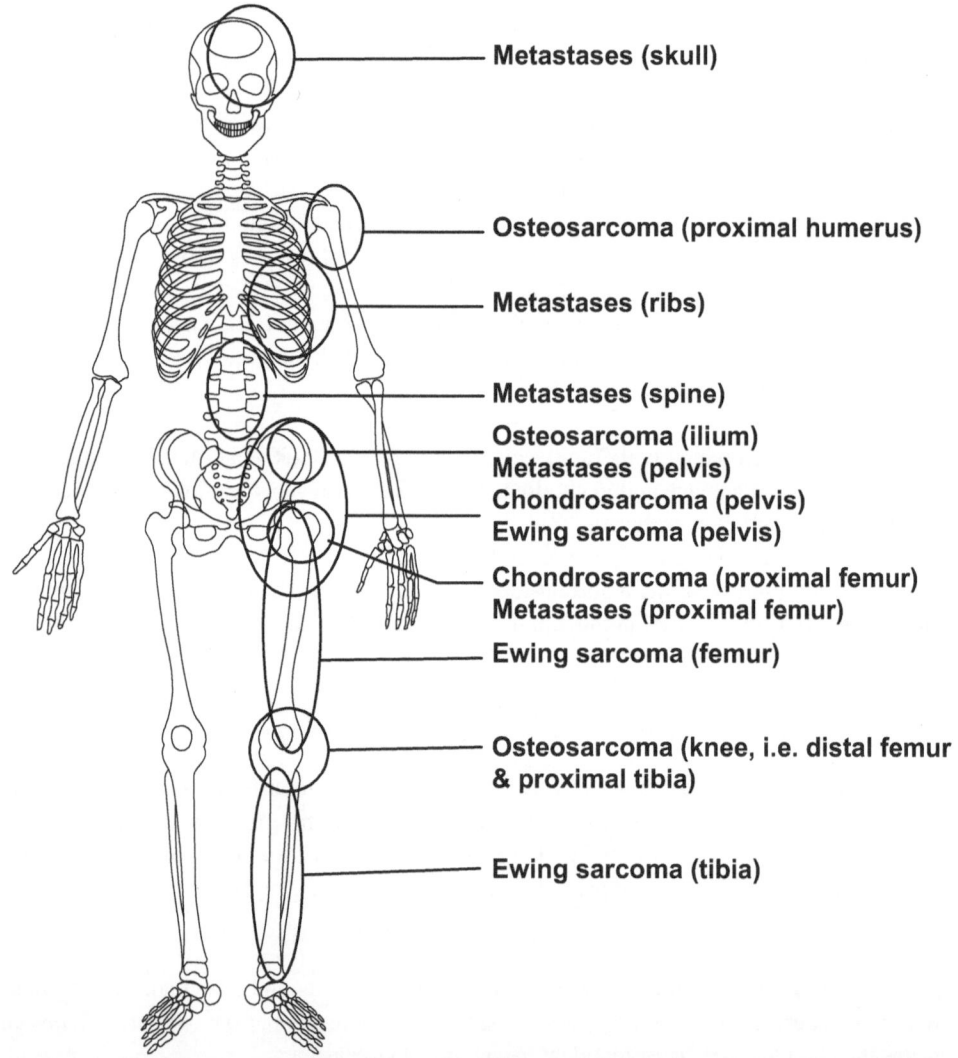

FIGURE 14.1 Commonest skeletal sites of bone cancers.

the affected bone. The tumour consists of sheets of small cells with round nuclei and very little cytoplasm. The cells often undergo cellular death, causing areas of necrosis.

About 85% of cases of Ewing sarcoma are linked to the gene translocation t(11:22) (q24;q12). This results in a fusion between the *EWSR1* gene (see 'Chromosome 22', Addendum, p. 360) and the *FLI1* gene (see 'Chromosome 11', Addendum, p. 353), that is, *EWSR1–FLI1*.

Bone secondary tumours (metastases)

The bone is the third most frequent site for metastatic spread after the liver and the lung (metastases are discussed in Chapter 6). Common sites of primary tumours that cause bone secondary deposits are lung, thyroid, breast, kidney, and prostate (Figure 14.2). Most bone metastases occur in the spine, pelvis, ribs, skull, and proximal femur.

Secondary bone tumours may interfere with the function of normal bone cells, that is, the **osteoclasts** (bone-absorbing cells) and **osteoblasts**[4] (bone-building cells) (see 'Bone tissue', Chapter 1, p. 12):

- **Osteolytic tumours** affect osteoclasts by increasing their reabsorption of bone, causing excess destruction of bone.[5] This creates cavities in the bone, weakening the bone, which then fractures easily, that is, pathological fractures. Osteolytic tumours cause thinning of the bone on X-ray examination, that is, increased **radiolucency**. Most osteolytic secondary tumours arise from primary cancers in the lung, thyroid, and kidney; multiple myeloma (see 'Multiple myeloma', Chapter 7, p. 138); or melanoma (see 'Malignant melanoma', Chapter 13, p. 247).
- **Osteoblastic tumours** affect osteoblasts, causing excessive bone growth. This results in a very dense, hard, brittle bone tumour which will appear dense on X-ray screening. The excess bone formation also raises the blood level of **alkaline phosphatase**. Osteoblastic metastases are usually the result of primary cancer of the prostate, lung, Hodgkin lymphoma (see 'Hodgkin lymphoma', Chapter 7, p. 143), or medulloblastoma (see 'Non-gliomas', p. 260).

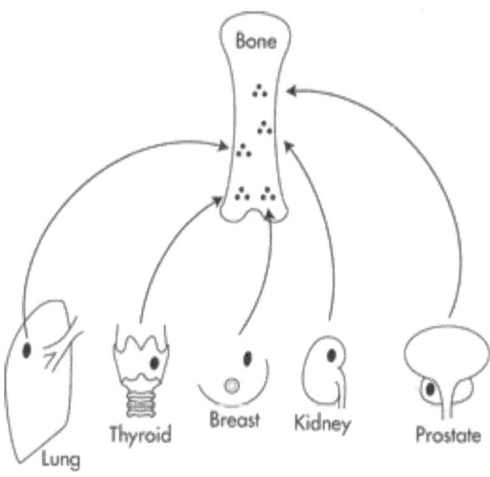

FIGURE 14.2   Bone metastases. The main sites for primary tumours are lung, kidney, breast, thyroid, and prostate.

- Mixed-bone secondaries are those that affect both osteoclasts and osteoblasts, resulting in some patches of bone resorption and other patches of excess bone formation. Mixed secondaries originate mostly from cancers of the breast, testicular and ovarian cancers, squamous cell skin cancers, or gastrointestinal and liver cancers.

Pain is a common feature of these tumours, and the patient will be at risk of pathological fractures, particularly because of osteolytic tumour activity. Bones become so weak they break very easily, with little pressure involved, and are poor at healing.

The brain

The functional cell of the brain is the **neuron** (see Figure 1.13, Chapter 1, p. 16). The supportive tissue of the brain is the **neuroglia**, or **glial cells**, of which **astrocytes** are by far the most numerous. Table 14.1 lists the different types of glial cells.

The nervous system is divided into the **central nervous system (CNS)**, consisting of the brain and the spinal cord, and the **peripheral nervous system (PNS)**. The PNS consists of the nerves coming directly from the brain (cranial nerves) or from the cord (spinal nerves). The function of nerves is to carry impulses, which are either **motor** (controlling muscles for movement) or **sensory** (taking sensations back to the brain) or mixed motor with sensory.

Between the blood and the brain is the **blood–brain barrier**, a system of tight junctions between epithelial cells of the blood vessel. These cells select what can and cannot pass through and enter the brain. They are the least permeable of all the body capillaries (Marieb and Hoehn 2022). This barrier may form a tough challenge for the entry of malignant metastases and may partly be the reason that most metastatic intracranial tumours do not occur inside the brain.

Tumours of the nervous system

CNS tumours are new growths of the brain and spinal cord. PNS tumours are new growths of the nerves and nerve coverings, both **cranial nerves**, directly from the brain, and **spinal nerves**, coming from the spinal cord.

TABLE 14.1 The cells forming the neuroglia (glial cells)

Glial cell	Notes
Astrocyte	Stabilises the tissue environment of the brain; provides nutrition to neurons; processes some neurotransmitters
Oligodendrocyte	Myelination of CNS neurons
Schwann cell	Myelination of PNS neurons
Ependymal cell	Lines the ventricles and ducts of the brain; assists in the formation and flow of CSF
Microglia	Phagocytic cells of the brain
Satellite cell	Nutrient supply to neurons and cushions neuron cells; binds some brain compounds

Note: CNS = central nervous system (brain and spinal cord); CSF = cerebrospinal fluid; PNS = peripheral nervous system (cranial and spinal nerves).

Nervous system tumours are classified according to the tissue they originate from; their location; their cellular, genetic, and molecular composition; and their growth and spread. They are identified as **primary**, that is, starting in the nervous system itself, or **secondary**, that is, arriving as metastases from a primary tumour elsewhere in the body. Intracranial tumours are those that arise inside the skull but outside the brain, that is, sandwiched between the brain and the skull, usually within the meninges.

Primary tumours of the central nervous system (CNS)

Gliomas (about 40–45% of tumours) are a large group of tumours which are derived from glial cells (neuroglia) (Table 14.1). The various types are based on the glial cell of origin:

- **Astrocytomas** are derived from **astrocytes** and are the second commonest form of tumour in the central nervous system (CNS) after glioblastoma. They are graded as:

  1. Grade 1 is slow-growing, well-differentiated, and non-invasive tumour occurring in several subtypes, for example, *pilocytic astrocytoma* and *pleomorphic xantho astrocytoma*.
  2. Grade 2 is a low-grade diffuse astrocytoma.
  3. Grade 3, called *anaplastic astrocytoma*, is a rare and aggressive tumour.
  4. Grade 4 is an aggressive, infiltrating tumour previously known as *glioblastoma multiforme (GBM)*, now usually called *glioblastoma*. It occurs more frequently in men over 60 years of age and carries a poor prognosis.

  Low-grade astrocytomas are more common in children or young adults and rarely spread outside the central nervous system to other tissues.
- **Oligodendrogliomas** are derived from **oligodendrocytes** (Table 14.1). These tumours are more common in childhood, and they often calcify, which means they may show up on X-ray examination. Most are grade 2, that is, slow-growing and responding well to treatment, or grade 3 (**anaplastic oligodendroglioma**), that is, malignant and aggressive, growing and spreading quickly and responding less to treatment.
- **Mixed glioma**, a combination of astrocytoma with oligodendroglioma.
- **Ependymal tumours (ependymomas)** arise from the cells lining the ventricles of the brain and the central canal within the cord. There are five main types of ependymoma in adults. Some of these types are further divided into subtypes based on gene mutations within the tumour. They are graded according to speed of growth, that is, most are grade 2 or 3, but subependymoma is grade 1 (slow-growing), The main types are:

  1. **Posterior fossa ependymoma** occurs in the lower rear part of the brain, the cerebellum and brainstem.
  2. **Supratentorial ependymoma** occurs in the upper part of the brain, the cerebrum.
  3. **Spinal cord ependymoma** occurs in the spinal cord.
  4. **Subependymoma** occurs in any part of the brain or spinal cord and is usually slow-growing, that is, grade 1.
  5. **Myxopapillary ependymoma** occurs in the lower part of the spinal cord and is slow-growing.

- **Paediatric-type diffuse low-grade and high-grade gliomas.** Diffuse *low-grade* paediatric glioma includes:

  1. **Diffuse astrocytoma *MYB* or *MYBL1* altered** is a low-grade tumour seen mostly in children and young adults, age range of 0–26 years. They occur mostly in the cerebral hemispheres, thalamus, hypothalamus, and brainstem. They are associated with mutations of the *MYB* gene (see 'Chromosome 6', Addendum, p. 348) or with mutations of the *MYBL1* gene (see 'Chromosome 8', Addendum, p. 349).

  2. **Low-grade polymorphic juvenile neuroepithelial tumour** is a solid or partly cystic growth of the cerebral cortex, notably the temporal lobe. It causes epileptic seizures that are resistant to anti-convulsant drugs. It is linked to *BRAF* gene mutations and fibroblast growth factor receptors 2 and 3. It has a good prognosis after surgical removal.

  3. **Angiocentric glioma** is a rare neuroepithelial growth in 3- to 14-year-old children. It consists of abnormal cells gathered around blood vessels. It is usually benign (grade 1) and causes seizures, headaches, vision disturbance, dizziness, and speech arrest.

  4. **Diffuse low-grade glioma with altered MAPK (mitogen-activated protein kinase) pathway**. These are infiltrative tumours that may involve astrocytes, or oligodendrocytes, or a mix of both cells. The tumour occurs anywhere in the central nervous system, but especially in the cerebral cortex. Identification requires molecular analysis and the presence of *BRAF* (see 'Chromosome 7', Addendum, p. 348) and *FGFR1* (see 'Chromosome 8', Addendum, p. 349) gene mutations. MAPK is a protein signalling pathway from cell surface receptor to the DNA in the nucleus. Mutations of any protein in this pathway can be a starting point for cancer.

  'Adult-type' and 'paediatric' diffuse gliomas are considered as distinct from each other, although occasional crossover in age range does occur. Because paediatric gliomas have different molecular characteristics from adult gliomas, analysis of the molecular genetics in paediatric gliomas is necessary for accurate diagnosis and treatment (Funakoshi et al. 2021).

  Diffuse *high-grade* paediatric gliomas, or **paediatric-type glioblastomas**, are grade 4 malignant brain tumours that grow and spread quickly. There are multiple subtypes, defined by various genetic mutations, for example, **diffuse midline glioma (DMG)**. This is a rare glioma caused by the H3-K27M mutation of the *H3F3A* gene (see 'Chromosome 1', Addendum, p. 343). This gene codes for part of histone H3.3 (see 'Epigenetics', Chapter 2, p. 36). This glioma occurs mostly in the pons, thalamus, and spinal cord and carries a poor prognosis.

  Non-gliomas are derived from all other brain tissues that are not neuroglia.

- **Embryonal tumours (ETs)**[6] are a group of CNS tumours that are derived from embryonic tissue and therefore occur mostly in children. There are some subtypes:

  1. **Medulloblastoma** is the most common high-grade, fast-growing tumour in children. It is rare in adults. The tumour forms in the **cerebellum**, the centre for many motor functions. Children with this tumour may present with movement difficulties, such as unsteady gait (**ataxia**). It can spread into other parts of the brain and into the CSF. It may cause obstruction to CSF flow, which would cause **raised intracranial pressure (RICP)** (see 'Symptoms of brain tumours', p. 268). Medulloblastomas are linked to *BRCA1* (see 'Chromosome 17', Addendum, p. 356), *BRCA2* (see 'Chromosome 13', Addendum, p. 354), *APC* (see 'Chromosome 5', Addendum, p. 346), and *TP53* (see 'Chromosome 17', Addendum, p. 356) gene mutations.

2. **ET with multilayered rosettes (ETMR)** (previously known as **ependymoblastoma**) are derived from ependymal cells (Table 14.1). They can happen at any age but are commonest in the first 20 years of life. Most develop within one ventricle of the brain. They can interfere with CSF flow, and in smaller children, they could be a cause of **hydrocephalus**, that is, fluid accumulation of the brain, causing the head to swell. Spread of these tumours often involves entry into the CSF within the subarachnoid space. ETMRs are characterised by *amplification* (see 'Mutation of genes', Chapter 2, p. 27) of the C19MC region of chromosome 19,[7] or DICER-1 mutations (see 'Chromosome 14', Addendum, p. 355). A variation of ETMR which was previously known as **medulloepithelioma** is a rare and aggressive tumour arising from primitive **neuroepithelium**, that is, tissue that forms the embryonic nervous system (Figure 14.3). They can occur anywhere in the CNS, but most often within the cerebrum.

- **Choroid plexus tumours** are rare tumours of the choroid plexus, the blood capillary structure that produces cerebrospinal fluid (CSF) into the ventricles of the brain. The three grades of choroid plexus tumour are:

1. **Choroid plexus papilloma** is a grade 1 tumour with good prognosis.
2. **Atypical choroid plexus papilloma** is a grade 2 tumour.
3. **Choroid plexus carcinoma** is a grade 3 tumour with poor prognosis.

- **Pituitary tumours (sella region)** are tumours of the pituitary gland at the base of the brain, below the hypothalamus. The pituitary gland is situated in the **sella turcica** of the **sphenoid bone** (Figure 14.6) and produces a range of hormones (see 'Pituitary gland', Figure 4.10,

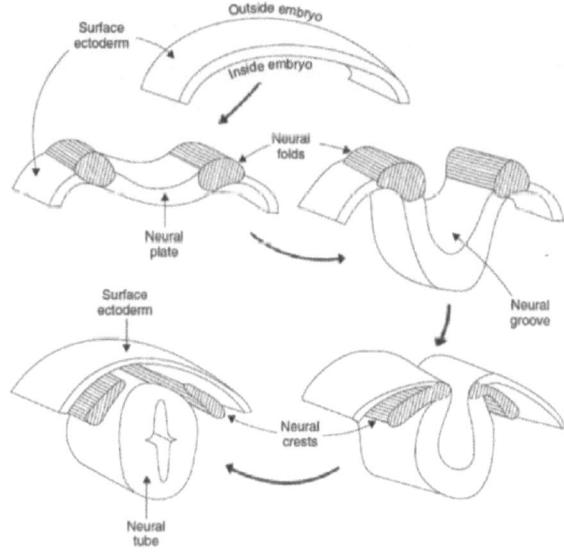

FIGURE 14.3 Embryonic brain development. Neuroepithelium forms the neural tube, a process called neurulation. This tube will develop from the neural plate and will form the brain and cord (the central nervous system). Neuroepithelium are the neural stem cells from which neurons and neuroglia form, first as progenitor cells, which then differentiate into neurons and glia through the process of neurogenesis. Cells of the neural crest will become the peripheral nervous system (PNS).

Table 4.2, Chapter 4, p. 71). Pituitary tumours either produce excessive amounts of any of the specific pituitary hormones or do not produce any excess hormones. Most are benign adenomas, that is, derived from glandular cells, and they tend to grow slowly, putting pressure on surrounding structures. As the cell numbers increase, they quite often produce too much hormone.

1. **Prolactinomas** produce excess prolactin hormone that stimulates excessive breast milk production. They can cause breast enlargement in both sexes and breast discharge in women. In males, they can cause low libido and erectile dysfunction.
2. **Somatotroph adenomas** produce too much **human growth hormone (HGH)**, also known as **somatotropin**. This normally regulates growth, but in excess, it causes acromegaly, an enlargement of the hands, feet, and face, or gigantism in children. It can also cause hypertension (high blood pressure), joint pain, and diabetes.
3. **Thyrotroph adenomas** produce too much **thyroid-stimulating hormone (TSH)**, which then overstimulates the thyroid glands, causing excessive thyroid hormone (**hyperthyroidism**), that is, goitre, tremors, palpitations, weight loss, nervousness, sweating, and an inability to tolerate heat.
4. **Corticotroph adenomas** produce too much **adrenocorticotropin hormone (ACTH)**, and this overstimulates the adrenal cortex to produce too much cortisol. Excess cortisol is a disorder known as **Cushing syndrome**, causing symptoms of weight gain, hypertension, diabetes, round face, and muscle weakness, as well as depression and mood changes.
5. **Functioning gonadotroph adenomas (FGA)** are a rare tumour producing excess follicle-stimulating hormone (FSH) and luteinising hormone (LH). The level of excess hormone produced is often too low to produce any symptoms. Symptoms caused by the pressure of the tumour on surrounding tissues are headache and visual disturbance. Menstrual irregularities and infertility can occur in women, low libido and infertility in men.
6. **Non-functioning adenomas** are pituitary tumours that do not cause excessive hormone production. Symptoms are due to pressure on surrounding structures as the tumour grows. These symptoms include visual problems, headaches, nausea and vomiting, and possibly a reduction in normal hormone production.
7. **Pituitary blastoma** was described for the first time in 2008. It is a rare anterior pituitary tumour occurring in infants less than 24 months old. It causes symptoms of Cushing syndrome (see 'Corticotroph adenomas', p. 262), increased intercranial pressure (see 'Symptoms of brain tumours', p. 268), diabetes, and reduced thyroid hormone (**hypothyroidism**). The tumour extends from the sella into the hypothalamus, and sometimes the optic chiasma. The indications are that it is caused by a *DICER1* gene mutation (see 'Chromosome 14', Addendum, p. 355).
8. **Craniopharyngiomas** are rare benign tumours occurring *near* the pituitary gland, contrary to pituitary adenomas that develop from the gland itself. Craniopharyngiomas are slow-growing but more aggressive than pituitary adenomas. They put pressure on surrounding structures, causing visual and hormonal problems. They occur more often in children but do sometimes affect adults. There are two subtypes: **papillary craniopharyngiomas (PCP)** and **adamantinomatous craniopharyngiomas (ACP)**. PCP has a specific gene mutation in the *BRAF* gene, called *BRAFv600E* (see '*BRAF* gene, chromosome 7', Addendum, p. 348). This mutation causes more gene activity, leading to increased cellular growth. This subtype is a solid tumour more commonly seen in adults 50–60 years

of age. ACP has a mutation in the *CTNNB1* gene (see '*CTNNB1* gene, chromosome 3', Addendum, p. 345). The tumour is cystic, that is, it has a cavitation appearance and is usually seen in children 5–15 years of age.

- **Pinealomas** are rare pineal gland tumours located deep within the brain and derived from the pineal gland (Figure 14.4). This gland produces **melatonin**, which is a hormone involved in the regulation of the 24-hour sleep–wake cycle. They can be graded according to how benign or malignant they are:

  1. **Pineocytomas** are grade 1, benign, and slow-growing tumours.
  2. **Pineal parenchymal tumours** (and possibly **papillary tumours**[8]) are grades 2 or 3. These have a good chance of returning after treatment.
  3. **Pineoblastomas** are grade 4 malignant tumours which are fast-growing and invasive.

  They can put pressure on surrounding structures, causing headaches, hydrocephalus, nausea, vision difficulties, and **Parinaud syndrome**, that is, a disorder of vision and eye movement, notably vertical gaze and pupillary function.

Vascular tumours (haemangioblastomas)

These are rare benign (grade 1) tumours of the blood vessels of the central nervous system. They can occur anywhere in the brain or cord but are more commonly found in the cerebellum and brainstem area. Since they are slow-growing, the symptoms are caused by the

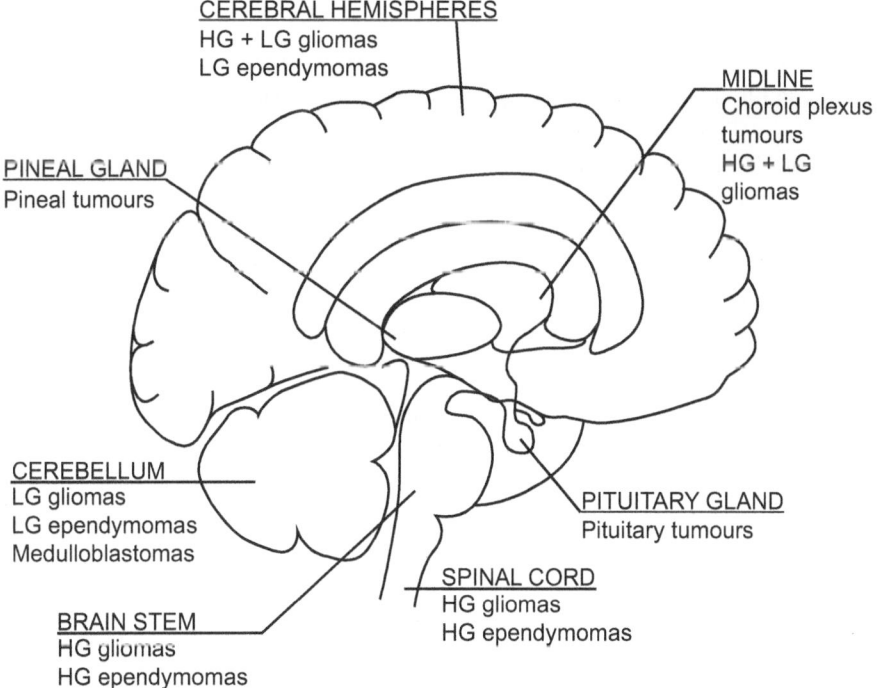

FIGURE 14.4 The sites of brain tumours. *LG* = low-grade; *HG* = high-grade.

increasing pressure it applies to surrounding structures. These symptoms include headache, nausea, difficulty with balance and coordination, visual disturbance, and motor weakness of the limbs.

Primary tumours of the peripheral nervous system (PNS)

PNS tumours arise from the nerves that leave directly from the brain, that is, cranial nerves, and those that arise from nerves that leave the spinal cord, that is, spinal nerves.

Cranial and paraspinal nerve tumours

- **Schwannoma**, or **neurilemmoma,** is a tumour that grows from **Schwann cells**, that is, cells that form the myelin sheath covering of peripheral nervous system (PNS) neuronal axons (Table 14.1). Most schwannomas are benign and slow-growing, with only the occasional tumour becoming malignant. The most frequent example of this tumour is the vestibular schwannoma that affects the eighth cranial nerve. This is the nerve of hearing and balance, connecting the inner ear to the brain. Symptoms include tinnitus, that is, a ringing sound in the affected ear, hearing loss on the affected side, headaches, dizziness, and disturbed balance. Schwannomas of other nerves produce symptoms dependent on which nerve is involved. These can be motor (movement) disturbance, sensory losses, and pain. Mutations of the *NF2* gene (see 'Chromosome 22', Addendum, p. 360) are often involved in the development of schwannomas.
- **Neurofibroma** is another type of tumour derived from the myelin sheath around nerves. The differences between this and schwannomas are:
  1. The *schwannoma* is purely Schwann cells, whilst the *neurofibroma* is a mix of Schwann cells with fibroblasts, mast cells (Figures 5.4 and 5.12, Chapter 5, p. 83 and 93), and neuronal axons (Figure 1.13, Chapter 1, p. 16).
  2. The neurofibroma encases the nerve root and can cause nerve compression or damage, but schwannomas do not do this.
  3. Schwannomas are often caused by mutations of the *NF2* gene (see 'Schwannoma', p. 264), but neurofibromas are linked to *NF1* gene mutations (see 'Chromosome 17', Addendum, p. 356).
  4. Although both are considered benign, there is a greater chance of the neurofibroma becoming malignant than the schwannomas.

- **Acoustic neuroma** is a tumour that begins from the acoustic nerve, which is also called the **auditory nerve**, and is part of the **vestibulocochlear nerve (cranial nerve VIII)**. It is the nerve of hearing and connects the cochlea of the inner ear to the auditory area of the brain. Acoustic neuromas are usually unilateral, benign, and slow-growing. They cause hearing problems, such as hearing loss and tinnitus,[9] and they can cause disturbance to balance and dizziness.
- **Ganglioneuroma** is a rare solid benign tumour of the autonomic nervous system axons originating from the neural crest cells in the embryo (Figure 14.3). They usually occur in the abdomen, for example, in the paraspinal retroperitoneum and adrenal gland, although they can grow anywhere. They are composed of ganglion and Schwann cells with fibrous tissue. Symptoms are associated with the location of the tumour, and some linked to glandular organs may secrete certain hormones.

Spinal cord tumours occur within or around the spinal cord. They may be primary or secondary, malignant or benign. They can interfere with spinal cord function, causing pain and loss of sensation or movement below the site of the tumour.

Brain secondary tumours

Brain metastases account for more brain cancers than any primary tumour, and they cause more than half of all brain tumours. They also mark a serious point in the cancer development, as they often carry a poor prognosis. The lung is one of the commonest sites for a primary tumour that gives rise to secondary brain metastases. Other primary sites are the breast and malignant melanomas (Figure 14.5).

Most brain metastases are seen in the elderly population. The lesions are usually well-demarcated masses, either singular or multiple, and may occur in the meninges as well as the brain itself. Early signs of brain involvement include developing neurological deficits, for example, limb weakness or speech difficulties, or psychiatric disturbance, for example, personality changes, fits, or depression, or physical symptoms associated with RICP.

The unique environment of the brain, that is, with neurons and neuroglia, provides a better support for tumour cell metastases than the rest of the body. The response of astrocytes to the invasion of tumour cells is a good example of this. In common with most other body cells, astrocytes, a major component of neuroglia (Table 14.1), have immune protein molecules, called **inflammasomes**. These are large multiprotein complexes, part of the innate (non-specific) immune system (see 'Innate (non-specific) immunity', Chapter 5, p. 78). Inflammasomes regulate the inflammatory response to cellular damage, tumour cells, and infections. There are several types of inflammasomes, including:

- **NLRP3 (NOD-like receptor pyrin domain containing 3)**
- **NLRC4 (NOD-like receptor family caspase-associated recruitment domain–containing protein 4)**
- **NLRP1 (NOD-like receptor pyrin domain containing 1)**
- **AIM2 (absent in melanoma 2)**

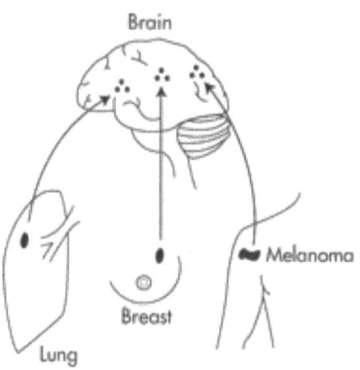

FIGURE 14.5 Brain metastases. The main sites for primary tumours are lung, breast, and melanomas.

They all have three components in common:

1. A sensor that detects a threat to the cell, such as infection or damage, and triggers an inflammatory response.
2. A **CARD (caspase activation and recruitment domain)**, which allows for the binding of inflammatory caspases to the complex.
3. The inflammatory caspases, which activate the inflammatory process. They are **zymogens**, which means they require cleavage, that is, cutting or trimming of the protein, in order to be activated.

Caspases are protease enzymes that are essential during apoptosis (programmed cell death). There are different types:

- **Initiator caspases**, that is, caspase 2, 8, and 9, start the apoptosis process.
- **Executioner caspases**, that is, caspases 3, 6, and 7, carry out extensive proteolysis (protein breakdown) during apoptosis.
- **Inflammatory caspases**, that is, caspases 1, 4, 5, 11, and 12, cause inflammation.

In brain metastases from breast cancer, the NLRP3 inflammasome and the cytokine IL-1β are highly expressed in peritumoral astrocytes. Together, the activation of NLRP3 and release of IL-1β from astrocytes contribute towards the progression of triple-negative breast cancer metastases in the brain (see 'Triple-negative breast cancer (TNBC)', Chapter 11, p. 210). The tumour cells cause upregulation and activation of NLRP3 and IL-1β in astrocytes.

In addition to inflammasomes, there are several other responses from astrocytes which promote cancer metastases in the brain. For example:

- Astrocytes release fatty acids, which activate the cancer cell's **PPAR gamma (peroxisome proliferator–activated receptor gamma)**[10] pathway, which provides conditions that allow the cancer cell to survive in the brain.
- Secretions from astrocytes that increase inflammation, such as IL-6, TNF-α, and CXCL10, promote malignant cell migration and proliferation.
- Combined astrocyte/tumour cell–derived matrix metalloproteinases (MMPs) greatly assist the tumour cell to get through the blood–brain barrier.
- Astrocytes will start to produce **type I interferons (IFNs)**, that is, **IFNα** and **IFNβ**, in a sustained, low-level manner. These normally have anti-tumour effects (see 'Cytokines and chemokines', 'Interferons (IFNs)', Chapter 5, p. 94), but some evidence suggests that they may promote brain metastases in a low-grade, chronic inflammatory environment. In this situation, type I IFNs become active at low levels over long periods, that is, becoming a chronic state of interferon activity, and this is causing the activation of a **chemokine** called **CCL2 (C-C motif chemokine ligand 2)** (see 'Cytokines and chemokines', 'Chemokines', Chapter 5, p. 94). This is involved in innate immunity (see 'Innate (non-specific) immunity', Chapter 5, p. 78), and it attracts **monocytic myeloid** cells to the tumour site. These cells are harmful to the brain by promoting tumour growth in breast- and melanoma-derived brain metastases, and possibly in other secondary brain tumours as well (Figure 14.6).

Some, if not most, of these processes can become targets for drug therapy designed to treat or prevent brain metastases.

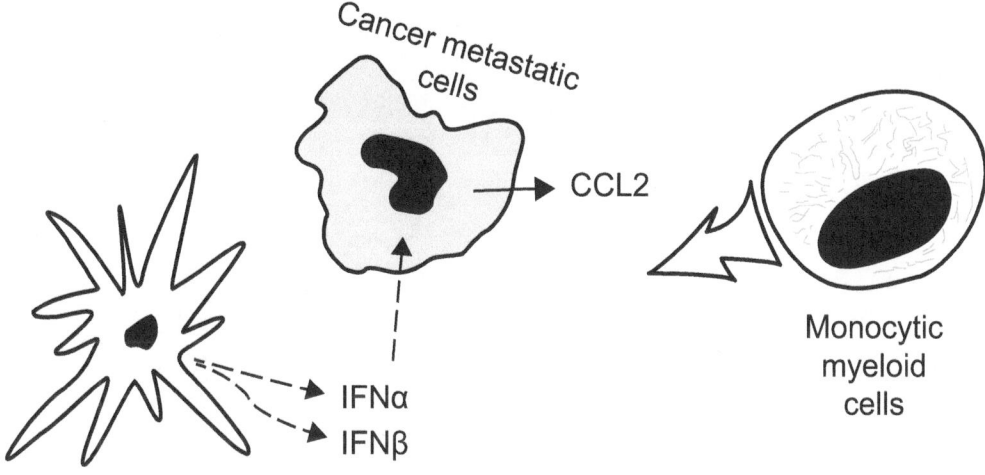

Astrocytes

FIGURE 14.6   A mechanism for secondary brain tumour survival. Astrocytes (left) react to brain meta-static tumour cells (centre) by producing type I interferons (IFNα and IFNβ) on a long-term, low-grade basis (broken arrows). In this chronic state, the interferons raise the production of a chemokine (CCL2) from the cancer cell, and this attracts (large arrow) monocytic myeloid cells (right). These monocytic myeloid cells promote secondary tumour growth.

The meninges

Between the brain and the skull are three coverings, the **meninges** (Figure 14.7). The inner membrane is the **pia mater**, the middle membrane is the **arachnoid mater**, and the outer membrane, lining the skull, is the **dura mater**. Between the pia and the arachnoid is the **subarachnoid space**, filled with **cerebrospinal fluid (CSF)**. CSF originates from blood plasma inside the brain cavities (called **ventricles**) and returns to the blood via the arachnoid mater. CSF has its own circulation, and malignant cells getting into this system can be washed to many parts of the **central nervous system (CNS)**, that is, the brain and the spinal cord.

- **Meningiomas** accounts for 10–15% of tumours. They are derived from the meninges and are classified as *intracranial* tumours, that is, inside the skull, but not strictly brain tumours, unless they spread into the brain. They put local pressure on the adjacent brain and can therefore interrupt the function of that brain area. They are most often associated with the **arachnoid mater** in adults, predominately women, and can arise from this layer within the spine as well as inside the skull. They are often well-demarcated solid tumours that can invade the skull or the brain beneath. Excision of the tumour improves the prognosis.

There are three grades of meningiomas:

- **Grade 1** are low-grade and slow-growing. They are the most common form of tumour.
- **Grade 2** are atypical,[11] mid-grade meningiomas. They have a high chance of coming back after surgical removal and can invade surrounding tissues.
- **Grade 3** are rare, anaplastic[12] meningiomas. They are malignant, fast-growing tumours.

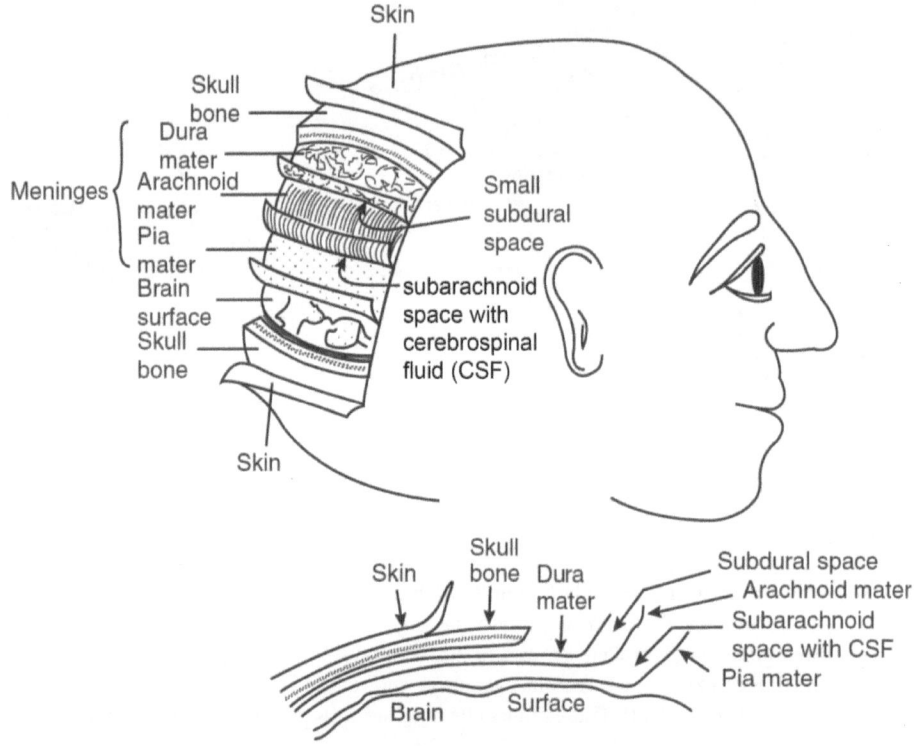

FIGURE 14.7 The meninges. The pia mater is the innermost layer, close to the brain, and the dura mater is the outermost layer, close to the skull. Between them is the arachnoid mater, below which is the subarachnoid space, filled with cerebrospinal fluid (CSF).

The genes involved with meningioma are all in the Addendum, as follows:

- *PDGFB* (see 'Chromosome 5', Addendum, p. 347)
- *SMARCB1* (see 'Chromosome 22', Addendum, p. 360)
- *BAP1* (see 'Chromosome 3', Addendum, p. 345)
- *AKT1* (see 'Chromosome 14', Addendum, p. 354)
- *SUFU* (see 'Chromosome 10', Addendum, p. 351)

Symptomology: the symptoms of intracranial tumours

Intracranial tumours cause their symptoms by a combination of:

1. Expansile growth putting pressure on surrounding tissues. The tumour creates what is called a **space-occupying lesion (SOL)**, demanding space from brain tissues, which are then pushed aside. This raises the pressure inside the skull, that is, raised intracranial pressure (RICP).
2. Infiltration into the surrounding brain tissue and disrupting neuronal functions (see 'Cancer neuroscience . . . the safe harbour hypothesis', p. 269).
3. Obstruction of CSF or blood flow through or around the brain. CSF obstruction leads to an accumulation of the fluid, adding to the RICP.

4. Oedema formation around the tumour, adding to the SOL and the RICP.
5. Irritation of neurons, which then fail to function properly. Fits are one product of cerebral irritation.
6. Release of products such as free radicals, cytokines, and electrolytes.

The main symptoms of intracranial tumours are:

1. Those associated with RICP, which are headache, nausea and vomiting, altered state of consciousness, dizziness, blurred vision, **diplopia** (double vision), pupillary changes, fits, disturbance to the pulse and blood pressure, **nystagmus** (involuntary rapid eye movements), and respiratory irregularities.
2. Those associated with the loss of neuronal function (called **neurological deficits**), such as **motor** (movement) weakness, memory loss, confusion, and speech disturbance.
3. Those associated with the brain's psychological functions, such as disturbance of behaviour, changes in personality or mood, and anxiety or depression (see 'Cancer neuroscience . . . the safe harbour hypothesis', p. 269).

Brain tumour vaccine

A vaccine called DCVAX-L, trialled in London, takes the patient's own dendritic cells (see 'Dendritic cell (DC) vaccines', Chapter 5, p. 108), then adds a biomarker from the patient's tumour, a glioblastoma (see 'Astrocytoma, grade 4', p. 259). This creates a vaccine which, when returned to the patient, will treat their cancer. The results are promising. Another promising vaccine, trialled in the USA, is also directed against glioblastomas. This vaccine uses CRISPR–CAS9 technology (see 'Gene editing, base editing, and prime editing', Figure 17.7, Chapter 17, p. 318) to gene-edit the cancer cells to become killer cells and, at the same time, prime the immune system to attack cancer cells (see 'Cancer vaccines', Chapter 5, p. 107).

Cancer neuroscience . . . the *safe harbour hypothesis*

Cancer neuroscience is the study of the relationship between malignant cells and the nervous system. An important outcome from these studies is that tumour cells in the brain may take advantage of the neurological tissue's ability to block or reduce the immune response to pathogens. The neurological tissue has this ability to preserve its own neurons and neuroglia from immune cell attack. Tumour cells can survive better in this environment, known as the *safe harbour hypothesis.* The closer the tumour cells get to neurons, the safer they will be from the immune system. Tumour cells positioned inside nerves not only hide from the immune cells but may also hide from the drugs used in chemotherapy, making them available to trigger a relapse later.

Tumours are like organs, that is, they grow, and as such, they need a blood supply to stay alive. Similarly, they also need to develop some degree of innervation.[13] To achieve this, tumour cells produce a protein called **ephrin B1** (see 'Chromosome X', Addendum, p. 361), and this causes neurons nearby to grow into the tumour. Once established, the nervous system integration into the tumour further reduces the immune system's attack on the tumour, and this increases the *safe harbour hypothesis*. This allows the tumour to grow in a protected environment. Tumours with strong innervations appear to have an increased tendency to produce metastases, and they relapse more often. Strong connectivity between the tumour and the brain also reduces life expectancy and suppresses language processing skills. Increased electrical activity in the brain language centre matches an increase in the electrical activity of the tumour. The tumour and the brain can be connected by direct innervation, by tumour invasion or compression of the speech area, or by sharing a common blood supply. In addition, tumour cells in direct contact with astrocytes can establish a pathway which acts as a conduit for the passage of mitochondria[14] from the astrocyte to the tumour cells. The tumour cells using stolen mitochondria from astrocytes grow and replicate better and quicker than tumour cells using their own mitochondria. This has been identified in glioblastoma.

Sensory nerve innervation of tumours creates a good immunosuppressed environment for the tumours due to the PD-L1 surface protein (see 'Monoclonal antibodies (MABs) known as immune checkpoint inhibitors (ICIs)', Chapter 5, p. 103), which is expressed not only on tumour cells but also on some sensory neurons. This suggests that sensory neurons may have the ability to effectively reduce the immune response to the tumour.

The brain is an ideal location for the integration of tumours into the nervous system. Tumour cells develop synaptic connections with neurons, and they get involved in the neurological circuitry. This also happens in peripheral nerves. These connections between the tumour and the nervous system allow for tumour growth, progression, and metastases in a safer environment. It does suggest, however, that possible pharmacological interventions, such as **perampanel**, an anticonvulsant drug, could be used to disconnect the nervous system from the tumour cells, and trials are underway to test this.

The integration of tumour cells into the brain circuitry is one reason for changes in mental health in brain tumours. Typical changes are depression and anxiety. Tumours with nervous system connections alter brain functions in several ways, including elevated electrical activity and increased sensitivity to pain. This may be due to the brain being linked to the acidic environment that is lacking oxygen within the tumour and not just the result of having a cancer diagnosis, possibly with a poor prognosis. There is a distinct biological process behind their mental health disturbance. These brain changes may last for some time after the cancer has gone.

Body-wide, brain–tumour connections may cause symptoms previously assigned to the cancer alone. Sleep disturbance is a good example. Insomnia could be caused by the brain–tumour connections anywhere in the body, and not just by the anxiety and worry of the diagnosis. This may be why sleep patterns change during the course of the disease and its treatment. It may become possible in the future to detect, with AI,[15] cancers anywhere in the body at an early stage just from the brain wave changes seen on electroencephalogram (EEG).

Key points

Skeleton

- There are 206 bones in the skeleton.
- The skeleton can be divided into the axial and appendicular skeletons.

Bone cancer

- Primary bone tumours fall into several types: osteosarcomas, chondrosarcomas, and Ewing sarcoma.

- Osteosarcoma often begins with a pathological fracture at the site, and an enlarged mass in the bone is seen on physical and X-ray examination.
- The bone is the third most frequent site for metastatic spread.
- Tumours may destroy bone (osteolytic tumours) or produce extra bone (osteoblastic tumours).

The brain

- The functional cell of the brain is the *neuron*.
- The supportive tissue of the brain is the *neuroglia*, or *glial cells*, of which astrocytes are by far the most numerous.
- Between the brain and the skull are coverings called the meninges.
- The inner covering is the pia mater, the middle covering is the arachnoid mater, and the outer covering is the dura mater.
- Between the pia and the arachnoid is the subarachnoid space, filled with cerebrospinal fluid (CSF).
- CSF originates from blood plasma inside the brain ventricles and returns to the blood via the arachnoid mater.
- Between the blood and the brain is the blood–brain barrier, a system of tight junctions between cells of the blood vessel epithelium.

Brain cancer

- Gliomas are derived from glial cells, mostly astrocytomas formed from astrocytes.
- Glioblastoma is the most aggressive fast-growing brain tumour.
- Non-gliomas are derived from neurons or neuronal myelin sheaths.
- Some tumours are outside the brain, for example, meningiomas occurring within the meninges.
- Brain and other intracranial tumours cause their symptoms by expansile growth creating a space-occupying lesion (SOL).
- SOLs cause raised intracranial pressure (RICP).
- Obstruction of CSF around the brain leads to an accumulation of the fluid, adding to the RICP.
- Irritation of neurons may cause fits.

Notes

1 *Chondrogenic* means 'cartilage-forming' cells.
2 *Epiphyses* are the ends of long bones that form the joints. They develop separately from the shaft (diaphysis) and fuse onto the ends during childhood.
3 *Vacuolated* means the cell cytoplasm has numerous vacuoles, that is, membrane-lined cavities.
4 The way to remember the two different bone cells is to say 'B' for *blast* is also 'B' for *build*.
5 *Lysis* or *lytic* (e.g. in osteolytic) means to 'break down'; *osteolytic* = bone breakdown.
6 The term PNET (primitive neuroectodermal tumours) was used until 2016 (Louis *et al* 2021) to encompass most of these tumour types. The new term is embryonal tumours (ETs). Also, there could be some confusion between PNET and pNET (pancreatic neuroendocrine tumours) and PitNET (pituitary neuroendocrine tumour).
7 Chromosome 19 MC (C19MC) region is a DNA segment consisting of a cluster of genes that encode for microRNAs. These are small RNA molecules that regulate the expression of other genes. The C19MC region is also involved in cell proliferation, differentiation, and apoptosis (see 'Chromosome 19', Addendum, p. 358).

8 Papillary tumours of the pineal gland are, as yet, ungraded.
9 *Tinnitus* is a constant buzzing or ringing noise in the ears.
10 Also known as NR1C3 (nuclear receptor subfamily 1, group C, member 3).
11 *Atypical* means not representative of normal cells; 'a' means 'without', that is, cells without being typical of the tissue.
12 *Anaplastic* means cells or tissues that have lost their specialised and mature features.
13 *Innervation* is the development of a nerve supply.
14 See Figure 1.1 and Table 1.1, Chapter 1, p. 3.
15 AI, artificial intelligence (see 'Artificial intelligence (AI) in cancer management', Chapter 17, p. 320).

15

PAIN AND ANALGESIA

- **Introduction**
- **The neurophysiology of pain**
- **Chronic pain in cancer**
- **Pain assessment and monitoring**
- **Pain in children**
- **Analgesia**
- **Key points**

Introduction

Pain and death are perhaps the two most frightening aspects of cancer to any patient. And not just pain from the cancer but also the pain associated with the medical investigations and treatments is also a major source of concern. But research has moved on, and the picture now is that with our greater understanding of the causes and effects of pain, the mechanisms of drug action, and of how to manage pain more effectively, prolonged suffering is no longer an inevitable consequence of cancer.

The neurophysiology of pain

There are several types of pain:

- **Acute pain** tends to be of sudden and relatively short duration. It serves a purpose in one sense, that is, it alerts the individual that something is wrong and needs attention, or it protects the individual against further tissue injury.
- **Chronic pain** has a longer duration than acute pain, often lasting for weeks, months, or even years. Some definitions put chronic pain as existing for longer than three months (Wood 2002) or longer than six months (see 'Symptomology: chronic pain', p. 279).

DOI: 10.4324/9781003389125-15

• **Intractable pain** is chronic pain unrelated to any detectable pathology. As such, it is very difficult to treat and offers a major challenge to healthcare professionals. Although there are some theories, there remains no underlying cause of intractable pain.

Localised pain is often caused by **inflammation** of the tissues involved. Inflammation is, in turn, caused by local trauma or irritation of the tissues, as seen in infections, mechanical injury, or tumour formation. It can also be caused by chemicals released locally from cells (see 'Anaphylatoxins (C3a, C5a)', Chapter 5, p. 93). Inflammation is a natural mechanism through which the **immune system** functions. We dislike inflammation because of the discomfort it causes, but the immune system could not function adequately without it.

Inflammation causes an increase in capillary wall permeability, thus allowing increased amounts of water to leak into the tissues from blood plasma. And not just water, but capillaries also allow the leakage of proteins from the blood and allow larger numbers of white blood cells to leave the blood and enter the tissues. The protein leakage makes the tissue fluid protein-rich, and this attracts more water from the capillaries. The result is a build-up of tissue fluid in the inflamed area, that is, a local **oedema** (see Table 10.1, Chapter 10, p. 198). The pain is generated almost as a side effect.

Pain mediators, that is, chemicals that cause pain, are released at the site, notably **histamine**, **prostaglandins**, and **bradykinins** (Figure 15.1). These mediators bind to receptors on **nociceptors**,[1] which are pain nerve endings. There are two types of nociceptors, **polymodal** and **mechanoreceptors**. Mechanoreceptors are pain receptors that respond to mechanical injury, whilst polymodal receptors respond with pain caused by many types of tissue insult. Nerve impulses generated by nociceptors are recognised as pain by the brain only after certain criteria are reached.

1. A sufficient level of irritation to the receptors is required. This may be in the form of pressure from a tumour increasing in size, or increasing fluid oedema, or it could be from increasing

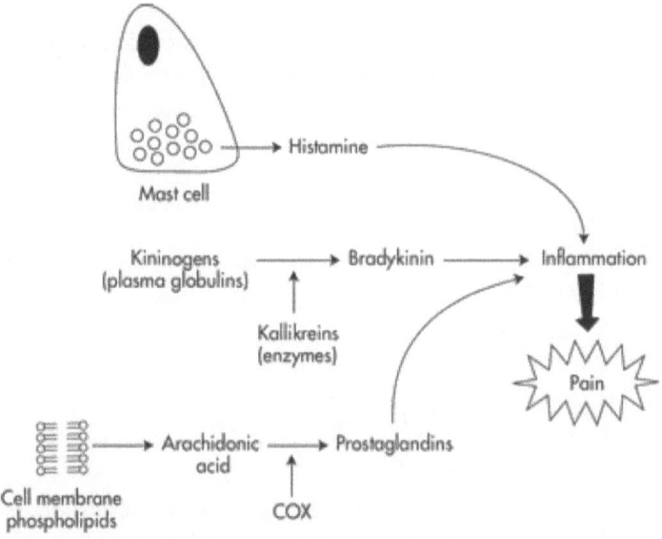

FIGURE 15.1 Pain caused by pain mediators. Histamine is released from mast cells (Chapter 5, Figures 5.4 and 5.11), bradykinins are derived from the plasma globulins kininogens, and prostaglandins are formed from arachidonic acid (Figure 5.12).

levels of chemical mediator released locally. Whatever is the cause, it must be sufficient to raise the level of nociceptor stimulation to **pain threshold** point or beyond. *Threshold* means the amount of stimulation necessary to generate strong-enough impulses from the nociceptors that are recognised as pain by the brain. With less stimulation, that is, below pain threshold level, impulses can still be generated from the nociceptor, but these are weaker and are recognised by the brain as **irritation**, rather than pain. **Itching** is one form of irritation caused by nociceptor stimulation below that needed to activate the pain threshold level (Figure 15.2).

2. Even if the threshold is exceeded, the nature, severity, and duration of pain conceived by the brain are dependent on the intensity of neuronal firing from the nociceptor. If the nociceptor firing is weak, that is, just above threshold level, the pain conceived by the brain will be significantly less than if the firing intensity was high. It is a simple relationship; the greater the intensity of impulses generated, the greater the perceived level of pain.

Pain impulses pass to the brain via the peripheral **sensory nervous system**. Two types of nerve, or neuronal pathways, that is, '**A' fibres**[2] ('A' neurons) and '**C' fibres** ('C' neurons), carry impulses destined to register as pain in the brain. 'A' fibres are further divided into various subtypes, of which the **Aδ fibre** carries pain. Aδ fibres are fast, that is, they convey impulses very quickly to the brain, whilst 'C' fibres are slower. The difference is the thickness of the fibres and the degree of **myelination** the fibre has. *Myelin* is the fatty covering along the axon of neurons (Figure 1.13, Chapter 1, p. 16). It has gaps that are involved in impulse conduction. The better the myelination, as in 'A' fibres, the faster the impulse will travel, that is, up to 25 m per second in 'Aδ' fibres. 'C' fibres are unmyelinated and transmit impulses at speeds considered as 'slow' in comparison, that is, up to 2 m per second. They are important, however, since 'C' fibres carry about 80% of pain impulses to the brain, and they are widely distributed throughout the body.

Nociceptors at the end of the Aδ fibres are found in the skin and mucous membranes, where they are in the 'front line' for warning the brain against sudden sharp pain due to trauma. Compare that to nociceptors of 'C' fibres, which are also in the skin but are found in most other body tissues as well.

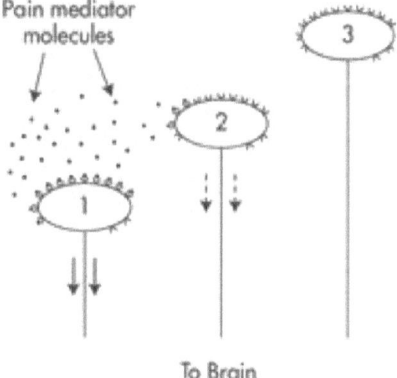

To Brain

FIGURE 15.2   Pain mediator molecules bind to nociceptors ('1', '2', and '3'): '1' has bound a lot of molecules and sends rapid impulses to the brain, and pain is experienced; '2' has fewer bound molecules and sends less impulses, which the brain may interpret as itching; '3' has no molecules bound and sends no impulses to the brain.

The pathway from the periphery to the brain is a three-neuronal system, that is, the impulse must pass through three **sensory neurons** to get from the nociceptor to the brain (Figure 15.3):

- *Neuron 1* passes from the nociceptor into the posterior part of the **spinal cord**. It is a specialised neuron, having the cell body on a branch just outside the cord. This cell body is called the **posterior root ganglion (PRG)**.
- *Neuron 2* synapses with the first neuron in the cord. The axon of neuron 2 first crosses the midline before passing up the cord to a part of the brain called the **thalamus**. The crossover (called a **decussation**) means that impulses from the left of the body will continue up the right side of the nervous system, and vice versa.
- *Neuron 3* synapses with neuron 2, the axon of neuron 3 passing from the thalamus to the **sensory cortex** of the **cerebrum**.

Synapses are connections that create microscopic gaps between neurons. Synapses use chemicals called **neurotransmitters** to bridge the gap that the synapse creates. This gap, the **synaptic cleft**, and the neurotransmitters found to fill the gap are important in pain transmission. Beyond the nociceptor, therefore, three main parts of the nervous system are involved in impulse transmission that leads to pain. These are the spinal cord, the thalamus, and the sensory cortex of the cerebrum.

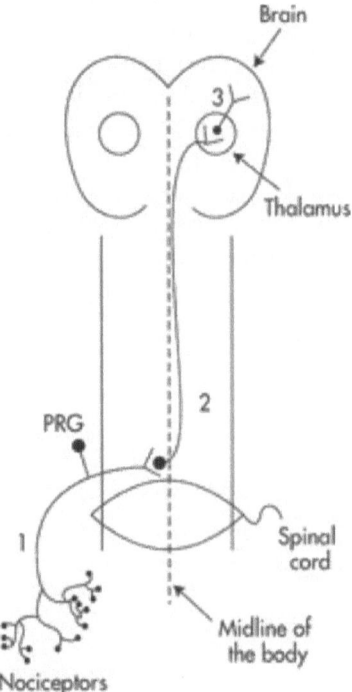

FIGURE 15.3 Three neural pain pathways. All sensations, including pain, use a three-neuronal system from periphery to the brain. Neuron 1 extends from the nociceptors in the periphery to the cord (*PRG* = posterior root ganglion, the cell body of neuron 1). Neuron 2 crosses the midline in the cord and extends to the thalamus. Neuron 3 relays the impulses from the thalamus to the cerebral cortex of the brain.

The spinal cord

Pain is *not* recognised as a conscious sensation at spinal cord level. All impulses pass through the cord and its synapses purely automatically at subconscious level. The posterior spinal cord is the site of the first synapse, between neurons 1 and 2 (Figure 15.3). This connection permits the formation of a pain **reflex arc**, a mechanism that allows pain impulses to trigger another impulse in the corresponding **lower motor neuron (LMN)** in the cord, which then causes muscles to contract and withdraw the affected part away from the source of pain. Here, also, is the location for a pain-blocking process, called the '**gate control theory**', which is illustrated and described in Figure 15.4. Anything that promotes 'A' fibre stimulus will help block pain at spinal cord level but activates the substantia nigra, and this may be how **TENS (transcutaneous electrical nerve stimulation)** or **acupuncture** works.

Also, what must not be overlooked is the fact that the 'gate control' mechanism is significantly influenced from above by the higher intellectual centres of the brain. Impulses descending from the **reticular formation** and other parts of the **brainstem**, or from the **hypothalamus** and the cerebral cortex, modify the events at spinal cord level. The brain does this because factors such as emotions, culture, personal beliefs, and learning are all involved in the total pain experience. Descending neurons from the brain create synapses in the cord that use a variety of neurotransmitters, such as **enkephalins**, **endorphins**, and **dynorphins** (see 'The opioid drugs', p. 288), to block further pain transmission up the cord (Clancy and McVicar 1998).

At a local level, one important neurotransmitter at the synapse between neurons 1 and 2 is **substance P**. This neurotransmitter is a facilitator for pain transmission at cord level, and anything that inhibits or prevents substance P will decrease pain impulses from reaching the brain. The release of substance P is inhibited by another naturally produced chemical called **enkephalin** (see 'The opioid drugs', p. 288).

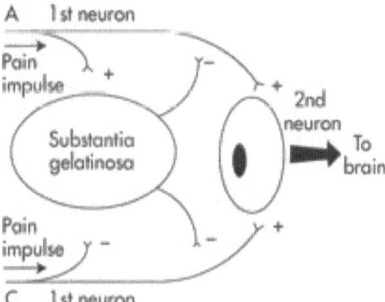

FIGURE 15.4   The gate control theory. The first neuron (from periphery to cord) is either an 'A' (fast) fibre or a 'C' (slow) fibre. Both carry pain impulses, and both stimulate (+) the second neuron in the cord. The 'A' fibre also activates the substantia gelatinosa, which then blocks impulses along both the 'A' and 'C' fibres using its own negative (−) (inhibitory) synapses. This closes the gate to pain impulses reaching the second neuron. 'C' stimulation shuts down the substantia gelatinosa using a negative (−) (inhibitory) side branch and therefore shuts down the inhibitory branches from the substantia gelatinosa and opens the gate to pain impulses reaching the second neuron. Generally, the 'gate' is neither fully open nor fully closed but varies between these two states and can be further influenced by impulses from the brain.

The thalamus

Pain impulses begin to become part of our consciousness as they pass through our brain. As impulses travel up neuron 2 and enter the brain, they first pass through the **brainstem**. Here, pain impulses are recognised as something different from other sensory impulses. On arrival at the thalamus, pain impulses are consciously recognised as unpleasant. As a sensory relay station, the thalamus is normally dealing with thousands of sensations every minute, all of which are still at subconscious level, except pain. The thalamus must pass sensory impulses onto the conscious part of the brain, the *sensory cortex* of the cerebrum (in the *parietal lobe*), via neuron 3. With pain impulses, this still happens, but the thalamus also communicates with the *motor cortex* of the cerebrum (in the *frontal lobe*) and thus influences movement in response to the pain (called a **thalamic response** to pain) (Figure 15.5). So both synapses in the three-neuronal system, that is, in the cord (spinal reflex arc) and in the thalamus (thalamic pain response), have motor connections facilitating responses to the pain impulses.

The cerebral cortex

Finally, the nociceptive impulses arrive at the sensory cortex of the cerebrum via neuron 3. This is the conscious brain, where the individual will become aware of the pain as a noxious and unpleasant sensation. The cells of the sensory cortex are laid out in a plan representative of the body (Figure 15.6), Having been 'relayed' from the thalamus, the pain impulses will arrive at that part of the cortex that represents that area of the body from where the pain has originated. Thus, pain impulses arising from the abdomen, for example, will arrive in that part of the cortex that specialises in the abdomen. Remember, there is also a crossover of the sensory neuron 2 in the cord, so pain impulses from the left of the body will arrive in the right cortex, and vice versa.

The conscious nature of the cortex allows for the individual to make decisions and to act on the pain, for example, to rest, to take pain-killing drugs, or to see a doctor. This is very different

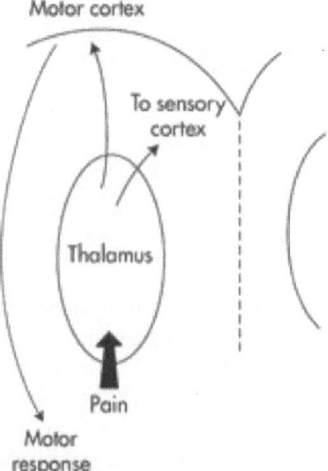

FIGURE 15.5   The thalamic pain response. Pain impulses are not only passed from the thalamus to the sensory cortex but the thalamus, by including the motor cortex, can also initiate a motor response to pain.

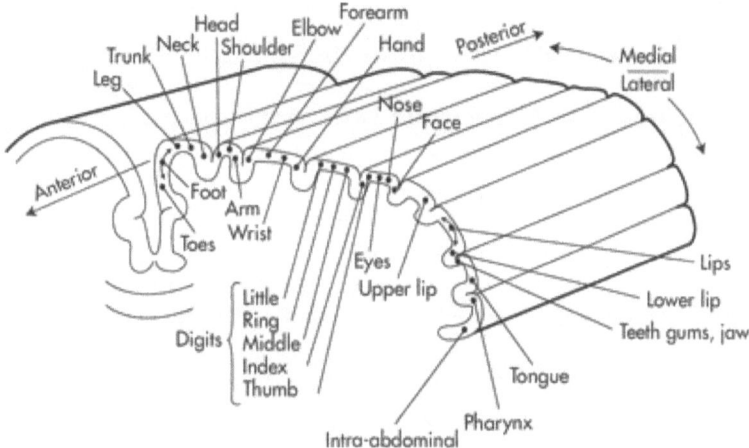

FIGURE 15.6 The sensory cortex of the brain is laid out as a body plan. Impulses from the body must be sent to the relevant part of the cortex, and directing these impulses to the appropriate part of the cortex is a function of the thalamus.

Source: From Blows (2024), Figure 11.5.

to the responses found at cord or thalamic levels, which are less sophisticated and are only there to save life and prevent further injury.

What is also interesting is that we are only conscious of the pain sensation when it reaches the cerebrum of the brain, but still we recognise the pain as arising from the body part affected. As an example, consider pain impulses arising from the bowel. These impulses are not conscious, and therefore not recognised as pain until they reach the brain. Yet as soon as we are aware of them in the cortex, we actually 'feel' the pain in the bowel, not the brain. This is because the cerebral cortex receiving the impulses is laid out in a body plan. So in our example, there is part of the cortex where the brain cells are representatives of the bowel. When these brain cells receive pain impulse, they make the person aware of pain in the bowel, *not* in the brain.

Endogenous opioids

These are chemicals produced naturally in the brain and cord which block pain impulses from entering the brain, thus providing some protection for the brain against noxious stimuli. They are produced at the time that pain is experienced. Further discussion of these substances is found in the section on analgesia (see 'Analgesia', p. 283).

Symptomology: chronic pain

Chronic pain affects between 7% and 30% of the population for a range of different reasons. Chronic pain changes the sufferer's lifestyle and personality, and it causes insomnia, depression, fatigue, and dependence on others for help.

Chronic pain can be **nociceptive** (see 'Nociceptors', p. 274) and can be severe. It may be from the main body structure (**somatic**) or from the internal organs (**visceral**). Alternatively, the pain may be **neuropathic**, that is, caused by an abnormal process of sensory nerve conduction, such as occurs in a nerve pathology. It is often described as burning, dull, aching, tingling, or shooting in character. The chronic pain in cancer may have any of these three causes:

1. Further advancement of the disease, which is the most common cause of the pain, where the cancer is growing into the surrounding tissues or spreading as **metastases** (Chapter 6). Such advancement puts pressure on surrounding structures, including pain nerve endings; it induces inflammation and can result in complications, such as obstruction.
2. The effects and side effects of cancer treatments.
3. The presence of any co-existing disease, that is, some other disorder the patient is suffering from that may not be related to their cancer but could be affecting the tumour.

Cancer specialists point to *chronic back pain* and *chronic chest pain* as being consistently associated with stage 4, advanced-stage cancers of various types. Whilst both back and chest pains are more commonly caused by other, non-cancerous conditions, the development of these symptoms in cancer patients is a signal of possible advancement of the disease (see 'Symptomology: Cancer-related fatigue (CRF)', Chapter 18, p. 335).

Pain assessment and monitoring

The question arises: 'How can you quantify and measure pain?' It is not difficult to identify when a person is in pain; they can usually tell you, and they may show the signs of pain (Figure 15.7). But how *much* pain are they suffering – that is, is it quantifiable? And is it getting better or worse? Pain is very much an individual (or subjective) concept: what is severe pain to one person would be mild to another.

Pain assessment requires judgement concerning the following factors:

1. Pain site, that is, where is the pain? Remember that not all pain occurs at the site of the pathology (or the cause of the pain). **Referred pain** occurs some distance away from the site of the cause (Figure 15.8). This is because pain impulses travel along nerve pathways and sometimes gives the brain a false impression of where the pain is originating from.
2. Pain intensity, which is very subjective and will vary between individuals and at different times in the same individual.

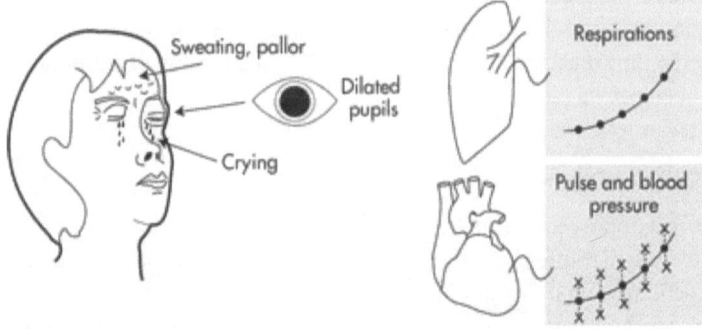

FIGURE 15.7   The signs of pain. The pulse, blood pressure, and respiration rates rise. The pupils dilate, and the person may show sweating, pallor, and may cry.

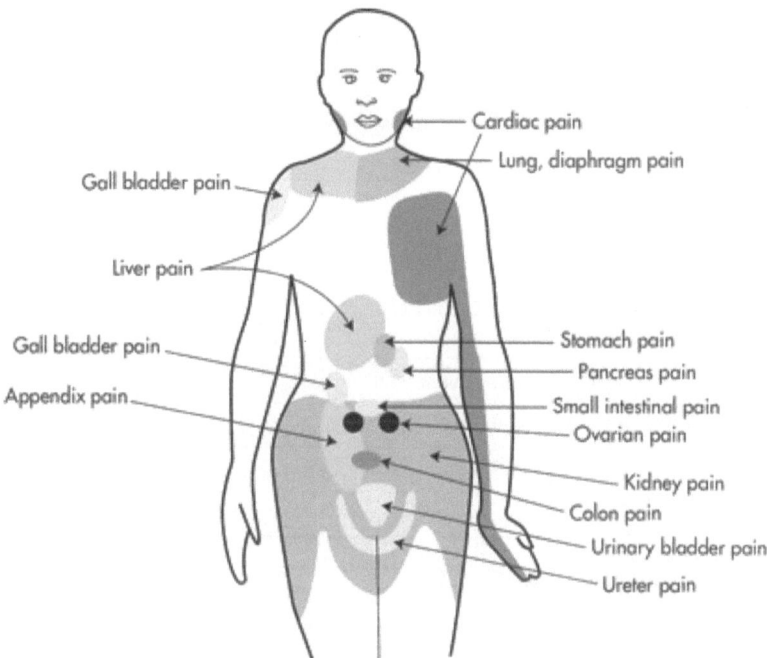

Cardiac pain

Lung, diaphragm pain

Gall bladder pain

Liver pain

Gall bladder pain

Appendix pain

Stomach pain

Pancreas pain

Small intestinal pain

Ovarian pain

Kidney pain

Colon pain

Urinary bladder pain

Ureter pain

FIGURE 15.8 The areas where referred pain is experienced and the organs the pain is derived from.

3. The nature of the pain, that is, is it sharp like a knife, a dull ache, or is it burning?
4. Is the pain associated with specific activities, like eating, vomiting, or urinating, or with a specific movement or position?
5. Duration of the pain, that is, is it sudden or acute, or is it chronic?

To be as objective as possible about such a subjective phenomenon, **pain assessment tools**, for example, **pain charts** or **pain scales**, have been devised. Pain assessment tools fall into three categories:

Verbal descriptor scales use words which may be appropriate to describe pain, ranked in order of severity, for example, *none (no pain)*, *slight pain*, *moderate pain*, *severe pain*, *agonising pain*. Patients indicate the word most applicable to their pain, and a numerical ranking alongside the words would aid in charting the response (Figure 15.9). The word list may provide rather limited choice when applied to some patients' pain, but it is easy to score and analyse.

Visual analogue scales consist of a line representing a pain continuum, with descriptive word 'anchors' at both ends. An example is the continuum that stretches from 'no pain' at one end of the line to 'pain as bad as it could be' at the other end. Patients must indicate where along this line their pain ranks. Additional word descriptions may be added along the line to aid the patient in their choice (Figure 15.10). They are relatively easy to use and do not rely heavily on the choice of wording. However, they may not be suitable for all patients, particularly the elderly and confused, or those with educational disabilities.

Description	Score
No pain	0
Slight pain	1
Mild pain	2
	3
Moderate pain	4
	5
Severe pain	6
More severe pain	7
Very severe pain	8
	9
Worst possible pain	10

FIGURE 15.9   Verbal descriptor scale for pain.

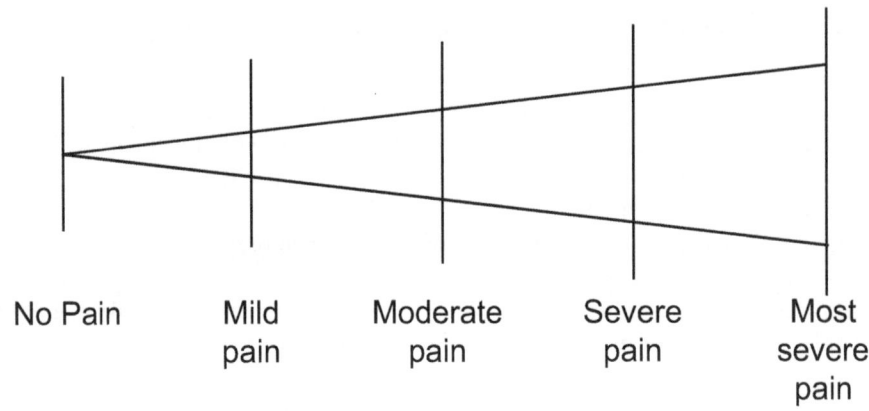

No Pain   Mild pain   Moderate pain   Severe pain   Most severe pain

FIGURE 15.10   Visual analogue scale for pain.

Pain behaviour tools are based on the understanding that patients in pain demonstrate certain behaviour patterns. These behaviour patterns are most likely to consist of:

- *Verbal responses to pain,* for example, crying or swearing
- *Pain-related body language,* for example, holding or rubbing the affected area
- Specific facial expressions
- *Certain behaviour changes,* for example, seeking analgesia or medical attention
- Changes in consciousness level
- *Pain-related physiological responses,* for example, mild pain causing a rise in blood pressure, severe pain causing a drop in blood pressure

These observations can be used on patients with communication problems, but they are more time-consuming and complex than the previous tools, and they exclude the patient's own subjective assessment (Manchester Triage Group 1997).

Numerous variations of these tools will be seen in clinical practice, where they have been combined or modified to suit specific patient needs.

Pain in children

In **neonates**, the first pain pathway to mature is the 'C' fibre, but slow myelination of motor pathways means that their responses to pain tend only to be generalised, for example, crying rather than specific to the site of pain. **Infants** can localise pain better after about 3 months of age and can produce more specific reactions. They still produce generalised reactions as well, crying and a change in facial expression being the most obvious. Some older children are better at discussing and describing pain. However, they often think in terms of extremes, that is, it is either very bad or gone. They are also very good at pinpointing precise locations of pain, but because they do not understand the cause of pain, or often how to stop it, pain can cause confusion, fear, and anger. Often, the cause will be obvious, for example, following a minor accident. But if the cause is less obvious, as in cancer, for example, they do not understand why they are suffering from pain or what to do about it for themselves. They become entirely dependent on their parents or guardians at first, and later on nurses and other healthcare professionals, to solve the problem of their pain.

Assessing pain in children is difficult, and to help overcome the problems, several pain charts have been developed specifically for children of any age, in some cases down to 4 years old. Some consist of a series of cartoon faces showing a range of expressions, from happy (experiencing no pain) to very sad or crying (experiencing severe pain). Beneath each face are words describing the pain intensity in terms (verbal and written) that a child is likely to understand, for example, the word 'hurt' instead of 'pain'. The most reliable indicator of pain in children is their verbal statements about the pain they are suffering and what the child is saying should always be believed.

But scales are only part of the story. **QUESTT** is an overall pain assessment that incorporates scales where required (Baker and Wong 1987). **QUESTT** stands for:

Question the child.
Use pain rating scales.
Evaluate behaviour and physiological changes.
Secure parent's involvement.
Take the cause of the pain into account.
Take action, and evaluate the results.

In children with severe pain, as in the later stages of cancer, the analgesic ladder can be employed to ensure adequate pain therapy. Remember that pain generates fear in a child, and for this reason, painful procedures must be reduced to the absolute minimum required. Full explanation is required from the parents and nurses for any procedures, especially if they are painful, including being honest about the possibility of pain. Children must not be left alone in pain.

Analgesia

Two important sciences, **pharmacokinetics** and **pharmacodynamics**, describe the events inside the body once drugs have been administered. Pharmacokinetics involves the way drugs move through the body, from absorption through to distribution, metabolism, and finally, excretion. Pharmacodynamics describe how drugs actually work, that is, how they achieve what they are given for.

Analgesia (*an* = without; *algesia* = increased sensitivity to pain) is the absence of pain *without* causing loss of consciousness (general anaesthesia) or loss of touch sensation (local anaesthesia). Two major groups of analgesic drugs exist: the **opioids** and the **non-steroidal anti-inflammatory drugs** (**NSAIDs**). Basically, they work very differently, not only in their mechanism of action, but also in the location of action within the nervous system. NSAIDs act in the tissues where pain originates from, that is, they work *peripherally*, while opioids work in the brainstem and spinal cord, that is, they work *centrally*.

The analgesic ladder and adjuvant therapy

The **World Health Organization (WHO) (1986)** introduced the concept of a stepped approach to pain management known as the 'analgesic ladder' (Figure 15.11 *left*). Since then, it has been modified to show that the steps taken to control pain can be reversed, and that a new top level of pain relief is sometimes indicated (Figure 15.11 *right*).

It works like this:

Step 1: The baseline treatment to start with is a *non-opioid* drug, for example, a **non-steroidal anti-inflammatory** agent, with or without **adjuvant therapy** (see 'Adjuvant therapy', p. 284). Such non-opioids include aspirin (except in children), paracetamol, or ibuprofen.

Step 2: If pain persists or increases, an **opioid drug** suitable for moderate pain is introduced, with or without the NSAID, and with or without the adjuvant therapy. Such an opioid drug is codeine, dihydrocodeine, pentazocine, dipipanone, or oxycodone.

Step 3: If pain continues to persist or increase, a stronger opioid drug is introduced, one reserved for severe pain, such as morphine, diamorphine, pethidine, or fentanyl (see 'Fentanyl', p. 290). The addition of the NSAID and adjuvant therapy remains an option as well.

Step 4: Surgery and other invasive procedures remain an option if pain persists.

Adjuvant therapy

This is non-drug treatment for pain and consists of a wide range of possibilities, such as simple massage techniques. The following is a summary of adjuvant therapies available.

- Local **radiotherapy** is very good for relief of symptoms, including pain (see 'Radiotherapy', Chapter 17, p. 310).
- **Epidural infusion** of local anaesthetic, perhaps given slowly via an infusion pump. Infusions are into the **epidural space**, that is, a space outside the **dura mater**, the outer of the three coverings of the central nervous system, within the spinal canal, and may be continuous or intermittent. Effectiveness is usually only for a few weeks, after which tolerance becomes a problem, but it is very good for acute pain control without paralysis or disturbance of the autonomic nervous system.
- **Transcutaneous electrical nerve stimulation** (**TENS**) is an electrical apparatus for the delivery of a small electrical charge across the skin surface, the purpose of which is relief of pain. It is effective, being used frequently in midwifery during labour, but its uses extend

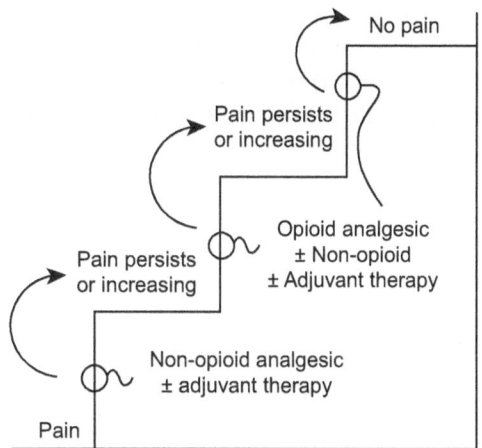

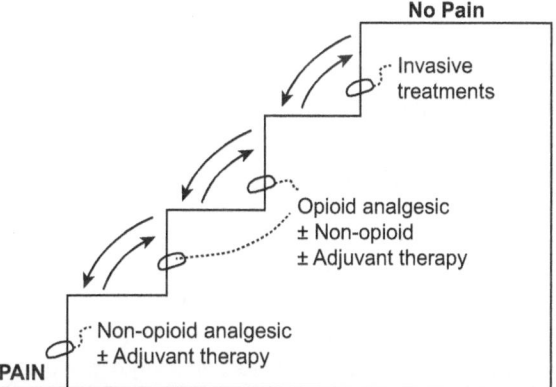

FIGURE 15.11 The analgesic ladder. Above: If pain persists or increases, the next level of analgesia must be attained. Below: Modified analgesic ladder to show that levels are reversible, and an additional level at the top.

to other causes of pain. The analgesia comes on about 20 minutes or so after starting and continues for a lengthy period after use has stopped. There are no significant side effects. Limitations of use are few, that is, it should not be used near the eye or over the heart if the patient has had a heart complication, not used on the head or neck in epileptic patients, and used with caution in pregnancy. It can interfere with the function of pacemakers and electro-cardiographs (ECG) or electroencephalograms (EEG). How it works is not known, but it may induce the closure of the spinal gate to pain (see 'Gate theory of pain', p. 277).

- Massage and **aromatherapy** can be used as adjuvant therapy.
- **Acupuncture**, the Chinese art of inserting needles into the skin to relieve pain and other conditions. Like TENS, the way acupuncture works is unknown, but it may prevent the flow of pain impulses through the gate control mechanism. The Chinese theory of *channels* and *collaterals* indicates the presence of 12 regular main trunks (*channels*) running horizontally and vertically across the body, connecting all the major parts of the body from inside out,

from top to bottom. Thinner and smaller channels (*collaterals*) run as branches to all other areas of the body. These connections maintain the integrity and harmonious union of the entire body. It may be possible that these pathways coincide with the nervous system, as Western medicine recognises it. There are more than 300 standard acupoints along the channels and collaterals. Acupuncture prescription includes two or more points selected according to the symptoms and cause of the disease, and the functions of the points themselves. Applying needle stimulation to the prescribed points is said to regulate the body and restore any imbalance. It may release hormones from the endocrine system, stimulate the immune system and release antibodies, and increase the body's resistance to inflammation (L. Zhang-Lheureux, personal communication).

- **Psychological support**, that is, staying with the patient, comforting, distracting their attention away from the pain, for example, reading to them. Distraction, like television or favourite games, is particularly useful with children in pain.
- **Nerve block** is carried out by injecting parts of the sensory nerves, for example, the **dorsal root**, or sympathetic nerves with phenol or alcohol, thus blocking pain sensations. The destruction of the nerve by the chemical is irreversible, so the procedure is not carried out until all other avenues have been tried.
- Surgery is a last resort because it is also irreversible. The aim is to divide the pain pathways permanently and therefore stop the passage of pain impulses to the brain.

Non-opioid analgesics 1: non-steroidal anti-inflammatory drugs (NSAIDs)

Linoleic acid is a natural fat-based component of the diet often found in margarines. In the body, linoleic acid is converted to **arachidonic acid**, and this becomes an important part of **phospholipids**, a major component of our cell membranes. In addition, arachidonic acid can be recovered from cell membranes if required, since arachidonic acid is the basic substance (or *substrate*) from which other substances can be made. One large group of these other substances are **prostanoids**, a major class of chemicals that includes **prostacyclins**, **prostaglandins**, and **thromboxanes** (Figure 5.13, Chapter 5, p. 96).

Prostacyclins, prostaglandins, and thromboxanes act like hormones, mostly locally, but sometimes systemically. Like hormones, they cause changes in the tissues generally close to where they are produced. Prostacyclins, for example, cause several tissue changes, including local **vasodilation**, that is, dilation of local blood vessels, bringing more blood to the area. Thromboxane A2 does the opposite by causing **vasoconstriction**. Prostaglandins are a large group of substances that have many effects, both locally and more widespread, including prostaglandin E (PGE) and prostaglandin F (PGF), which cause pain. These prostaglandins are very important pain mediators which increase the sensitivity of nociceptors, making them respond more to other pain mediators, that is, lowering the threshold to pain.

To produce all these chemicals from arachidonic acid requires the enzyme **cyclo-oxygenase** (**COX**), which occurs in two forms: COX-1 and COX-2. COX-1 is found in most cells most of the time (i.e. it is *constitutive*), whilst COX-2 is found in inflammatory cells when activated during inflammation (i.e. it is *induced*). NSAIDs work primarily by temporarily[3] blocking (or *inhibiting*) COX-1 in peripheral tissues where the pain is generated (Figure 15.12).

The best-known drug in this group is **aspirin** (a **salicylic acid**), which causes irreversible blockage of COX-1, thus preventing the formation of the prostaglandin pain mediators.

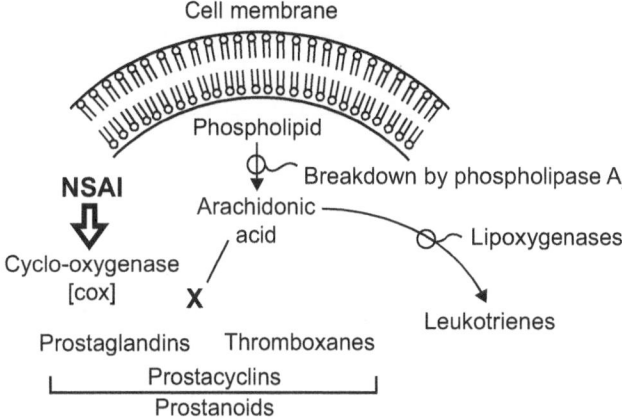

Cell membrane

Phospholipid

Breakdown by phospholipase A$_2$

NSAI

Arachidonic ─── acid

Lipoxygenases

Cyclo-oxygenase [cox]   **X**

Leukotrienes

Prostaglandins   Thromboxanes
Prostacyclins
Prostanoids

FIGURE 15.12   The action of NSAI drugs. NSAIs block the enzyme COX so prostaglandins cannot be produced from arachidonic acid.

Indomethacin also inhibits COX-1, **diclofenac** and **naproxen** inhibit COX-1 and COX-2 equally, and **nabumetone** preferentially blocks COX-2.

Gastric *intolerance* is a problem, mostly for the ingested COX-1 inhibitors, and these should not be given to patients with a current gastric problem or a history of gastric disorder, for example, ulceration. They could cause gastric irritation, bleeding, and ulceration of the gastric mucosal lining, especially in higher dosage. Drugs that are selective for COX-2 inhibition have greater gastric *tolerance* when given by mouth.

The NSAIDs often have a combination of several drugs in one tablet, and sometimes with **caffeine** added, as this is said to enhance the analgesic property of the NSAIDs. Aspirin and other NSAIDs can be used in cancer pain control, especially in the very early stages and as a backup measure when stronger drugs are in use (see 'Analgesic ladder', Figure 15.11, p. 285). They are a very good means of controlling mild pain, but for severe pain, there is often a need for an additional stronger analgesia: the opioids.

Non-opioids 2: paracetamol

Paracetamol, a well-known and popular analgesic drug, is only a weak inhibitor of both COX-1 and COX-2, so its mode of analgesic action is still somewhat unknown. What is known is that some metabolites of arachidonic acid caused by the action of COX are **hydroperoxides**, and these, in turn, then further stimulate COX to produce more cytokines. Paracetamol blocks this feedback pathway, therefore inhibiting COX indirectly by stopping the activity of hydroperoxides. Paracetamol is active in the brain (centrally acting), where it has an analgesic and an antipyretic effect but practically no anti-inflammatory effect. Therefore, paracetamol is not generally considered to be an NSAID because of its absence of anti-inflammatory activity. It has been used in palliative care in combination with opioid drugs, but its stand-alone use in cancer care is not yet established (Wood et al. 2018).

Nefopam acts in the brain and spinal cord to relieve pain by affecting the activity of neurotransmitters such as glutamate.

TABLE 15.1 The NSAIDs related to cancer pain treatment

Non-steroidal anti-inflammatory drug (NSAID)	Notes
Aspirin	Mild to moderate pain; contraindicated in gastric disorders, for example, peptic ulceration, and bleeding disorders.[4]
Aspirin with codeine	Mild to moderate pain; contraindicated in gastric disorders, for example, peptic ulceration, and bleeding disorders.
Dexketoprofen	Mild to moderate pain; contraindicated in gastrointestinal disorders, for example, peptic ulceration, and bleeding disorders.
Flurbiprofen	Mild to moderate pain; contraindicated in gastrointestinal disorders, for example, peptic ulceration, and bleeding disorders.
Ibuprofen	Mild to moderate pain; contraindicated in gastrointestinal disorders, for example, peptic ulceration, and bleeding disorders.
Mefenamic acid	Mild to moderate pain; contraindicated in gastrointestinal disorders, for example, peptic ulceration, and bleeding disorders.
Nabumetone	Mild to moderate pain; contraindicated in gastrointestinal disorders, for example, peptic ulceration, and bleeding disorders. It is a prodrug of little activity, but its metabolite (6-methoxy-2-naphthyl acetic acid) preferentially blocks COX-2.

TABLE 15.2 Paracetamol and nefopam hydrochloride

Non-opioid drug (centrally acting)	Notes
Paracetamol (acetaminophen)	Mild to moderate pain and pyrexia. Serious liver damage can occur in overdose. Often combined with other analgesics.
Nefopam hydrochloride	Persistent moderate pain that does not respond to other non-opioid drugs. It acts centrally in the brain and spinal cord. It does not cause any respiratory depression.

The opioid drugs

Opium, the natural product of the opium poppy plant, is a powerful analgesic and psychoactive drug. Its use in pain management, and also for sedation and even recreation, has been important for many years. It was used extensively in the last century as **'tincture of opium'** (known then as **laudanum**), which contained **morphine**, an opium derivative. Laudanum is no longer used, but morphine is still used along with other opium derivatives, and these are a major means of solving the pain problem.

Unlike the NSAIDs, the opioid drugs work *centrally* within the central nervous system (CNS, that is, the brain and the spinal cord). They bind to special receptors within the brain and cord to provide a degree of analgesia at spinal cord level, called **spinous analgesia**, or brainstem level, called **supraspinous analgesia**. There are three main kinds of receptors on the surface of cells in the CNS that bind opioid drugs: the **mu (μ) opioid receptor (MOR)**, **kappa (κ) opioid receptor (KOR)**, and **delta (δ) opioid receptor (DOR)**. These receptors are referred to as **metabotropic**, that is, their activation changes the metabolism of the cell through a G protein mechanism (Figure 2.2, Chapter 2, p. 28). The mu receptor is found mostly in the brainstem and is the one mostly associated with supraspinous analgesia, respiratory depression, euphoria, and dependence. This is the receptor that morphine and other opioids mostly bind to. The kappa receptor is found in the upper spinal cord and provides spinous analgesia by blocking substance P (see 'The spinal cord', p. 277). The delta receptor is found in the brain and spinal cord and some tissues outside of the CNS. It does have a role in pain control, but this is complex with many factors, such as receptor location, affecting the result.

All cell receptors bind naturally to products called **ligands**. In the case of the opioid receptors, the ligands are products of the CNS called **endogenous opioids**. The endogenous opioid group of ligands consists of **endorphins**, **enkephalins**, **dynorphins**, and **endomorphines**. In addition, some less well-known small peptide ligands also exist, for example, **dermorphins** and **morphiceptins**.

Endorphins are the largest peptide molecules of the group. They come in various forms, called **alpha** (α) **endorphin**, **beta** (β) **endorphin**, and **gamma** (γ) **endorphin**. They tend to be produced in the brain in response to severe pain and provide some degree of analgesia for around 4 hours or so.

Enkephalins are smaller peptide molecules. There are two types: **met-enkephalin** (*met* = **methionine**) and **leu-enkephalin** (*leu* = **leucine**). They are present in the ratio of about 4 met to 1 leu. They are produced in response to more mild pain and provide analgesia for around 2 minutes or so. A neurotransmitter called **substance P** (see 'The spinal cord', p. 277) is a facilitator for the passage of pain impulses across the synapse between neurons 1 and 2 of the pain pathways. Substance P is therefore a pain mediator at spinal cord level. By binding to kappa receptors in the spinal cord, enkephalin inhibits the release, and therefore the function, of substance P, thus reducing pain impulses at spinal cord level.

Dynorphins occur in two known types, **dynorphin A** and **dynorphin B**. They are also small peptide molecules. Endomorphins are small peptide molecules that also occur in two forms: **endomorphin-1** and **endomorphin-2**.

The principal members of the opioid drug group (Table 15.3) include morphine, diamorphine, pethidine, codeine, and fentanyl. **Morphine** remains the major drug for pain relief in this group. It is the analgesic against which all others are compared. It is a potent analgesic for the management of severe pain, but it does cause respiratory depression (see 'Titration', p. 291), nausea, vomiting, and constipation as side effects. It has found an important role in palliative care for the maintenance of a pain-free state. Morphine also causes a state of euphoria, the reason for morphine addiction, and some degree of mental detachment, which is useful in reducing the psychological response to pain.

Morphine has variable absorption when taken by mouth and undergoes considerable first-pass metabolism in the liver, making injection more efficient as a route of administration. **First-pass metabolism** is the alteration of the drug in the liver after absorption from the bowel. These changes occur prior to the drug entering general circulation and carrying out its pain control activity. The liver reduces the amount of drug available for pain control, that is, the **bioavailability** (see 'Pharmacokinetics', p. 294). These changes do not apply to the injected drug, since only the drug delivered by the oral route is taken first to the liver by the hepatic portal vein. Injected drugs have 100% bioavailability. The metabolism of morphine in the liver results in a metabolite called **morphine-6 glucuronide** (**M6G**), which has a greater analgesic effect than morphine itself, and it crosses the blood–brain barrier.[5] It has been used in research as a very effective analgesic, but it can accumulate in the kidneys, causing the potential for renal failure. **Morphine-3 glucuronide** (**M3G**) is also produced from morphine metabolism, but conversely,

TABLE 15.3 The opioid drugs

Opioid drugs	Notes
Buprenorphine	Moderate to severe pain
Co-codamol	Moderate to severe pain
Codeine phosphate	Moderate pain
Diamorphine hydrochloride (heroin hydrochloride)	Acute and chronic pain
Dihydrocodeine tartrate	Moderate to severe pain
Dihydrocodeine with paracetamol	Moderate to severe pain
Dipipanone hydrochloride with cyclizine	Acute pain
Fentanyl	Chronic severe pain and breakthrough pain (see text).
Hydromorphone hydrochloride	Severe pain in cancer
Meptazinol	Moderate to severe pain
Morphine	Moderate to severe pain, chronic pain, and pain in palliative care
Oxycodone hydrochloride	Moderate to severe pain; used in palliative care and as patient-controlled analgesia (PCA)[6]
Oxycodone with naloxone	Severe pain
Pentazocine	Moderate to severe pain
Pethidine hydrochloride	Acute pain
Tapentadol	Moderate to severe pain
Tramadol hydrochloride	Moderate to severe pain
Tramadol with dexketoprofen	Moderate to severe acute pain
Tramadol with paracetamol	Moderate to severe pain

its pharmacological significance is complex and has not been fully evaluated. For example, M3G has very little binding to MOR and cannot cross the blood–brain barrier. Morphine glucuronides are excreted through the urine, but also through the biliary system, to the bowel, where the morphine component is largely reabsorbed. The duration of pain control activity for morphine is about 3 to 4 hours.

Diamorphine (heroin) is a powerful analgesic. It is more soluble than morphine, and this is useful in palliative care to allow the injection of effective doses in smaller volumes. Diamorphine is converted to morphine in the body, although diamorphine itself is more active as an analgesic than morphine. Diamorphine has greater powers than morphine in crossing the blood–brain barrier and therefore enters the brain faster, especially when given intravenously (IV). This makes it attractive as a drug of illicit use. Diamorphine is active in the body for about 2 hours.

Pethidine provides rapid but short-lasting analgesia. It is less potent than morphine, even in higher doses, but it is less constipating. Severe pain on a long-term basis is better managed with drugs other than pethidine. Pethidine is metabolised in the liver to **norpethidine**, a metabolite with hallucinogenic and convulsant properties.

Codeine is made from morphine (codeine is **3-methylmorphine**) but is better absorbed when given by mouth than morphine, although it has only about 20% of the analgesic effect. Codeine is effective for treating mild to moderate pain but is not advisable for long-term use due to its side effect of causing constipation. It causes little to no euphoric effects and is therefore rarely addictive.

Other opioid analgesic drugs include **fentanyl**, a drug with similar but shorter-lasting actions to morphine and is available in transdermal skin patches for the prevention of 'breakthrough' pain, that is, transient periods of pain not prevented by other drugs. **Hydromorphone** has similar efficacy to morphine, but with fewer side effects, especially nausea and vomiting.

The dosage of opioid analgesics is calculated accurately to combine a complete pain-free state without excessive drug administration, which would lead to unwanted side effects. Finding the right dosage level is called **titration**. Opioid drug *titration* is defined as 'calculating the least amount of the drug required in circulation to achieve full analgesia'. A serious side effect that must be avoided is **respiratory depression**, that is, the reduction in breathing caused by some opioid drugs binding to receptors on the respiratory centre in the brainstem. Respiratory depression is particularly dangerous in the elderly, due to their reduced lung capacity, and in those with pre-existing respiratory disease, and both criteria apply to cancer. The elderly suffer cancers more commonly than the young, and if this is lung cancer, it will already be seriously affecting the patient's breathing. Additional respiratory depression caused by the drugs could result in unnecessary serious complications. Opioid titration relies on feedback from the patient on their pain status and any side effects, and this is where a pain assessment tool is of value. If they are still in pain, then they require more analgesia whilst considering any side effects. Top-up doses are given until a pain-free state is achieved (see 'Analgesic ladder', Figure 15.11).

Key points

Pain

- Acute pain tends to be sudden and of short duration. Chronic pain has a longer duration of weeks, months, or even years. Intractable pain is chronic pain unrelated to any detectable pathology.
- Localised pain is often caused by inflammation of the tissues involved.
- Pain mediators are released at the site, for example, histamine, prostaglandins, and bradykinins.

Pain pathway

- Nociceptors are pain nerve endings occurring in two types: mechanoreceptors and polymodal receptors.
- Two types of sensory nerve pathways carry pain impulses to the brain: fast 'A' fibres and slower 'C' fibres.
- The A and C fibres are the first neurons of a three-neuronal system from the periphery to the brain.
- The 'gate control theory' describes a pain-blocking process in the spinal cord.
- The thalamic response to pain is to initiate movement to help overcome the pain.

Pain assessment

- Pain assessment tools fall into three categories: verbal descriptor scales, visual analogue scales, and pain behaviour tools.
- Child pain assessment tools often consist of a series of cartoon faces showing a range of expressions, from happy (experiencing no pain) to very sad or crying (experiencing severe pain).

- Referred pain occurs some distance away from the site of the cause.
- The chronic pain suffered in cancer is caused by one or more of three effects: further advancement of the disease, the pain involved in treatment, or pain from co-existing disease.

Analgesia

- The World Health Organization (WHO) introduced the concept of a stepped approach to pain management, known as the 'analgesic ladder'.
- Adjuvant therapy is non-drug treatment for pain and consists of a wide range of treatments, from simple things like massage, TENS, acupuncture, and aromatherapy to nerve block and surgery.
- *Analgesia* is the absence of pain without causing loss of consciousness or loss of touch sensation.
- There are two major groups of analgesic drugs: the opioids and the non-steroidal anti-inflammatory drugs (NSAIDs).
- NSAIDs act in the peripheral tissues where pain originates, while opioids work centrally in the brainstem and spinal cord.
- Opioid drugs bind to the mu (μ), kappa (κ), and delta (δ) receptors within the brain and spinal cord.
- A drug acting on receptors at spinal cord level is called spinous analgesia, and at brainstem level is called supraspinous analgesia.
- The opioid receptors mu, kappa, and delta are there to bind the naturally produced endogenous opioids called endorphins, enkephalins, dynorphins, endomorphins, dermorphins, and morphiceptins.
- Palliative care is used for those patients where further treatment options are not possible. *Palliative care* indicates the management of symptoms, like pain, to allow comfort and improved quality of life.
- Morphine is the major opioid drug for pain relief, against which all others are compared. It is a potent analgesic for the management of severe pain, but it does cause respiratory depression, nausea, vomiting, and constipation as side effects.
- Finding the right dosage level of analgesia is called titration.
- Opioid drug *titration* is defined as calculating the least amount of the drug required in circulation to achieve full analgesia.
- A serious side effect that must be avoided is respiratory depression.
- Respiratory depression is particularly dangerous in the elderly (owing to reduced lung capacity) and in those with pre-existing respiratory disease.

Notes

1 The word **nociception** is often used as another word for *pain*.
2 *Fibre* is another term for the axon of a neuron (Figure 1.13, Chapter 1, p. 16).
3 Temporarily, in the sense that new COX will be produced to replace the COX blocked by the NSAID.
4 Low-dose aspirin taken on a long-term basis has provided some protection against colorectal cancers by increasing the immune response to the tumour. Low-dose aspirin shows an increase in important biomarkers required by the immune system and a decrease in the risk of metastases.
5 The blood–brain barrier is the endothelial interface between the blood and the central nervous system which allows the passage of nutrients into the brain but prevents the passage of toxic substances.
6 Patient-controlled analgesia (PCA) is used in palliative care to achieve a pain-free state. Patients can control their own drug administration with an IV pump.

16

THE TREATMENT OF CANCER 1

Pharmacology and chemotherapy

- **Introduction**
- **Basic principles of pharmacology**
- **Chemotherapy**
- **Nanodrug technology**
- **Key points**

Introduction

The treatment of cancer is multifaceted, meaning, that several different ways of tackling the problem are employed, often at the same time, to give the maximum possible benefit to the patient. These treatment methods include not only the mainstream therapies of surgery, radio-therapy, and chemotherapy but also other important and developing scientific approaches, such as immunotherapy. Mixed in with this cocktail of treatments is the need for pain control and management of the stress and anxiety that a diagnosis of cancer will bring.

Basic principles of pharmacology

Pharmacology is the study of drugs and is divided into several sciences:

- **Pharmacokinetics**, the study of how drugs are moved through the body, from entry to exit. It is divided into absorption, distribution, metabolism, and excretion.
- **Pharmacodynamics**, the study of how drugs work.
- **Pharmacotherapeutics**, the study of drugs in clinical use, that is, storage, dosage, routes of administration, monitoring drug effects and side effects, drug allergies, etc.
- **Pharmacogenetics**, the study of how drugs interact with the patient's genetic profile to give the best possible outcome. This is part of the modern approach of targeted and personalised treatment.

A useful way to distinguish pharmacokinetics from pharmacodynamics is to say the former is the way the *body handles the drug*, and the latter is the way the *drug handles the body*.

DOI: 10.4324/9781003389125-16

Pharmacokinetics

Most drugs are administered by mouth, but this route requires the drug to be able to survive digestive enzymes and changes in pH,[1] from gastric acidity to bowel alkalinity. Some drugs must be given by injection, for example, insulin, because these drugs would not survive digestion. Drugs injected into a muscle, that is, intramuscularly, will be absorbed slowly, and that delays their activity. Drugs injected directly into the blood, that is, intravenously, bypass absorption entirely and is the fastest route for instant drug delivery.

Oral drugs are transported to the liver via the hepatic portal vein[2] prior to release into general circulation. The liver carries out some metabolism, called **first-pass metabolism**, on the drug prior to its release into the general circulation. This reduces the **bioavailability** of the drug dose, that is, the amount of active drug arriving in the general circulation. As an example, if the oral dosage of a drug as 100%, first-pass metabolism may reduce this by 15%,[3] with 85% leaving the liver unchanged, that is, the bioavailability. Most drugs are transported in the blood bound to proteins, notably **albumin**, the commonest blood protein.

Metabolites are the products of drug metabolism. Most metabolites are no longer active as a drug and have been prepared for excretion via the kidneys. They are transported to the kidney via the hepatic vein (see footnote 2) and the general circulation. Sometimes a drug metabolite is still active and becomes part of the bioavailability. In a few cases, the original drug is not active until it has been metabolised. The original (inactive) drug is called a **prodrug**, and the active metabolite is the drug itself.

How long drugs are active and remain in the blood depends on their **half-life** (Figure 16.1). The *half-life* is the time it takes for the kidney to excrete half the circulating dose of the drug. This varies a lot for different drugs and is best explained by an example. Consider drug X has a

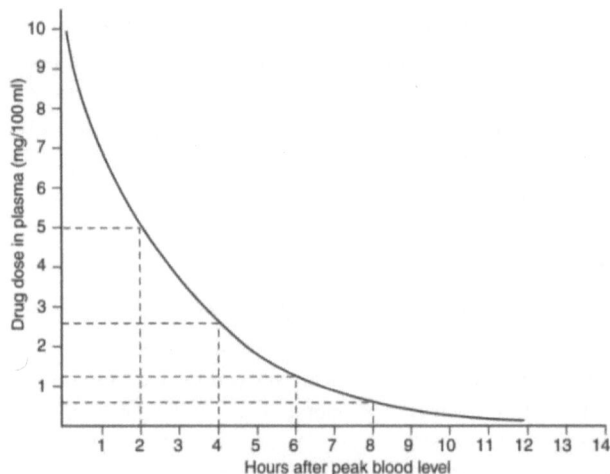

FIGURE 16.1 Drug half-life. This drug has a half-life of 2 hours, which means 50% of the dose carried by the blood is removed from the blood in the first 2 hours, a further 25% is removed in the second 2 hours, a further 12.5% is removed in the third 2 hours, and so on. Different drugs have different half-lives. Those with short half-lives may need repeated doses during the day to maintain a reasonable blood level. Long half-life means that repeat dosage may be required less often.

half-life of 2 hours, and the initial bioavailability peak in circulation is 100%, then 2 hours later, the dosage in circulation is reduced to 50%. After a further 2-hour period, the blood level of the drug is further reduced by half to 25%. After a third 2-hour period, the blood level is reduced further by half to 12.5%, and so on. Two things are shown by this:

1. The excretion of the drug gradually slows down so only half of each of the preceding 2-hour period is removed from circulation.
2. Because each 2-hour period removes only half of the preceding bioavailability, it becomes impossible to determine when zero is reached. Given enough time periods, the values reached are incredibly small, far below the levels required to be active.

Pharmacodynamics

This is the mechanism by which drugs work. Some drugs bind to receptors on cell surfaces. These are either **agonists**, that is, they stimulate the receptor, or **antagonists**, which block the receptor so the receptor fails to work. The natural substance which normally binds to the receptor is the **ligand**. The ligands are a wide range of natural chemical agents, such as a hormones and cytokines (see 'Cytokines and chemokines', Chapter 5, p. 94). There are many different receptors for different ligands. Agonist drugs act like the ligand, but antagonist drugs prevent the ligand from binding. This mode of action applies to the anti-oestrogen drugs (see 'Hormonal treatment of cancer', Chapter 4, p. 71).

Pharmacotherapeutics

This is the way drugs are used in clinical practice. It covers many aspects of clinical drug usage, including dosage, storage, prescribing, drug calculations, routes of administration, side effects, drug interactions, and record-keeping.

The prescribed dose of a drug is based on the **therapeutic window** (Figure 16.2). This is the window of dosage that will benefit the patient whilst creating the least amount of side effects. The lowest point of the window is the smallest dose that will have a beneficial effect in the body, below which the effect is so small as to be of value. The highest point of the window is the dosage that has the maximum effect, above which side effects, and possibly toxicity, will become a problem. It is the safe dosage window for prescribing any drug. The ideal regime is to prescribe the drug at the lower end of the window so there is opportunity to raise the dose if required, but this depends on what drug is involved and the condition being treated.

Chemotherapy

Chemotherapy is the main approach to anti-cancer treatment, usually after the initial surgery. This is changing, as new treatments are becoming available. There is a range of drugs used in the treatment of cancer, and some are of the type that prevents the reproduction of cells, that is, cell division. The faster the rates of cell division, the more the cells are susceptible to drug therapy, including tumour cells, many of which divide rapidly. Cells that divide quickly are those that are constantly passing around the cell cycle in quick succession (Figure 1.6, Chapter 1, p. 7). In normal tissues, the cells of the bone marrow; the gonads, that is, sperm in males and ova in females; mucous membrane; and those of stratified epithelium, for example, the outer layer of

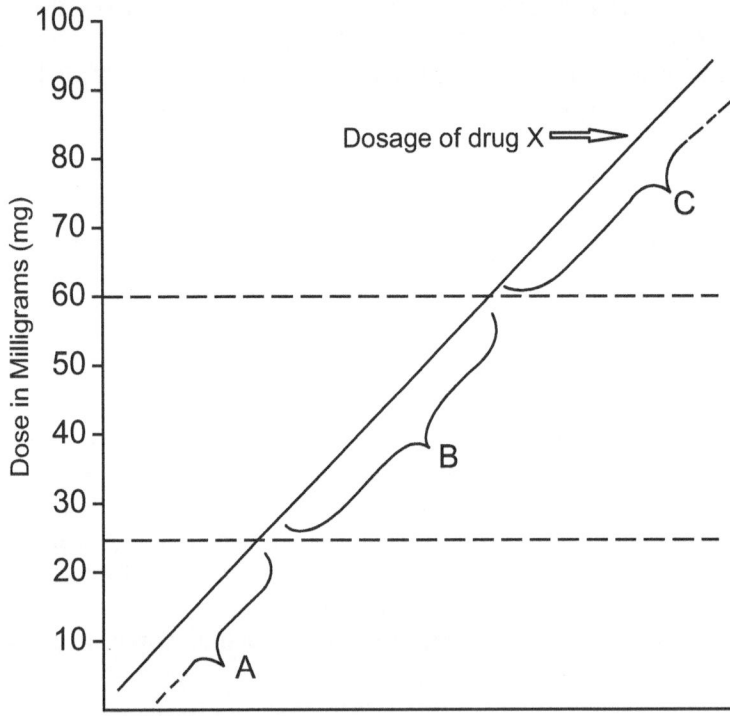

FIGURE 16.2 *Therapeutic window* is the dose range in which a drug is both safe and effective. In this example, drug X has a therapeutic window between 25 mg and 60 mg (zone B). Below 25 mg (zone A), the dose is too low and is unlikely to be effective. Above 60 mg (zone C), the dose is too high and is likely to cause unwanted side effects or may even be dangerous to life. Different drugs will have different therapeutic windows.

the skin (Figure 13.1, Chapter 13, p. 242), have the fastest cell division and are therefore the cells most affected by these drugs.

Chemotherapy is expanding to include therapy that targets the cancer microenvironment (see 'The tumour and its microenvironment', Chapter 6, p. 120), as this is key to the metastatic spread around the body that causes 90% of cancer deaths (Sounni and Noel 2013).

The main groups of chemotherapy drugs are (Figure 16.3):[4]

1. Alkylating agents, for example, cyclophosphamide
2. Anthracycline antibiotics, for example, daunorubicin
3. Antimetabolites, for example, methotrexate
4. Cytotoxic antibiotic, for example, mitomycin
5. Plant alkaloids

   • Topoisomerase I and II inhibitors, for example, irinotecan and topotecan
   • Podophyllotoxin, for example, etoposide
   • Taxanes, for example, cabazitaxel
   • Vinca alkaloids, for example, vincristine

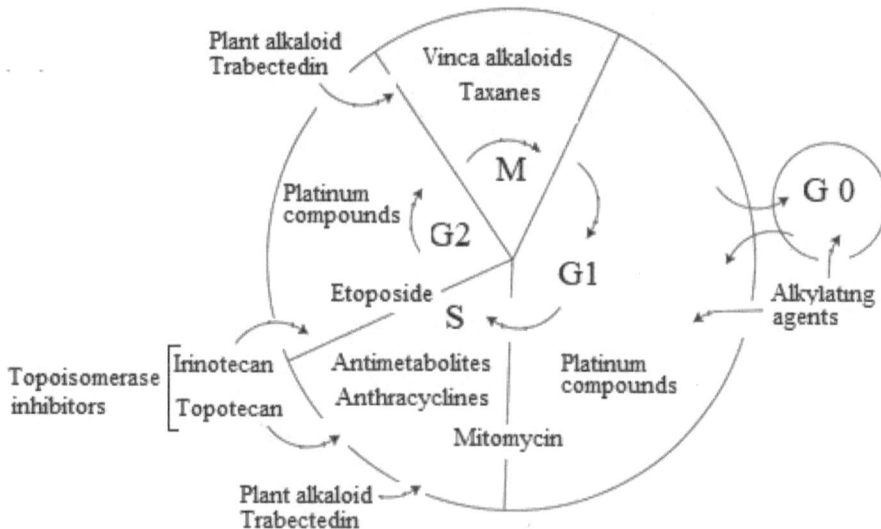

FIGURE 16.3   Overview of the cell cycle and the phases where the major anti-cancer drugs act. These drugs interfere with cell division and stop cell mitosis. Since cancer cells pass through mitosis frequently, they are more vulnerable to these drugs. Some drugs are *cell cycle specific*, meaning, they act at certain phases as shown, but others act more widely around the cycle, that is, they are *cell cycle non-specific*. The alkylating agents are generally non-specific but appear to act more often in G_0 and G_1. The plant alkaloid trabectedin acts during the S phase to slow the cycle down, and again in the G_2/M phase to halt the cycle. The topoisomerase inhibitors are irinotecan, which blocks topoisomerase 1 in the S/G_2 phase, and topotecan, which blocks topoisomerase 1 in the S phase. The antimetabolites and the anthracyclines act mostly in the S phase. The cytotoxic antibiotic mitomycin acts in the late G_1 and S phases, and the podophyllotoxin etoposide acts in late S and early G_2 phases. The vinca alkaloids and taxanes act in the M phase, and the platinum compounds are cell cycle non-specific. M = mitosis; G_0 = leaving the cell cycle; G_1 and G_2 = growth phases; S = synthesis phase (see Figure 1.6, Chapter 1, p. 7).

6. Platinum compounds, for example, cisplatin
7. Protein kinase inhibitors
8. Proteasome inhibitors
9. Others (see 'Other cytotoxic drugs', p. 303)

Alkylating agents (Table 16.1)

The original drug (**chlormethine**, also called **mustine**) was developed from sulphur mustard gases used as a weapon in First World War trenches.

The group consists of five subgroups of drugs based on function: (1) **nitrogen mustards**, (2) **ethylenimines**, (3) **alkyl sulphonate**, (4) **nitrosoureas**, and (5) **triazenes**. Examples of each are shown in Table 16.1.

TABLE 16.1 The alkylating cytotoxic drugs used in the UK

Alkylating agents	Nitrogen mustards	Ethylenimines	Alkyl sulfonates	Nitrosoureas	Triazenes	Bif	Mon
Bendamustine	√						√
Chlorambucil	√						√
Chlormethine	√						√
Cyclophosphamide	√						√
Estramustine phosphate	√						√
Ifosfamide	√						√
Melphalan	√						√
Thiotepa		√					√
Busulfan			√				√
Treosulfan			√				√
Carmustine				√			√
Lomustine				√		√	
Streptozocin				√		√	?√
Dacarbazine					√		√
Temozolomide					√		√
Trabectedin	Classified as a tetrahydroisoquinoline alkaloid, a non-traditional alkylating agent, with some of its structure similar to the triazenes.				√		

Note: Columns 2 to 6 indicate the subgroup each falls into. *Bif* = bifunctional; *Mon* = monofunctional (see 'Alkylating agents', p. 297). There is some controversy concerning streptozocin, with most sources saying it is bifunctional, but some are saying monofunctional.

Mechanism of action of alkylating agents

Alkylating agents have an alkyl group which is highly reactive with DNA (called **alkylation**), causing irreversible bonds linking the two strands of the DNA molecule (called **intercalation**). This results in the two strands being unable to separate for replication. Guanine is especially susceptible to alkylation. These drugs are called **bifunctional** ('Bif' in Table 16.1) because they affect two bases. **Monofunctional** ('Mon' in Table 16.1) drugs bond to one base, causing it to separate from its partner, and this results in a single-strand DNA breakage (Figure 16.4). Both bifunctional and monofunctional drugs lead to the death of rapidly reproducing cells, such as cancer cells. These drugs function in all the cell cycle stages but affect G_1 and S phases the most and kills the cell during G_0 and G_1 (Figure 16.3; see also Figure 1.6, Chapter 1, p. 7).

Nitrosoureas undergo an additional reaction, called **carbamoylation**, where a **carbamoyl group** (NH_2CO) is added to amino acids. This binding reduces cancer cells' ability to repair the damage from alkylation.

Cells can employ mechanisms to overcome the damage caused by these drugs. These tactics include repair of DNA, decreasing the amount of the drug entering the cell, and mechanisms employed by the cell to inactivate the drug.

The alkylating agents have two main complications associated with their prolonged use. First, they may interfere with **gametogenesis**, the formation of sperm or ova, and this can lead to infertility. Second, again, on a long-term basis, they have been linked to **acute non-lymphocytic leukaemia**, especially if used in combination with radiotherapy. However, this does not appear to be a problem with short-term use of these agents.

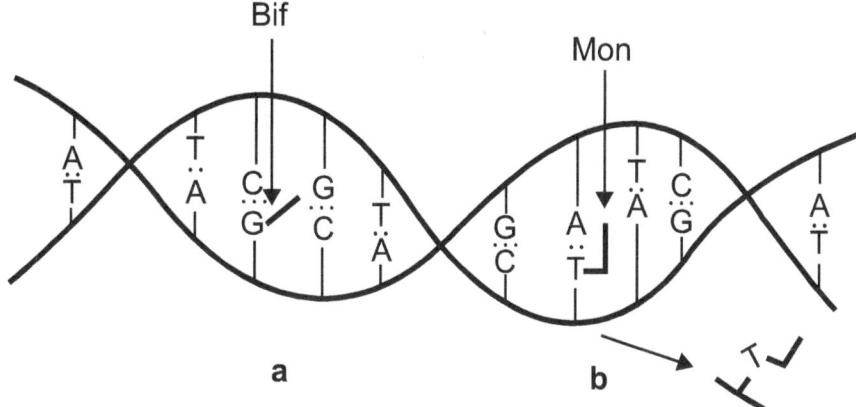

FIGURE 16.4   DNA alkylation by alkylating agents: (a) Bifunctional (Bif) drug causes irreversible cross-linked base bonding between two bases (guanine to guanine is shown) and between strands (interstrand, or intercalation), preventing the two strands from separating during DNA replication in cancer cells. (b) Monofunctional drug bonds to a single base on one strand, causing it to separate from its partner and break free from the DNA, that is, single-strand breakage.

Anthracyclines (cytotoxic antibiotics)

These include **doxorubicin hydrochloride, epirubicin hydrochloride, mitoxantrone, idarubicin**, and **daunorubicin**. They are derived from the *Streptomyces* bacterium. They act in the S phase of the cell cycle, with the death of the cell occurring in early G_2 phase (Figure 16.3). They are used in the treatment of leukaemia, lymphomas, and lung, stomach, ovarian, bladder, and breast cancers.

Mechanism of action of anthracycline drugs

These drugs act in three ways:

1. They prevent DNA synthesis and RNA transcription by causing intercalation (see 'Mechanism of action of alkylating agents', p. 298) and strand breakages between the two DNA strands (Figure 16.4). There is also some exchange of genetic bases between the sister chromatids (see 'The nucleus, chromosomes, and genes', Chapter 1, p. 3).
2. They create **free radicals**, which are highly reactive molecules. These include superoxide anion radicals,[5] for example, H_2O_2, NO, and OH-, that damage DNA. They interact and damage other cellular structures and cell energy production.
3. They interact with cell membranes, causing lipid peroxides (see footnote 5). Lipid peroxides are fat molecules with additional oxygen atoms. Such lipid peroxides cause adverse membrane damage and change membrane function within the cell.

The cells cannot survive this degree of intracellular destruction and loss of function and will die. They have the general side effects of all cytotoxic drugs (see 'Side effects of cytotoxic therapy', p. 304), but they may also cause cardiac complications, known as **cardiac toxicity**.

Antimetabolites

These drugs work by mimicking essential molecules, that is, the metabolites, that are part of normal cellular DNA metabolism. The drugs are often similar in structure to the normal metabolite. Cancer cells replace the normal metabolite with the drug in the construction of its genetic material, which then does not function, causing DNA synthesis to fail. Some drugs even block the enzyme that normally acts on it. The cell is no longer able to survive.

Antimetabolites fall into two main groups:

1. Folate antagonists (Figure 16.5)
2. Purine or pyrimidine base analogues (Figure 16.6)

A **folate antagonist** is a **folate** (or **folic acid**) **analogue**, that is, the drug very closely resembles the structure of folic acid, a vital component of metabolism, but being slightly altered, the drug

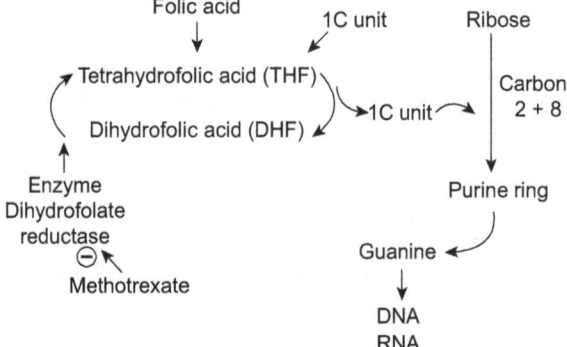

FIGURE 16.5 The action of methotrexate. Folic acid is converted to THF, which receives units containing one carbon (1C). THF then donates these units to the sugar ribose as part of the formation of the purine ring (Figure 16.6a). THF contributes two such 1C units to the ring, and these become the carbons at positions 2 and 8 of the ring. By donating a 1C unit, it becomes DHF, and to receive further 1C units, it must be converted back to THF by the enzyme DHF reductase. Methotrexate inhibits the function of DHF reductase, and this prevents THF conversion and thus blocks the purine ring synthesis. The purine ring forms the basis of guanine, a vital component of both DNA and RNA, and without the ring, guanine and DNA/RNA synthesis stops.

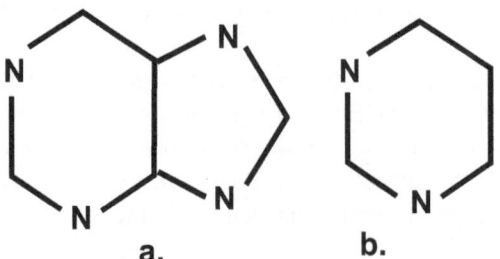

FIGURE 16.6 (a) The purine ring (adenine and guanine). (b) The pyrimidine ring (cytosine and thymine).

TABLE 16.2 The antimetabolite drugs

Antimetabolite	Folate analogue	Purine analogue	Pyrimidine analogue
Azacitidine			√
Cladribine		√	
Clofarabine		√	
Cytarabine			√
Decitabine			√
Fludarabine phosphate		√	
Fluorouracil			√
Gemcitabine			√
Mercaptopurine		√	
Methotrexate	√		
Pentostatin		√	
Tioguanine		√	

does not act as folic acid. The drug **methotrexate** gets incorporated into the folic acid metabolic pathway and inhibits the enzyme **dihydrofolate reductase**. Folic acid is essential for the formation of DNA, and when the metabolism of folic acid fails, the cell dies (Figure 16.5).

Purine base analogues closely resemble the purine bases, that is, **adenine** and **guanine** (Figure 16.6a), and **pyrimidine base analogues** closely resemble the pyrimidine bases, that is, **cytosine** and **thymine** (Figure 16.6b), all major components of DNA.

Antimetabolites cause similar side effects to those seen generally for cytotoxic drugs (see 'Side effects of cytotoxic therapy', p. 304).

Cytotoxic antibiotic (non-anthracycline antibiotic)

Mitomycin is one of the three products, **mitomycin A, B**, and **C**, all derived from *Streptomyces caespitosus*. The name used on its own refers to mitomycin C. Although this is an antibiotic, it is not classified as an anthracycline. It functions as an alkylating agent, causing bifunctional and trifunctional cross-linking of DNA strands that prevents DNA replication and gene transcription. Mitomycin is cell cycle non-specific but works best during late G_1 and early S phases (Figure 16.3).

Plant alkaloids

These drugs are all derived from plants, but they are divided into four groups:

1. **Topoisomerase I and II inhibitors.** The enzymes **topoisomerase I (IA and IB)** and **II (IIA and IIB)** are required to maintain DNA structure and resolve DNA topological problems, such as supercoiling and entanglement. Type I enzymes cut and rejoin one of the two DNA strands. Type II enzymes cut both strands at the same time, which allows for disentanglement of strands that are tangled up during replication. If this process were to fail, this would cause cell death. The product camptothecin (CPT) was isolated from the tree *Camptotheca acuminata*, and the drugs **irinotecan** and **topotecan** are synthesised from camptothecin. Topotecan works by blocking the function of topoisomerase I. It forms a bond with the DNA/

topoisomerase I complex, causing breaks in the DNA strand, leading to cell death (apoptosis). Irinotecan has a similar mode of action. These drugs prevent DNA strand repair by topoisomerase I, and therefore, both DNA and RNA syntheses cannot take place, killing the cell. Side effects of these drugs are similar as for all cytotoxic drugs (see 'Side effects of cytotoxic therapy', p. 304) but also include **myelosuppression**, that is, reduced production of cells in the myeloid blood cell line (see Figure 7.2, Chapter 7, p. 131), and gastrointestinal effects, such as **diarrhoea**.

2. **Podophyllotoxin. Etoposide** is derived from the root of the **wild mandrake** (*Podophyllum peltatum*), and it binds to the complex formed by the joining of DNA and the enzyme **topoisomerase II**. This enzyme is involved in the cleavage, uncoiling, recoiling, and repair of the DNA double helix during DNA replication and works with topoisomerase I. The drug blocks DNA repair (re-ligation) after topoisomerase II has cut the double strands, and this prevents DNA replication, mostly whilst the cell is in G_2 of the cell cycle (Figure 16.3). Accumulated unrepaired cuts in the DNA will cause the cell to die. It may cause the usual side effects (see 'Side effects of cytotoxic therapy', p. 304). Etoposide is protein-bound in circulation, and excretion is via the kidneys.

3. **Taxanes.** The drugs **paclitaxel**, **cabazitaxel**, and **docetaxel** are derived from the coniferous tree *Taxus*. They bind to the microtubules of the cytoskeleton, and they stabilise the tubulin component. The resulting stabilised microtubules cannot be removed or broken down by the cell. Cells need to dismantle the cytoskeleton for the purpose of cell division, including breakdown of the mitotic spindle, which should normally disappear after mitosis. This means the cell cannot complete mitosis and will die. The main activity occurs during G_2 and mitosis (Figure 16.3). They can cause the general side effects of most cytotoxic drugs (see 'Side effects of cytotoxic therapy', p. 304), but also **neutropenia**, that is, low blood levels of **neutrophils** (see 'Blood cell types', Chapter 7, p. 131), **arthralgia** (joint aches), and **myalgia** (muscle aches).

4. **Vinca alkaloids.** The vinca alkaloids, for example, vincristine, vinblastine, and vindesine, are drugs derived from the periwinkle *Catharanthus roseus*. They are similar to taxanes because they also bind to tubulin and disrupt the microtubules of the cell cytoskeleton, including the mitotic spindle. It is the binding to tubulin of the mitotic spindle that causes failure of cell division, and the cell will die. Therefore, the drug is active during mitosis (Figure 16.3). The vinca alkaloids are especially useful drugs in the treatment of lymphomas (see 'Lymphatic cancers', Chapter 7, p. 143) and leukaemia (see 'Leukaemia', Chapter 7, p. 133). They can cause the general side effects of cytotoxic drugs (see 'Side effects of cytotoxic therapy', p. 304), as well neurotoxicity symptoms, such as peripheral neuropathy, that is, *in motor nerves*, for example, weakness, restlessness of the limbs, or *in sensory nerves*, for example, tingling, burning sensation, pain, or numbness of the limbs.

Platinum compounds

The drugs in this group include cisplatin, carboplatin, and oxaliplatin. Similar to the alkylating agents, these drugs cause cross-linked intercalation of the DNA bases during G_1 of the cell cycle (Figure 16.3) (see also 'Mechanism of action of alkylating agents', p. 298). This renders DNA unavailable for RNA/DNA synthesis, and this causes the cell to die. Platinum drugs are used in the treatment of lymphomas, sarcomas, and breast, colorectal, ovarian, lung, gastro-oesophageal, and bladder cancers. They are excreted by the kidneys but can be a cause of renal toxicity, and the patient should drink well to aid in the drug's safe elimination. This may conflict with some of the side effects (see 'Side effects of cytotoxic therapy', p. 304), such as nausea and vomiting. They can also cause ototoxicity, that is, damage to the ears, causing hearing losses and tinnitus, that is, continual noises, buzzing, or whistling sounds heard in the ears. Peripheral neuropathy, that is, damage to the nerve tissues in the extremities, is another possible complication of these drugs, causing tingling or burning sensations felt in the feet or hands.

Protein kinase inhibitors

Protein kinases are enzymes that add a phosphate group (PO_4), that is, phosphorylation, to a protein. This affects the way proteins function. Kinase inhibitor drugs (Table 16.3) prevent this process, and the kinase loses control of cellular growth. Tyrosine kinases are important for growth and cell signalling regulation, and they are also regular targets of kinase inhibitors. In cancer cells, this loss of phosphorylation leads to cell death. Bruton's tyrosine kinase is produced by B cell lymphocytes and some other immune cells, except T cells. It is essential for B cell development. In B cell cancers, this enzyme facilitates cancer cell replication. Ibrutinib (Table 16.3) blocks this enzyme and reduces B cell cancer proliferation whilst having less effect on other normal immune cells.

Proteasome inhibitors

These are drugs that block the action of proteasomes, which are a complex of proteinases, that is, enzymes that break down the proteins found inside the cell. Many proteins are encoded from genes into long chains, and these usually need to be cut up and folded. Drugs that block proteasomes prevent this protein processing, and the resulting long protein chains cannot function. In cancer, these inhibitors prevent growth and spread of malignant cells, and they die.

Three proteasome inhibitors are available to treat multiple myeloma: bortezomib, carfilzomib, and ixazomib.

Other cytotoxic drugs

Some other drugs available for anti-cancer therapy are listed in Table 16.4.

TABLE 16.3 Selected protein kinase inhibitors

Drug	Malignancy treated
Abemaciclib	Breast cancer
Alectinib	Non-small-cell lung cancer
Asciminib	Chronic myeloid leukaemia
Binimetinib	Melanoma
Crizotinib	*ROS1*+ non-small-cell lung cancer (see 'ROS1-positive lung cancer', Chapter 9, p. 188)
Ibrutinib	Chronic lymphoid leukaemia
	Mantle cell lymphoma
Entrectinib	Solid tumours
	Non-small-cell lung cancer
Pemigatinib	Cholangiocarcinoma

TABLE 16.4 Other cytotoxic drugs

Drug	Mode of action	Used for
Amsacrine	Binds to DNA, causing intercalation between base pairs, especially between A and T bases. It causes double-strand breaks in DNA. It is also a topoisomerase II inhibitor in the S phase.	Acute adult leukaemia and malignant lymphomas
Asparaginase	Breaks down the amino acid asparagine, which is essential for cellular survival and growth. Normal cells can make their own asparagine, but cancer cells rely on a supply from the blood, which becomes depleted by this drug.	Acute lymphoblastic leukaemia (ALL) and lymphoblastic lymphoma
Crisantaspase	Another form of asparaginase.	As for asparaginase
Procarbazine	A 'non-classical' alkylating agent, it prevents DNA and RNA syntheses. It has action similar to alkylating agents, although its function is not well understood.	Hodgkin lymphoma and brain tumours
Eribulin	A 'non-taxane' microtubule inhibitor. It stops the formation of the mitotic spindle and prevents cell replication.	Breast cancers and liposarcoma
Raltitrexed	Inhibits the enzyme thymidylate synthase, which is essential for the formation of thymidine triphosphate (TTP), a nucleotide required specifically for DNA synthesis. Loss of TTP causes DNA break-up and cell death.	Colorectal cancer and malignant mesothelioma
Mitotane	Adrenal cortex inhibitor that kills adrenal cortical cancer cells by mitochondrial damage.	Adrenocortical carcinoma
Arsenic trioxide	Causes apoptosis in blood cancer cells by an unknown mechanism.	Acute promyelocytic leukaemia (APL)
Hydroxycarbamide	Antimetabolite of poorly understood function.	Chronic myelogenous leukaemia and cervical cancer
Pegaspargase	Modified version of asparaginase (this table) that depletes asparagine in the blood.	Acute lymphoblastic leukaemia (ALL)
Panobinostat	Histone deacetylase (HDAC) inhibitor. It blocks the function of HDAC, which removes acetyl groups from histones, that is, proteins which package DNA in the chromosome. An excess of acetyl groups on histones prevents normal gene expression and leads to cancer cell apoptosis.	Multiple myeloma

Side effects of cytotoxic therapy

1. Distressing nausea and vomiting accompanied by **anorexia** (loss of appetite).
2. Intolerance to oral fluids makes the patient reluctant to drink.
3. Bone marrow suppression, where bone marrow produces too few cells, leading to low numbers of red blood cells, causing **anaemia**, and white blood cells in circulation.

4. **Alopecia** (hair loss), which will grow back in most cases after treatment is stopped.
5. **Teratogenesis**, that is, the ability of the drug to cross the placenta during pregnancy and affect the developing foetus.
6. **Hyperuricaemia**, higher than normal levels of uric acid in the blood. It is extracted by the kidneys, where it can form crystals and may inhibit kidney function (see 'Urine formation', Chapter 10, p. 195).

Oncogenic emergency

This is a rapid deterioration in the patient's condition due to a catalogue of metabolic changes which happen because of aggressive treatment of large rapidly growing cancers. Many chemical substances are released from dying tissues, and these result in a massive metabolic disturbance from which the body may not recover (Figure 16.7). The effects are dependent on:

- The size of the tumour, with the largest tumours having the greatest effect
- The rate of cancer cell growth and cell turnover within the tumour, with the fastest-growing tumours having the greatest effect
- The response of the tumour to treatment

The consequences of oncogenic emergency can be life-threatening, as the chemical changes may cause, amongst other things, acute renal failure. The effects of the metabolic changes typically occur about 24 to 48 hours after starting the treatment and comprise hyperuricaemia, hyperkalaemia, and hypherphosphataemia (Figure 16.7).

Hyperuricaemia (high levels of blood **uric acid**) is caused by cell death and breakdown, which releases the nucleic acids **DNA (deoxyribonucleic acid)** and **RNA (ribonucleic acid)**. These are converted, first, to **hypoxanthine** and **xanthine**, then to uric acid. Normally, uric acid is excreted in the urine, and in hyperuricaemia, the excess uric acid filtered from the blood may crystallise in the urinary tract and obstruct urine flow, a step towards renal failure.

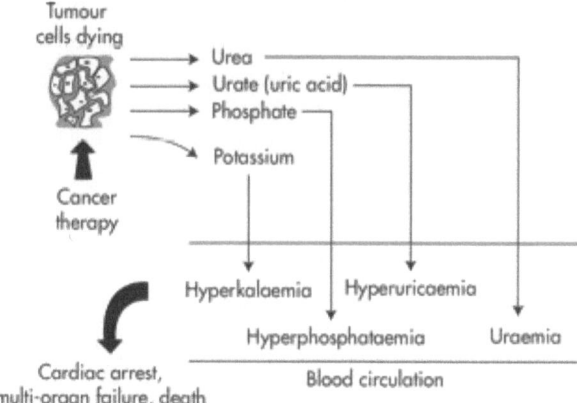

FIGURE 16.7   Oncogenic emergency, sometimes called cell lysis syndrome. This is caused by the massive destruction of tumour cells by cancer treatment. The cells release a cocktail of chemicals that, in circulation, can be life-threatening.

Hyperkalaemia, that is, excessive **potassium (K⁺)** levels in the blood, is caused by potassium coming from the dying and dead cells. About 98% of the K^+ in the body is stored inside cells and will be liberated if the cell dies. Potassium is excreted via the kidneys, but this removal mechanism may be impaired if the kidneys are damaged or begin to fail (see *hyperuricaemia* earlier), allowing the blood level to rise. Excess potassium in the blood and extracellular fluid reduces cardiac function, slowing the heart rate (called **bradycardia**) and causing **heart block**, that is, the inability of the impulse within the heart to travel from the atria to the ventricles properly. The ultimate result could be **cardiac arrest**, when the heart stops beating.

Hyperphosphataemia, that is, excessive phosphates in the blood, is caused by phosphates being released from dying cells. More than 99% of the body phosphates are inside the cells, and some malignant cells have higher than average phosphate levels. Large quantities are released from tumour cells when the drugs act to kill these cells. An increase in blood serum phosphates causes a corresponding loss of blood serum calcium, since the two substances have interrelated balances, and **calcium phosphate** molecules form. The resulting **hypocalcaemia** (low blood calcium) causes increased excitability of nerve tissue, **tetany** (severe muscle contractions linked to reduced calcium levels), and low conduction of impulses through the ventricles of the heart. The accumulation of calcium phosphate in the tissues precipitates the onset of organ failure, including the kidneys (Figure 16.7).

Nanodrug technology

One way to overcome the side effects of chemotherapy may be through **nanodrugs**, that is, extremely small anti-cancer medicines, 50,000 times smaller than an ant, that is, too small to be seen by the human eye. The drugs are delivered to the cancer cells by nanocarriers which attach to the malignant cells. These drugs are under development, but early tests are showing promise.

Key points

Pharmacology

- *Pharmacology* is the study of drugs, and this is broken down into separate topics.
- *Pharmacokinetics* is the study of the way drugs move through the body, from absorption, through metabolism and distribution, to elimination.
- *Pharmacodynamics* is the study of the way drugs work.
- *Pharmacotherapeutics* is the study of the way drugs are used in clinical practice.
- *Pharmacogenetics* is the study of the interactions between drugs and the human genome.

Chemotherapy

- The drugs used in the treatment of cancer (i.e. chemotherapy) prevent cell division. The cells mostly affected by the drugs are those with faster rates of cell division.
- The main groups of chemotherapy drugs are the alkylating agents, the platinum compounds, the topoisomerase I and II inhibitors, the cytotoxic antibiotics, the antimetabolites, and the drugs that disrupt microtubule function.
- The side effects of cytotoxic therapy are nausea and vomiting with anorexia (loss of appetite) and fluid intolerance; bone marrow suppression, causing anaemia and low white blood cells

in circulation; alopecia (hair loss); teratogenesis (the drugs cross the placenta during pregnancy and affect the foetus); and hyperuricaemia (high levels of uric acid in the blood).

- *Oncogenic emergency* is a rapid deterioration in the patient's condition due to a massive release of metabolic substances from dying cells because of aggressive treatment of large, rapidly growing cancers.

Notes

1   *pH* is the acid–alkaline scale, with pH 1 being the strongest acid and pH 14 being the strongest alkaline. pH 7 is neutral. Notice the *pH* term is always small 'p' and capital 'H'. This is important even at the start of a sentence. The capital 'H' is the chemical symbol for hydrogen, which means that *PH* and *ph* are incorrect and meaningless.
2   The hepatic portal vein (HPV) should not be confused with the hepatic vein (HV). The HPV takes blood, the products of digestion, and oral drugs to the liver from the gut. The HV takes blood and the products of liver metabolism, including drug metabolites, from the liver into general circulation. Two portal veins exist in the body: the large HPV from the gut to the liver, and the tiny hypothalamo-hypophyseal portal vein from the hypothalamus to the pituitary gland.
3   This is an arbitrary value in this example, since the actual amount differs between different drugs.
4   There is some variation in the way these drugs are classified, for example, some classifications put the vinca alkaloids and plant alkaloids together since the vinca drugs are derived from the vinca plant. The classification used here is based mostly on BNF 86 (2023).
5   *Radicals* are molecular structures that are free to interact with many other molecules, causing them damage. *Superoxides* are molecules that have acquired excess oxygen and act as free radicals, for example, molecules such as H_2O_2, which is hydrogen peroxide, and NO, which is nitric oxide. Lipid peroxides are fat molecules derived from cell membranes that have also gained oxygen and act as damaging free radicals.

17

THE TREATMENT OF CANCER 2

Other therapies and screening

- **Surgery**
- **Radiotherapy (RT)**
- **Stem cell therapy**
- **Gene therapy**
- **RNA interference therapy**
- **PROTAC therapy**
- **Histotripsy**
- **Adjunct therapy**
- **Artificial intelligence (AI) in cancer management**
- **Blood and saliva screening, liquid biopsies, and organoids**
- **Key points**

Surgery

Surgical removal, that is, **excision**, of new growths, wherever possible, is important for several reasons:

1. Surgery removes as much of the malignancy as possible, to reduce further growth and spread.
2. Surgery can often reduce the bulk of a tumour, which otherwise is a burden to the body. The tumour will consume energy and nutrients, may produce unwanted amounts of hormones (see Table 4.1, Chapter 4, p. 66) or other harmful substances that will have wide-ranging consequences for the rest of the body, and may obstruct, squeeze, or infiltrate surrounding tissues.
3. Surgery may be able to reduce tumour growth in circumstances where it cannot be entirely removed, for example, it may be possible to reduce the blood supply to a tumour, and this will cause it to regress.
4. Surgery can often correct the defects that are caused by the tumour, for example, creating a bypass around the obstruction can often relieve the symptoms of obstructions that cannot be cleared.

DOI: 10.4324/9781003389125-17

5. Surgery can be a major component in pain relief. Many surgical procedures can make the patient more comfortable and improve their quality of life and reduce the need for large doses of analgesic drugs.
6. Surgery may offer the patient some hope towards a future cure. It is not usually a cure in itself; in most cases, surgery needs follow-up treatment of secondary growths. But surgery will often make the postoperative treatment period shorter and with a much greater chance of success.

Surgery is a vital first step in many cases. But surgery has its own set of problems, and some of the important problems are:

1. Cancer is more frequently a disease of the older-aged population than any other age group, that is, those who are least well equipped physically to withstand surgery. Cancer surgery is often extensive, putting an enormous burden on the older person, particularly during the days immediately after the operation. Many of the elderly may not have the optimum respiratory fitness to tolerate an anaesthetic, especially those who had a lifetime of smoking. Alongside this is the fact that this older person may have been ill for quite a while and is therefore not at their peak physical condition. Surgery, and the accompanying anaesthetics, puts yet another burden on the patient's health, and it may be, in many cases, a burden too far.
2. Surgery is not, even today, entirely safe, at any age. Whilst every effort is made to reduce the risks, complications can and do arise, and this will add a further burden on the patient's health and quality of life. Complications are numerous and varied, including problems such as haemorrhage and infections, and these may be enough to cause the patient to deteriorate, especially if they are elderly.
3. Surgery may cause disfigurement. Here, too, great efforts are made to prevent any such disfigurement, but sometimes it is unavoidable. Facial disfigurement, for example, following surgery for facial, mouth, or jaw cancers, is one of the hardest for patients to come to terms with, and the follow-up reconstructive surgery only adds to their physical and psychological burden. Other forms of disfigurement, such as loss of a limb, are also major traumas for the patient to live with. It involves a rapid reassessment of one's own body image by the patient after many decades of being used to the way they look and feel. The burden is increased when the patient has to re-learn a basic function, such as feeding, walking, or elimination, for example, following a **colostomy** (see Figure 8.16, Chapter 8, p. 172), or the patient faces the rest of their life in a wheelchair.

Postoperative care following cancer surgery means not only for the physical care needed, for example, the pain relief, but also for the psychological support these patients will need. This is particularly important when the surgery is **palliative**, that is, it only relieves the symptoms or improves the quality of life, or when further postoperative treatment is required or complications occur.

The success of other subsequent treatments will often depend on the results of surgery. Like all therapies, it needs to be considered carefully in all cases, on an individual basis, looking at all the known facts about the patient's diagnosis, prognosis, current health status, the risks involved, and the patient's own desires and concerns.

Radiotherapy (RT)

Radiotherapy is the use of ionising radiation to kill cancer cells. Nearly 50% of people with cancer receive radiotherapy. Radiation was reviewed as a potential cause of cancer in Chapter 3 (see 'Environmental factors: radiation', Chapter 3, p. 51), and this is because radiation damages DNA, causing mutations. But it is because of this DNA-damaging effect that it can also be used to treat cancers, for two reasons:

1. The damage is dose-related; the higher the dose, the more damage is incurred and, therefore, the less chance of the cell surviving. Short exposures of higher dosage can therefore be used to kill cancer cells, while the prolonged exposure to lower dosage can cause cancers.
2. The damage to DNA occurs mostly in cells undergoing mitosis, that is, cell replication. The rapid rate of cell replication that occurs in many tumours makes them particularly vulnerable to radiation (Figure 17.1).

Radiotherapy affects cells during their most vulnerable point of the cell cycle, mitosis, when DNA is exposed and being manipulated. Consequently, as with chemotherapy, those cells passing around the cell cycle rapidly, and dividing at a fast rate, are most susceptible to this treatment, that is, they are more often going through mitosis. Cancer cells are particularly affected by this treatment, but also some normal cells that divide quickly, that is, the skin, bone marrow, and mucous membrane. Of these, the skin, or more accurately, the **epidermis** (see 'Structure and function of skin', Chapter 13, p. 241), is particularly vulnerable to the effects of radiation

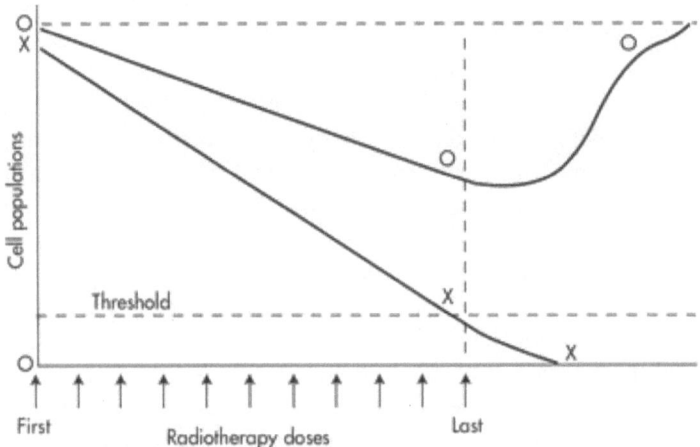

FIGURE 17.1 A diagrammatic representation of the separation of normal cells from cancer cells by radiotherapy. The arrows along the base line are the individual daily doses of radiation over the selected treatment period. At the start of the treatment, the cancer cells (X) and the normal cells (O) are mixed in the tissue. As a result of radiotherapy, both populations of cells decline, but because the cancer cells are reproducing quickly, they are more vulnerable to the radiation and decline faster than the normal cells. The cancer cells reach threshold first, that is, the point where the number and quality of the cells are so poor that survival is no longer possible. From here they go on to extinction. The normal cells have not reached threshold at this point and are able to recover.

therapy. To reduce the problem, it became regular practice to break up the total dose into separate daily doses, known as **fractionation**, spread over a period of about 10 or more days, maybe up to 25 days, per episode. Sometimes, several episodes like this are planned, with breaks in between to allow normal tissue to recover. Figure 17.1 shows arrows along the base of the graph, indicating separate doses of treatment.

Radiotherapy is delivered in several ways:

- **Intensity-modulated radiation therapy (IMRT)**, which uses a moderate- or high-intensity radiation beam matched to the shape of the tumour to protect surrounding tissues.
- **Volumetric modulated arc therapy (VMAT)** is similar to IMRT but delivered in an arc around the patient, thus distributing the dose over a wider area (Figure 17.2).
- **Stereotactic ablative radiotherapy (SABR)** uses high-energy doses of radiation delivered in fractions to destroy (i.e. ablate) the tumour at an early stage, when the tumour is small. To prevent damage to surrounding organs, the radiation beam is targeted precisely on the tumour using various imaging techniques.
- **Image-guided radiation therapy (IGRT)** uses **computerised tomography (CT)** or **magnetic resonance imaging (MRI)** to guide the treatment to the tumour only, missing the vital organs.
- **Proton therapy** uses **protons**, which are positively charged particles, instead of electromagnetic energy. Protons have the advantage of delivering their energy at a specific depth, known as the **Bragg peak**. This means that when the Bragg peak is set to coincide with the tumour, the surrounding normal tissues and organs can be preserved. In this way, high levels of energy can be accurately targeted to deliver protons directly to the tumour. There are few side effects, and it is useful for treating children and young adults.
- **Brachytherapy** is a surgical implantation of a radioactive substance within or near the tumour.
- **FLASH-RT** briefly delivers ultra-high radiation levels, that is, 40 Gy (gray) per second, to a tumour. It has been shown to cause less harm to surrounding normal tissues than standard radiotherapy that delivers 0.5–5 Gy per minute (see 'Measuring radiation and the magnetron', p. 312) (Matuszak et al. 2022).

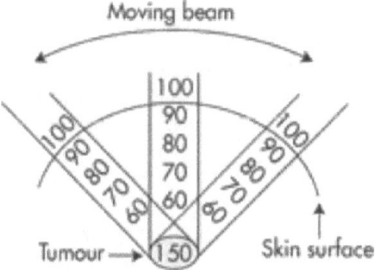

FIGURE 17.2　A diagrammatic representation of the principle behind VMAT. If this tumour needed a dose of 150, a single beam aimed at the tumour would have to deliver a dose much higher than 150 because the beam strength drops as it penetrates the tissues. The skin at the point where the beam enters would suffer from a very high radiation dose. VMAT spreads this dose as a moving beam which is constantly focused on the tumour from above. The beam delivers a lower dosage so the skin suffers less, but the focus point at the tumour receives the full combined strength.

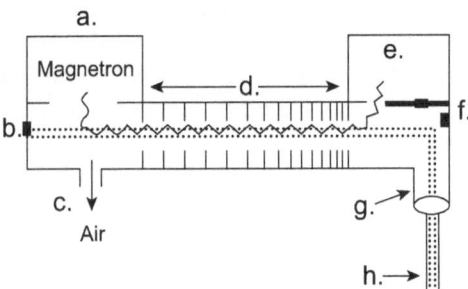

FIGURE 17.3 A diagrammatic view of a linear accelerator (LINAC). Microwaves are produced by a magnetron (a), and these microwaves pick up electrons (b) at one end of a vacuum tube (air is pumped out). (c) Baffles positioned along the tube (d) at decreasing intervals shorten the wavelength and therefore increase the energy. This energy is transferred to the electrons, which reach very high speeds. At the other end of the tube, the microwaves are removed (e) and the high-speed (high-energy) electrons are directed (f) onto a target (g), which then generates a high-energy beam of X-rays (h). The longer the tube (d), the higher the energy.

The usual method of delivering an external source of high-energy X-rays is by a **linear accelerator (LINAC)** (Figure 17.3). As a guide, a standard diagnostic X-ray procedure would use around **50 kV** (**kV** is **kilovolts**). Therapeutic X-rays used in radiotherapy require voltages up to **30 MV** (**MV** is **megavolts**), that is, perhaps 600 times greater power than the standard X-ray. The standard 50 kV X-ray has a relatively long wavelength (see 'Environmental factors: radiation', Chapter 3, p. 51), but an increase in the voltage causes shorter wavelengths, which penetrate the body better. The very high voltages used in radiotherapy have great penetrating and cell-killing power to reach and destroy the deep-seated solid tumours that standard X-rays could not even pass through.

Measuring radiation and the magnetron

X-ray radiation is measured in the **rad** or the **gray (Gy)**. The gray is the **Système International unit**, or **SI unit**, for radiation, and the relationship between the gray and the rad is 1 Gy = 100 rad. This is a measure of the total absorbed dose by the tissues. The **centigray** (100th of a gray) is often used since this is an equal term to the rad (1 centigray = 1 rad). A linear accelerator (Figure 17.3) works, first, by using a **magnetron** to produce microwaves. These microwaves are fed past a source of electrons and on into a vacuum tube called a **waveguide**. The microwaves now carry the electrons along, speeding them up to a point, in some cases, close to the speed of light. The tube is long, and this length is important to the power of the radiation beam produced, that is, the longer the tube, the greater the electron speeds, and therefore the greater the power. As the electron-laden microwaves speed down the tube, they encounter baffles with ever-shorter distances between them. This has the effect of shortening the wavelength, and the shorter the wavelengths, the greater the tissue-penetrating power. At the end of the tube, the microwaves are removed, leaving a beam of extremely fast, high-energy electrons which hit a tungsten target, causing a very powerful X-ray beam emission. This X-ray beam is very precise and can be aimed accurately at a tumour; it also produces very little harmful X-ray scatter, thus reducing the risk to patients and staff. The ability to create a narrow accurate beam means that the lower-dose, and therefore potentially carcinogenic, outer rim of the beam, that is, the **penumbra**, is reduced to a minimum.

If the skin does suffer the effects of the radiotherapy, this will become evident by the following early changes in the epidermis:

1. The skin becomes red, known as **erythema**.
2. Dry or moist **desquamation**, that is, loss of epidermis by scaling, occurs.
3. Increased pigmentation.
4. Loss of sweat gland function.
5. **Epilation**, that is, loss or removal of hairs by their roots.
6. Formation of tissue **oedema**, that is, fluid collection in the tissues, causing swelling.
7. The area affected will become very painful.

On a long-term basis, the irradiated skin may also show the following developments:

1. Formation of fibrous tissue (called **fibrosis**)
2. Pigmentation loss (i.e. opposite to that seen in the early stages)
3. **Telangiectasias**, which are localised red spots made from dilated capillaries
4. Loss of connective tissue from the dermis, with hair loss and even nail loss

Bone morphogenetic protein and activin membrane–bound inhibitor (BAMBI) is a key pseudoreceptor that negatively regulates[1] the cytokine **transforming growth factor β (TGF-β)** (see Table 5.2, Chapter 5, p. 94). RT suppresses BAMBI, thus allowing TGF-β to increase. RT also activates **myeloid-derived suppressor cells** (**MDSCs**) that suppress the immune response to cancer. MDSCs secrete several proteins, notably TGF-β. Both of these activities will raise TGF-β, increasing the cancer's ability to grow and progress, while reducing the immune system's ability to fight the cancer. This is likely to be the reason that some tumours show resistance to RT. This suggests that increasing BAMBI may improve radiotherapy, as shown in animal models.

Radioimmunotherapy (RIT) (Figure 17.4)

Radiotherapy can also be delivered internally. Radiolabelled antibodies, that is, antibodies given a mild radioactive component (see 'Monoclonal antibodies (MABs)', Chapter 5, p. 102) which delivers radiation directly to the cancer cell. Some can be detected by a scanner, that is, **scintigraphic imaging**, and may be used in diagnosis and monitoring tumour spread. These antibodies bind to specific cancer antigens, and the tumour is then highlighted on the scanner screen. RIT has proven to be a useful treatment in haematological malignancies, and the treatment of solid tumours has met with some difficulties (Parakh et al. 2022).

Some drugs in use, or in development, in the UK are:

- **Ibritumomab tiuxetan**, for some types of non-Hodgkin lymphoma (see 'Lymphatic cancers', Chapter 7, p. 143)
- **Tositumomab**, also for some types of non-Hodgkin lymphoma (see 'Lymphatic cancers', Chapter 7, p. 143)

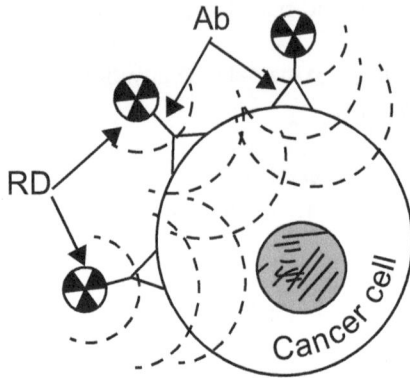

FIGURE 17.4   Radioimmunotherapy. A low-dose radioactive drug (RD) is added to an antibody (Ab) which binds only to cancer cell receptors, leaving the normal cell untouched. The radioactive component then kills the cancer cell by waves of very small radioactive beams (broken lines).

- **Lutetium-177 PSMA-617**, for advanced prostate cancer (see 'Prostate cancer', Chapter 12, p. 235)
- **Actinium-225 PSMA-617**, also for advanced prostate cancer (see 'Prostate cancer', Chapter 12, p. 235)
- **Radium-223 dichloride**, for bone metastases from prostate cancer (see 'Bone secondary tumours', Chapter 14, p. 257)

Stem cell therapy

Stem cells are those that can develop into any of the various cell types found in the body. They are called *undifferentiated* until they become specialised into a particular cell type, such as blood cells, endocrine cells, or neuronal tissue, that is, they become *differentiated* (see 'Blood cellular differentiation' and Figure 7.1, Chapter 7, p. 130). The early embryo is mostly composed of stem cells which become differentiated as they develop into organs and tissues. But stem cells exist into adult life, as they are required for normal tissue replacement and damage repair.

Apart from differentiation, stem cells can also renew themselves indefinitely and form clonal populations derived from a single cell (Chu et al. 2020). Various types of stem cells occur, and some could be used in cancer treatment (Figure 17.5, Table 17.1).

Stem cells could be used from several sources, as follows:

- **Autologous** are cells taken from the person who will receive them back.
- **Allogeneic** are cells donated from another compatible person.
- **Syngeneic** are cells taken from an identical twin, should the patient have an identical twin.

Stem cells can be used in cancer treatment in the following methods:

- Bone marrow transplant, where HSCs are used as part of the treatment of leukaemia, that is, restoring bone marrow after extensive chemotherapy and/or radiotherapy.

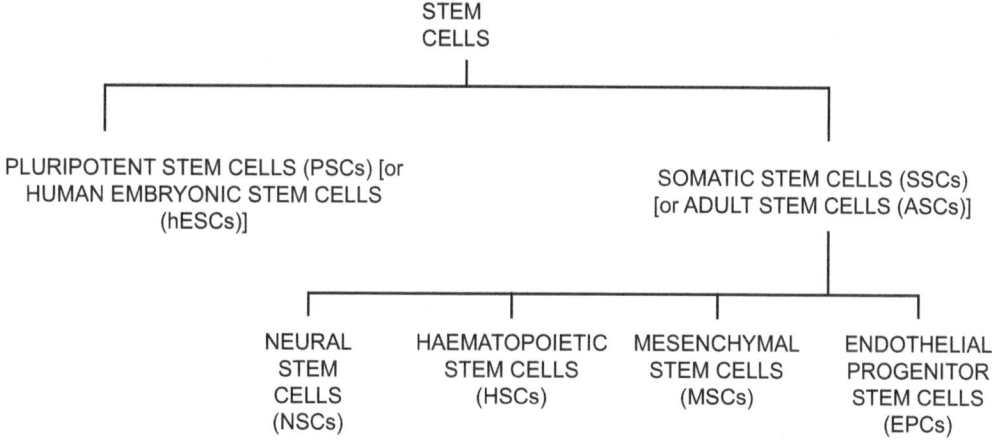

FIGURE 17.5   Classification of the major types of stem cells.

TABLE 17.1 Major types of stem cells

Stem cell type	Source of stem cell	Relevance to cancer
Pluripotent stem cells (PSCs) (human embryonic stem cells [hESCs])	From undifferentiated embryonic tissues and capable of becoming any body tissue type[2]	hESCs are a type of PSC. They are being developed for cancer vaccines.
Somatic stem cells (SSCs), also known as adult stem cells (ASCs)	Broad term for stem cells found in many adult body tissues	Many types are used in cancer (see *HSCs*, *MSCs*, *EPCs*, and *NSCs*).
Haematopoietic stem cells (HSCs)	Found in bone marrow and can differentiate into all blood cell types	A type of SSC used as part of the treatment of leukaemia.
Mesenchymal stem cells (MSCs)	Found in most tissues as a source of new cells for tissue repair and regeneration	A type of SSC used in cancer treatment.
Endothelial progenitor stem cells (EPCs)	From vascular tissue and the main cell in angiogenesis	A type of SSC used rarely in cancer treatment.
Neural stem cells (NSCs)	Found in the central nervous system (CNS) producing new neurons and glial cells	A type of SSC used in cancer treatment.
Cancer stem cells (CSCs)	Derived from epigenetic mutations in normal stem cells	Found in tumours, promoting cancer growth, metastasis, and relapse.

- Following intensive cancer treatment that has reduced the normal stem cells, MSC infusion helps restore the undifferentiated cell status and thereby improve tissue recovery. MSC and HSC can be given together with little or no adverse effects.
- Using MSCs and NSCs to carry therapeutic genes and drugs to the tumour. This reduces side effects of the drug and prevents the drug from being metabolised too quickly. It also improves the amount of drug reaching the tumour because of the intrinsic tumour-targeting nature of MSC stems cells.[3]

- Using genetically modified MSCs and NSCs to convert an inactive prodrug to an active drug inside a tumour rather than in general circulation (see 'Pharmacokinetics', Chapter 16, p. 294).
- Using stem cells to increase the generation of new immune cells for killing tumours.
- Whole-cell vaccine production using hESCs and iPSCs.

One problem has been identified. About 22% of stem cells used for research have been found to harbour mutations, which could go on to produce cancers. Although no stem cell treatments for patients have been licenced, unregulated use of stem cells in some countries has gone on to develop cancers in the recipient.

Gene therapy

Gene therapy is the manipulation and modification of genes, either DNA or RNA, in order to correct a genetic defect, as treatment or prevention of a disease caused by that defect (Figure 17.6). Cancer is a prime target for this approach, but it is useful for other diseases where genetic errors are a known cause. Gene therapy can:

- Reduce the number of disease-causing proteins being produced
- Increase the level of disease-fighting proteins
- Produce modified or new proteins beneficial to the cell

Gene therapy can involve:

- Gene silencing, where mutated and unwanted genes are 'switched off', that is, they become dormant
- The addition of new beneficial genes
- Gene editing (see 'Gene editing, base editing, and prime editing', p. 316)

Gene therapy can be carried out by one of the following routes (Figure 17.6):

- *In vivo*, that is, within the body, when the new genes are delivered to the cells by a transport mechanism called a vector. This is often a harmless virus, for example, adenovirus, but other methods are also used
- *Ex vivo*, that is, outside the body, where cells that are collected from the patient are genetically manipulated before being returned to the patient

Gene editing, base editing, and prime editing

Gene editing is a mechanism for removing the abnormal gene structure and replacing it with a normal gene sequence. The genetic scissors to do this are engineered nucleases, for example:

- **Zinc fingers** are nuclease proteins that can modify and regulate genes. A new tool using artificial intelligence (AI), called ZFDesign, can both widen the scope for zinc finger editing and increase its speed of action.

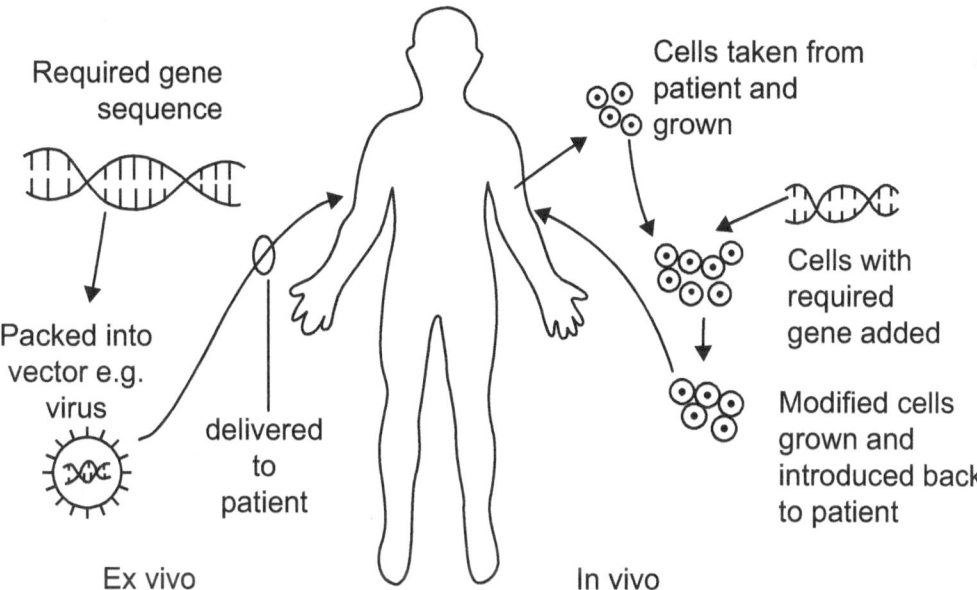

FIGURE 17.6 Gene therapy. Left: Ex vivo, where the required gene is packed into a vector, usually a harmless virus, and delivered to the patient. Right: In vivo, where cells taken from the patient are modified with the required gene before being delivered back to the patient.

- **TALEN**s (transcription activator–like effector nucleases) are engineered enzymes that make precise changes in DNA within living cells.
- **CRISPR (clustered regularly interspaced short palindromic repeats)** are a family of DNA segments consisting of short repetitions of base sequence found naturally in the immune defence genes of bacteria. They have associated proteins called **Cas** (**CRISPR associated protein**), which are numbered endonuclease enzymes. The combined system using Cas9, that is, CRISPR–Cas9, is used by bacteria to cut up and destroy the DNA of harmful viruses invading the bacteria. CRISPR–Cas9 is now being used in **gene editing** to cut and edit human DNA for the purpose of removing or adding genes (Figure 17.7). CRISPR–Cas9 is the easiest and cheapest method from other nucleases.

As a cancer treatment, the CRISPR–Cas9 system is being developed to modify immune cells that attack the tumour cells (see 'Gene therapy', p. 316). First, these immune cells are obtained from the patient's blood. CRISPR–Cas9 is added to the cells in a laboratory. It is guided to the required DNA sequence by a short, artificially prepared 'guide RNA' that fits the DNA sequence that needs to be removed. Then, the Cas9 enzyme acts like scissors to cut out the DNA (Figure 17.7). The guide RNA can be modified to target a wide range of DNA sequences as required. The cell then tries to repair the cut in the G_1/S phases of the cell cycle (Figure 1.6, Chapter 1, p. 7), and if the correct gene is introduced along with the CRISPR–Cas9, the cell will insert this. The cell can then be grown into large numbers before being returned to the patient.

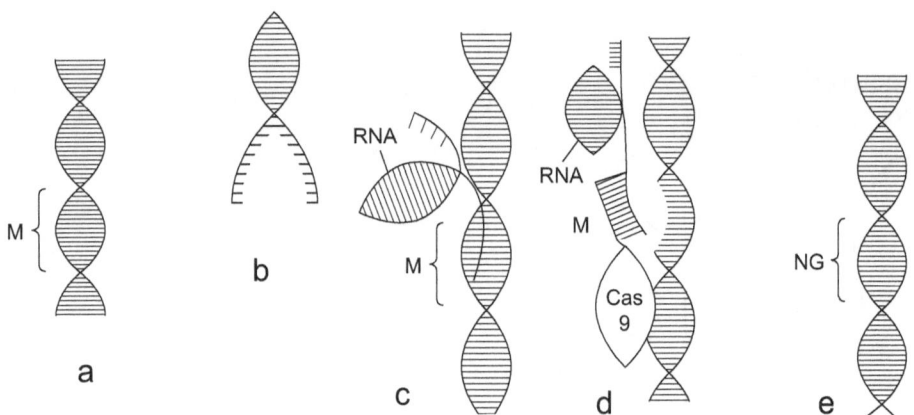

FIGURE 17.7 CRISPR–Cas9 gene editing: (a) the gene mutation (M) is identified; (b) a guide RNA that fits the mutation is created; (c) the guide RNA finds and identifies the mutation; (d) Cas9 cuts the mutation out; (e) the cell will either repair the cut, with a new gene (NG) supplied to the cell, or repair the mutated gene by base substitution (see 'CRISPR base editing', p. 318) or prime editing (see 'Prime editing', p. 318) or just silence the gene, that is, render it inactive.

Cas origins

Cas9 was isolated from the bacterium *Streptococcus pyogenes*, but other organisms have since provided Cas proteins which have different DNA-cutting abilities and easier targeting, for example, Cas12a from *Francisella novicida* and Cas13 from *Leptotrichia shahii*.

CRISPR base editing

This is a modified version, where individual bases, that is, adenine (A), guanine (G), thymine (T), and cytosine (C) (see Figure 1.3, Chapter 1, p. 4), can be removed if incorrect and swapped for the correct base. This changes the DNA gene sequence to code for the correct protein, with the correct amino acid, rather than a faulty protein with the wrong amino acid (Figure 2.3a, Chapter 2, p. 29). This simplifies the process since it does not cut the entire DNA.

Prime editing

Further modifications can made to the system, for example, **prime editing**, where Cas9 is changed so it does not do a full DNA cut; it just creates a tiny cut in one of the strands which permits a short DNA sequence to be deleted or added.

New versions of CRISPR gene editing

One problem with the original Cas9 enzyme is the number of 'off-target' interactions it makes, that is, targeting the wrong section of DNA. A new version of the Cas9 enzyme, which is just as efficient as the original enzyme but causes 4,000 times less 'off-target' DNA cuts, is called **'SuperFi-Cas9'**.

Another new version is **multiple effector guide arrays CRISPR (MEGA-CRISPR)**, which shuts down the proteins that are causing immune cells to become exhausted. MEGA-CRISPR uses Cas13d instead of Cas9 (see 'Cas origins', p. 318). Cas13d cuts RNA instead of DNA and destroys the mRNA that promotes these debilitating proteins. One type of cell treatment that benefits from this update are CAR T cells (see 'Chimeric antigen receptor T cell (CAR T or CART)', Chapter 5, p. 99).

RNA interference therapy (RNAi)

Small RNA interference (siRNA) molecules occur naturally after gene transcription. They bind to messenger RNA (mRNA) and promote its destruction. These siRNA can stop almost any gene from being transcribed, that is, they are effectively 'gene silencing'. There is a good opportunity to use siRNAs to silence cancer cell protein production, which would lead to the cancer cell dying. Once inside the cancer cell, siRNA combines with proteins to form an **RNA-induced silencing complex (RISC)** which breaks up the mRNA. Trials are underway using receptor-targeted nanoparticles (RTNs) as a delivery mechanism for siRNA. RTNs can target malignant cells specifically and therefore deliver siRNA only to cancer cells, avoiding normal cells.

PROTAC therapy

PROTAC (proteolysis-targeted chimera) therapy targets the cellular protein waste disposal system, called the **ubiquitin–proteasome system (UPS)**. Normally, cells dispose of unwanted proteins by first labelling them with an enzyme tag called **ubiquitin** (Figure 17.8). This is done by an E3 ligase attached to an E2 molecule that is part of the ubiquitin/E2 complex. When the E3 ligase and the target protein come in close association, E2 adds its ubiquitin to the waste protein. More ubiquitin is added to the target protein, forming a polyubiquitin chain. Any protein attached to this ubiquitin chain is destined for destruction and disposal by **proteosomes**,

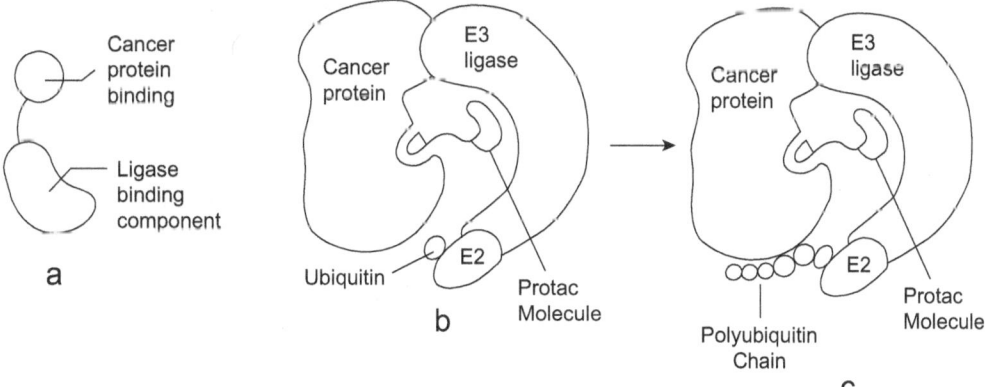

FIGURE 17.8   The PROTAC mechanism for degrading cancer-causing proteins: (a) PROTAC molecules have a component for binding to an E3 ligase enzyme at one end and a target (cancer) protein binding component at the other end. (b) In combination, the PROTAC molecule brings the E3 ligase and the cancer protein close together. The E3 ligase has a ubiquitin-conjugating enzyme (E2) attached which passes the ubiquitin to the target protein. (c) Further ubiquitin proteins are added by the same mechanism, forming a polyubiquitin chain, and the cancer protein is degraded to amino acids in the proteasome of the cell.

which reduce the protein to amino acids. PROTAC molecules are designed to bind to both cancer-causing proteins and the E3 ligase enzyme, bringing the unwanted protein and the E3 ligase together so the polyubiquitin process can begin (Figure 17.8). PROTAC has a target protein binding site linked to an E3 ligase binding site. After use, the PROTAC molecule is recycled to repeat the process. Currently, two PROTAC drugs are in clinical trials.

Histotripsy

This is the use of sound waves which are targeted on a tumour to kill it. The sound waves cause microbubbles to form inside the tumour. As these microbubbles expand and collapse, they damage the tumour and kill cancer cells by breaking down their outer membrane. The remaining tumour debris is subject to further immune system processing and finally eliminated from the body. Some heat is generated in the body, which may affect normal tissue close to the tumour. So far, this has proved successful in liver tumours and may progress to include renal and pancreatic tumours.

High-intensity focussed ultrasound (HIFU) is being used to treat pancreatic cancers. Ultrasound waves have greater frequency than 20 kHz (see 'Electromagnetic radiation, Hertz (Hz)', Chapter 3, p. 52); 20 kHz is the highest frequency detectable by the human ear, so all frequencies above that are ultrasound.[4] HIFU concentrates an ultrasound beam on the tumour, generating heat that destroys the cancer cells. The normal tissue, where the ultrasound beam is unfocussed, remains unaffected.[5] Tests using HIFU in combination with chemotherapy are proving to be promising.

Adjunct therapy

Apart from the main treatments of surgery, drugs, and radiation, patients may choose to follow various other courses of additional (**adjunct**) therapies. These are mostly introduced into the treatment regime by the patient themselves according to their own wishes and desires. Such special adjunct therapies, such as herbal medication, acupuncture, and aromatherapy, may not be a cure for cancer but can provide some symptom relief, help overcome stress, and ease pain. They give psychological comfort to the patient. If such therapies are considered by a patient, they should first be discussed with the medical staff to check to see if anything the patient wants to use contradicts their regular treatment, for example, some herbs may interact with the drug treatment. Massage and acupuncture are simple adjunct therapies that provide comfort and perhaps pain relief and are unlikely to interfere with the patient's main treatment regime.

Artificial intelligence (AI) in cancer management

Artificial intelligence (AI) is the advancement of computer technologies that mimic human intelligence in the fields of data analysis, prediction, and decision-making. **Machine learning** is the application of AI computers to problem-solving. In cancer research, AI is already employed in many ways, for example, data set analysis, screening for disease, assisting with diagnosis, and treatment planning. Research into breast, lung, and prostate cancer, especially, is employing AI to advance the work. AI can:

- Speed up analysis of large data sets collected from clinical trials from weeks to just hours
- Increase the efficiency of zinc finger genetic editing (see 'Gene therapy', p. 316)

- Increase accuracy of diagnosis from radiograph examinations and from histological examination of tissue samples
- Select the molecules from thousands which are likely to be the best drug candidates for each tumour
- Simulate how cancer cells would respond to specific therapies and predict the tumour responses to selected drugs
- Assist with targeted therapy such that the best treatment can be selected for each individual patient
- Analyse long-term trends and make accurate predictions of future trends
- Track down the primary sources of metastases where the primary is unknown (see 'Cancer of unknown primary (CUP)', Chapter 6, p. 128)

Blood and saliva screening, liquid biopsies, and organoids

Blood and saliva tests and **liquid biopsies** (**LB**s) are done for the following purpose:

- To measure hormones, proteins, or other substances linked to the cancer, not just for the initial diagnosis, but also to monitor any spread of the disease and the effect of treatment over time. Among the important agents to monitor are biomarkers (see 'Immunotherapy', Table 5.4, Chapter 5, p. 97).
- Blood also contains minute fragments of DNA released from cells, called **cell-free DNA** (**cfDNA**), especially from tumour cells (**circulating tumour DNA, ctDNA**). The difference between normal and tumour DNA is that the DNA from cancer cells contains the mutations that cause the cancer. This allows researchers to separate cancer DNA from normal DNA and to identify the range of genetic mutations that have occurred within that tumour. This is the basis for targeted therapy: to know exactly what mutations are present within the tumour so the best treatment can be selected to attack all the cancer cells present.
- Liquid biopsies can also collect **circulating tumour cells** (**CTCs**), that is, obtaining cancer material from blood and other biofluids, for example, cerebrospinal fluid (CSF), and these may one day replace the need for surgical biopsies.
- **Saliva tests** are in late-stage development. Saliva provides data on changes to the glycoprotein levels that indicate the presence of cancer. Lung and breast cancers have, so far, shown positive changes in saliva-based glycoprotein levels. Clearly, an advantage is that the test is non-invasive, but it also provides on-the-spot instant results, thus avoiding the delay with laboratory tests.

In addition, minute tumours grown in the laboratory, from tumour cells collected from liquid or surgical biopsies, are called **organoids**. These organoids can offer a wealth of information about the specific cancer each individual patient has, from genomics and epigenomics to multiomics (see 'A revolution in multiomics', Chapter 1, p. 20), and this will guide the treatment that each individual needs.

And this technology is being researched for a range of disorders, not just for cancer.

The future for cancer management is looking good. With all the new screening techniques, accurate and fast diagnosis down to the molecular level, and the use of targeted drugs, cancer therapy is gaining ground rapidly.

Key points

Surgery

• Surgery is a life-saving vital first step in many cancer treatment regimes, and the success of other subsequent treatments will often depend on it.

Radiotherapy

• Radiotherapy comes in several forms. The usual method is to deliver high-voltage X-rays from a linear accelerator.
• Radiation works by killing rapidly reproducing cells, and cancer cells usually reproduce quickly.
• The skin suffers the effects of the radiotherapy because the epidermis has rapidly dividing cells.
• The skin may become red (erythema), dry, or moist, with desquamation (loss of epidermis), loss of sweat gland function, epilation (loss of hairs), tissue oedema, swelling, and pain.

Radioimmunotherapy

• The use of radiolabelled antibodies to deliver radiotherapy directly to the cancer cells.

Gene therapy

• Gene therapy involves cutting out unwanted genes or nucleotide sequences from DNA and sometimes replacing them with normal genes.

Artificial intelligence (AI)

• AI is assisting with improvements to data analysis and accurate screening, diagnosis, and treatment planning.

Blood (liquid) biopsies

• Blood screening will allow fast and accurate analysis of tumour content for targeted therapy.

Notes

1 *Negatively regulates* means it reduces activity.
2 The collection of hESCs from human sources was restricted by ethical issues. Artificially induced PSCs (iPSCs) overcome the ethical considerations.
3 MSCs are attracted to the tumour microenvironment due to secreted factors, such as IL-6, TNF-α, and IL-1β (see Table 5.2 and Table 5.3, Chapter 5, p. 94).
4 It is important to note that these are sound waves, not radiation.
5 Ultrasound is safe on normal tissues, as used in pregnancy scans, when the beam is not focussed on a small area.

18

NUTRITION AND THE CANCER PATIENT

- **Introduction**
- **Nutritional considerations in cancer**
- **Foods as a cause or prevention of cancer**
- **A strategy for reducing cancer risk**
- **Final word . . . space**
- **Key points**

Introduction

Food is important in restoring good health during and after illness. This applies to cancer as much as any other illness. Nutrition is required for the provision of energy and for establishing resistance to infection, maintaining the healing process, and ensuring that the metabolic processes of the cells continue to function normally. Without these, the body would soon succumb to the disease process and die. Central to this need for nutrition is water. Without it, the body becomes dehydrated, and all the cellular activities fail. Patients with problems that affect the normal intake of food, for example, vomiting, will have disturbance of fluid balance as well (see 'Fluid balance', Figure 10.5, Chapter 10, p. 197).

The 'well-balanced diet' contains seven major categories of nutrients. They are **proteins**, **carbohydrates**, **fats**, **vitamins**, **minerals**, **fibre**, and **water**. Of these, the proteins, carbohydrates, and fats need some degree of digestion in order to render them available for absorption into the blood. Vitamins and minerals, however, need no digestion, as they will be absorbed into the blood as they are. Fibre also needs no digestion, simply because it is not absorbed; instead, it remains in the gut and forms the bulk of faecal waste. This does not mean it is unnecessary to humans, as it forms the bulk of the colonic contents and is processed by microorganisms in the gut, the **intestinal flora**, to produce substances that are absorbed and used. Water, of course, also needs no digestion but is absorbed into blood (see 'Water balance', Chapter 10, p. 196).

DOI: 10.4324/9781003389125-18

Electrolytes

Minerals are inorganic substances, some of which can take on an electrical charge, either positive or negative, to create **ions**. This happens when mineral compounds present in the diet, like **sodium chloride (NaCl)**, are dissolved in water, as in the blood and tissues. The mineral compound splits to form sodium (that takes on a positive charge → **Na⁺**) and chlorine (that takes on a negative charge → **Cl⁻**). The reason they take on these charges is that the sodium donates a negative electron to chlorine, which accepts it. Having lost a negative electron, sodium's positive and negative balance is changed, and it becomes overall positive. Chlorine gains a negative electron, and that causes a greater overall negative charge. Similar effects happen to **potassium chloride (KCl)** in the body, to form **K⁺** and **Cl⁻**. Positive ions are **cations**, whilst negative ions are **anions**. The word **electrolyte** is a term used for *ions in a solution*, as in body fluids. It is important for electrolytes to balance in the body, that is, positives with negatives, for the normal function of body cells and tissues (Figure 18.1). Electrolyte imbalance causes serious changes in health. Our electrolytes are mostly derived from our diet, for example, sodium chloride (= table salt) and calcium (**Ca²⁺**). Notice how calcium, like some others, takes on a double-positive charge (i.e. it loses *two* electrons).

Nutritional considerations in cancer

Progressive cancer causes a loss of weight (both fat and muscle losses); plus, it causes **anorexia** (loss of appetite) and, eventually, **cachexia** (see 'Kwashiorkor and cachexia', p. 327). All this is aggravated by the presence of nausea and vomiting associated with radiotherapy and chemotherapy treatments and the emotional stress ill health causes. If the patient undergoes surgery, this further debilitates them, putting additional energy demands on their nutritional status, for example, for wound healing, during the recovery period. The removal of the patient to a hospital, an unfamiliar environment, away from the family puts further stress on the mind and body. The picture can easily become one of uncontrolled tumour growth whilst the patient wastes away emotionally and physically.

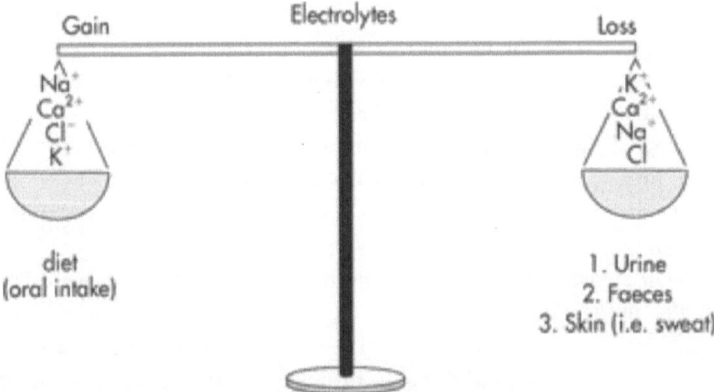

FIGURE 18.1 Electrolyte balance. Electrolytes, that is, charged particles, such as sodium (Na⁺), calcium (Ca²⁺), chloride (Cl⁻), and potassium (K⁺), in the diet must balance those lost in urine, in the faeces, and through the skin.

Traditionally, the patient has been encouraged to eat as well as possible to make good these losses. A high-protein diet, for example, may help replace wasting muscles, whilst additional carbohydrates should help replace the body's energy. However, a fast-expanding tumour will also use nutrients supplied from food for energy and growth.

Patients should try to achieve optimum nutrition to ensure the maximum possible resistance to the effects of the malignancy and the debilitation caused by the treatment. This can become an uphill struggle for the patient, particularly in patients who find eating undesirable due to their anorexia, nausea, and general weakness. Generally, the tumour's growth increases demand for two major nutritional components:

1. Nitrogenous amino acids derived from proteins, which may cause depletion of the muscle stores of amino acids and weight loss
2. Energy, derived from carbohydrate and fat stores in the body

Reinstating these stores to as near to normal as possible improves the patient's general condition, so they feel better and can respond more favourably to treatment. Symptoms such as **ascites**, that is, oedema in the abdomen that is causing the abdomen to swell, may also improve under better nutritional conditions, because low plasma proteins is one cause of oedema. Plasma proteins are made in the liver from amino acids derived from dietary protein. Part of their role is to attract fluid from the tissues, that is, **extracellular fluid (ECF)**, back into the blood. Low plasma proteins will allow fluid to accumulate in the tissues, that is, **oedema**. This is only one of several causes of oedema (see 'Fluid balance', Table 10.1, Chapter 10, p. 198), any of which may occur because of cancer.

Metabolism and energy

Metabolism is the term used to include all the chemical processes taking place in the body. Of course, most of these processes occur inside the cells, but many also take place in body fluids, for example, blood, and body cavities, for example, the bowel. Metabolism falls mainly into two forms: the building-up processes and the breaking-down processes. Those that start with simple substances, for example, amino acids, and build these into more complex structures, for example, proteins, are called **anabolism**. Those that start with complex substances, for example, polysaccharides, and break these down to form simple substances, for example, monosaccharides, are called **catabolism**. Metabolism uses **enzymes** as agents of chemical change. They are proteins that promote change to take place without themselves becoming chemically involved in the change. Metabolism requires the raw material on which to act, and these raw materials are mostly the nutrients in our diet, delivered to our cells by the blood. Metabolism also generates wastes, such as **carbon dioxide (CO_2)** and **urea**, which must be removed and excreted. Metabolism is ultimately responsible for all cellular activities, including **energy** production.

Energy is produced in cells in the form of **adenosine triphosphate (ATP)**, a high-energy molecule that can store energy until required by the cell. Many foods are said to have an energy value because they contain carbohydrates, fats, or protein, that is, the nutrients that can fuel energy production in the cells. Carbohydrates have an energy value of 4 **kcal (kilocalories)** per gram (g), lipids have an energy value of 9 kcal/g, and proteins have an energy value of 4 kcal/g. One kilocalorie is 4.186 kJ **(kilojoules)**, a standard international (SI) unit for energy, so the values for the three food types stated here in kilojoules are: carbohydrates, $4 \times 4.186 = 16.744$ kJ; lipids, $9 \times 4.186 = 37.674$ kJ; and proteins, $4 \times 4.186 = 16.744$ kJ. This final figure for protein is the same as for carbohydrates, and this is because when the time comes for protein to act as an energy source, the amino acids are converted to glucose. **Alcohol** also has some limited nutritional value because it provides energy, having an energy value of 7 kcal/g ($7 \times 4.186 = 29.302$ kJ). However, alcohol does *not* provide any other nutrients.

Metabolism has its lower limits, below which cellular chemistry must not fall. The **basal metabolic rate (BMR)** is described as the *minimum* rate of internal energy expenditure whilst *awake* but at *rest*. This means that if metabolism falls below this specific level, it endangers health, and even life. This level is 1.25 kcal per minute for males of 65 kg weight and 0.9 kcal per minute for females of 55 kg weight. Sleep induces metabolic rates about 10% lower than the BMR, whilst physical exercise, as would be expected, drives metabolism higher than the BMR, although the BMR itself is raised in exercise.

Energy balance is a comparison between energy intake (in the form of food) and energy use by the cells. **Neutral energy balance** indicates that the energy intake and cellular expenditure match exactly. However, energy intake and expenditure often do not match. **Positive energy balance** is the consumption of more energy in food than is used by the cells. On a long-term basis, this results in excess energy storage in the body, in the form of fats (**adipose tissue**), increasing the risk of becoming overweight (**obese**). The opposite is **negative energy balance**, where there is consumption of less energy in food than is used in the cells. The long-term effect is gradual loss of stored energy, with ensuing weight loss.

Energy, of course, is needed for the process of growth, both in height and in weight. Measuring weight and height provides very good indicators of positive or negative energy balance. However, a third indicator is the **body mass index (BMI)**, which compares weight with height. If you know the patient's weight (in kilograms) and their height (in metres), then you can calculate their BMI.

The formula is:

$$BMI = weight (kg) \div [height (m)]^2$$

What this means is that the BMI is the weight divided by the height squared, that is, the height is multiplied by itself. For example, if the weight is 55 kg and the height is 1.5 m, the BMI will be $55 \div 1.5^2$, or $55 \div (1.5 \times 1.5)$, or $55 \div (2.25)$, which equals 24.4. Notice there are no *units* – it is just 24.4 – hence, it is an *index*. The ideal BMI falls between 20 and 25, whilst 30 or above is considered to be overweight.

Whilst normal growth represents a healthy *anabolic state*, the cancer patient in the latter stages of the disease may be in a *catabolic state*, that is, the forces of tissue breakdown are dominant over any tissue growth or repair. The BMI in cancer patients is at risk of falling below the ideal levels.

Starvation is very much an undesirable state for anyone, but the cancer patient may be propelled into this condition if the disease is not controlled and the patient's nutritional status falls into decline. As the body loses its oral intake of food, it quickly uses up the carbohydrates in the blood (i.e. glucose), which are replaced from stored glucose in the liver, that is, **glycogen**. Muscle also has stored glycogen, which is available for the muscle's own use. These stores allow glucose levels to remain relatively steady for much of the patient's illness, but it may decline as the disease progresses to an advanced stage.

Carbohydrates are the first source of energy in the body, and a lack of glucose from the diet also increases a metabolic process called **gluconeogenesis**. This means the creation (= *genesis*) of new (= *neo*) glucose (= *gluco*), new in the sense that the glucose comes from *non-carbohydrate* sources, notably fats at first, and ultimately proteins. Fats, that is, adipose tissue, are therefore broken down to release **glycerol**, which is taken to the liver via the blood and converted to glucose. Fats are the second source of energy in the body, coming into play when glucose intake is getting low. Along with glycerol, adipose breakdown releases additional **fatty acids** into circulation, some of which can be used to drive energy production, but much of which will be converted to **ketones** by the liver. Under normal nutrition, ketones are produced in small quantities, and these are taken up by the muscles as an energy source; hence, none are found in normal urine. But in starvation, when fatty acid levels in the blood are raised and muscle itself is likely to be deteriorating, excess ketones are produced. These cannot be used by the muscle, and they are therefore filtered into the urine through the kidneys, creating a **ketonuria**. Ketones are acids, and this means that significantly raised amounts in the blood reduce the blood **pH** (the measure of the **acid–base balance**) from the normal pH 7.4 (which is just slightly alkaline). This pH change due to ketones causes a serious complication, called **ketoacidosis**. Once all the fat stores in the tissues are exhausted, the body is in crisis. There is little option but to turn to protein as an energy source.

In the long term, therefore, proteins (especially muscle) will suffer a similar fate as fat, that is, they will be broken down to form glucose, if the glucose shortage continues. Protein is the third and final source of energy, and when it is depleted, the body has no further energy stores. Amino acids from muscle proteins are also broken down in the liver, and later by the kidneys, a breakdown process called **deamination**, to produce glucose and **urea**, the waste product containing nitrogen. **Lactic acid** is also a potential source of glucose energy made available by the liver once it is delivered to the liver by the blood from muscles. Lactic acid is a by-product of **anaerobic metabolism** in muscles, that is, cellular chemical processes taking place without adequate oxygen. Muscles cannot themselves convert lactic acid to glucose – only the liver can do this – thus, large quantities of lactic acid can seriously affect muscle activity, unless the blood removes it quickly. Lactic acid, like ketones, is acidic, that is, it has a low **pH**, and is therefore going to seriously reduce the pH of the muscles, if it is allowed to accumulate there, or may contribute to a lower blood pH in circulation, leading to acidosis. The deamination of amino acids causes difficulties with fluid balance due to the elimination of increased levels of nitrogenous urea and acidic wastes, both of which require ample water to dissolve in – water which is lost along with the wastes. The picture becomes one of profound weight loss, dehydration, and acidosis, all of which seriously affect tissue function, leading to organ malfunction. Ultimately, the patient is likely to die from cardiac, renal, or other organ failure, combined with a ketoacidosis, a profound hypoglycaemia, and protein deficiency. The time taken to reach this end varies with the amount of stored adipose tissue the starved patient started with, but typically around eight weeks, unless nutritional support can be maintained.

Kwashiorkor and cachexia

Protein insufficiency combined with other factors leads to a condition called **kwashiorkor** (Figure 18.2). Mild kwashiorkor is likely to be present to some degree in cancer patients who are stressed by their removal to the unfamiliar environment of a hospital and are in pain, are nauseated, and may be fearful of their future. It is a debilitated physical state coupled with psychological stressors.

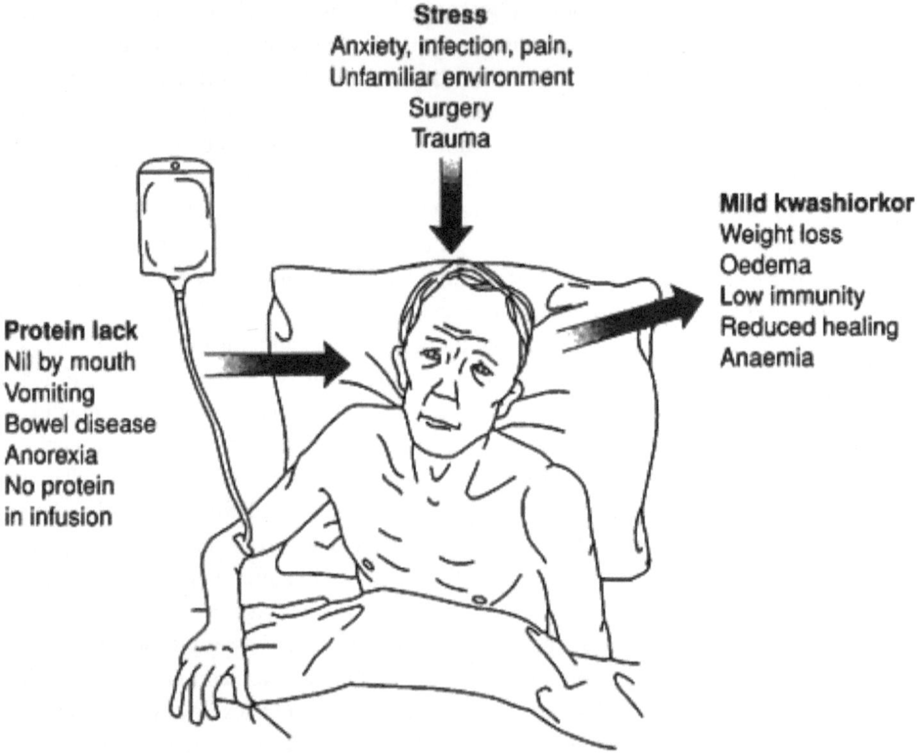

FIGURE 18.2   Mild kwashiorkor. This is caused by a lack of protein coupled with stressors of various kinds. The result is a set of symptoms shown by the right-hand arrow.

Source: Reproduced from Blows (2024).

Cachexia

This is a *syndrome*, a collection of symptoms that mark a particularly bad stage of a disease, which may occur during the end stage of the patient's life or be demonstrated by a slow decline throughout. It marks the onset of specific biochemical changes that begin the process of cellular and tissue breakdown. The syndrome is identified by:

- Significant **muscle wasting**, or **muscle atrophy**, that is, loss of muscle tissue, leading to reduced muscle bulk and strength
- **Adipose atrophy**, that is, a **lipolysis**, or fat breakdown, causing a loss of fat tissue
- A profound loss of weight
- A profound **weakness**

Muscle wasting can be partly caused by a cytokine called **OSM (oncostatin M)** (see 'Chromosome 22', Addendum, p. 360), which is frequently released from tumours. OSM binds to its receptor, **OSMR (oncostatin M receptor)** (see 'Chromosome 5', Addendum, p. 347), and directly causes muscle loss (Figure 18.5). In addition, the combination of OSM with OSMR also triggers increased genetic transcription of another receptor, **EDA2R (ectodysplasin A2 recep-tor)** (see 'Chromosome X', Addendum, p. 361). This receptor binds **EDA2 (ectodysplasin A2)**. Excess numbers of EDA2R binds additional EDA2, and this triggers increased gene transcription of two enzymes, **Murf1** and **Atrogin1**, which also break down muscle (Figure 18.3).

Muscle wasting and adipose atrophy together indicate that the patient is entering a serious *catabolic state*, **catabolism** being a metabolism characterised by tissue breakdown. The effect of these changes causes the patient to become extremely thin, with little flesh over the bones. They are so weak they become immobile, and therefore they are at risk of skin breakdown and multiple infections.

The patient suffers a severe loss of appetite (**anorexia**) and starts the metabolic process of survival based on their body reserves of fat and muscle. As these dwindle, the patient sinks to a physical low point, from which recovery is difficult or impossible (see 'Symptomology: cancer-related fatigue (CRF)', p. 335). Add to this a sense in the patient that the *end is near* – that is, they take on a mental attitude that death is inevitable, and they are basically giving up on life – then the risk of death for this patient becomes obvious. They move from a state of anxiety, through depression, then to the point of being resigned to their fate. The process is gradual, per-haps taking weeks rather than days for many patients, depending on the rate of growth of their tumour. Cachexia is not confined to cancer patients but sometimes can also be found in other terminal conditions, such as **AIDS** and **tuberculosis**.

What happens in cachexia is complex and not fully understood. A substance called **tumour necrosis factor** α (**TNF-α**, also called **cachexin**) is produced by activated **macrophages**. TNF-α, in conjunction with another chemical called **interleukin 1 (Il-1)** (see 'Cytokines and chemokines', Chapter 5, p. 94), has some *valuable* functions. Together they activate **lympho-cytes, eosinophils**, and **natural killer (NK)** cells (see 'Natural killer cells', Chapter 5, p. 91) to attack the tumour, and it may damage the tumour directly by harming its blood supply. However,

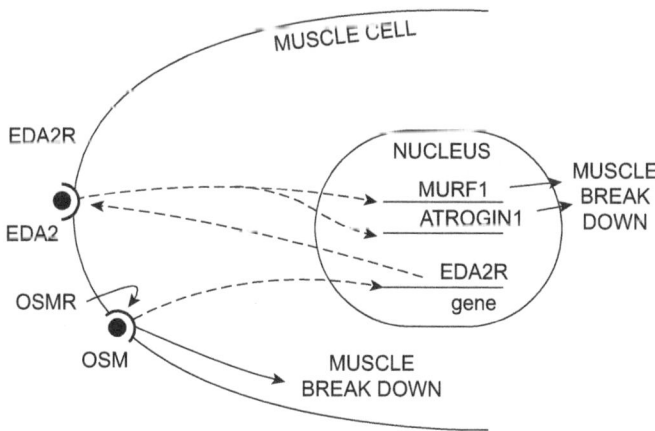

FIGURE 18.3   The mechanism of muscle loss in cachexia. OSM binds to OSMR, causing muscle wasting and increased production of EDA2R. Too much EDA2R binds additional EDA2, and this triggers a signalling pathway that leads to gene transcription of the muscle protein breakdown enzymes Murf1 and Atrogin1.

it also has some *harmful* effects on the body, especially in the long term. These unwanted effects include:

1. An increase in the adhesion of **granulocytes** (see 'Blood cells types', Chapter 7, p. 131) to **endothelium** (the inner surface cells of blood vessels), where these granulocytes then **degranulate**, that is, they discharge their granules. Chemicals from the granulocytes form **free radicals** (see 'Chemical agents', Chapter 3, p. 42), which then attack healthy tissues around the body and can induce circulatory collapse.
2. Endothelial cells losing their usual anti-coagulant properties, thus allowing increased deposits of fibrin on blood vessel walls. This leads to **diffuse intravascular coagulation**, that is, many small blood clots forming throughout the circulatory system. Blood clotting factors may become low, and this leads to bleeding.
3. In the short term, combined TNF-α and Il-1 (see 'Cytokines and chemokines', Chapter 5, p. 94) re-route nutrients away from the periphery to the liver, promoting an acute response to tumour formation, but in the long term, they cause abnormal carbohydrate, protein, and fat metabolism.
4. Anorexia is a consequence of long-term TNF-α and Il-1 activity and may be increased by a dietary zinc deficiency, lost or abnormal taste of food, or the presence of liver metastases.

Other cytokines involved in cachexia include **interleukin 6** and **interferon gamma (γ-interferon)**. *Interleukin 6* normally initiates a non-specific inflammatory response to infection, including NK cell activation, and thus helps mediate natural immunity. *Interferon γ* is a growth inhibitor in normal and malignant cells and activates inflammatory cells, including NK cells and macrophages, against viral-infected and tumour cells. In cachexia, however, these cytokines have been identified as playing an important role in abnormal fat breakdown (interferon γ) and protein breakdown, that is, muscle wasting (interleukin 6). The picture is complicated by a cascade effect involving other cytokines, which make it difficult to assess which cytokine is responsible for the clinical state. In addition, some products released by the tumour itself contribute to the overall effects, for example, some **lipolytic hormones**, which break down fats and cause anorexia and a negative **nitrogen balance**. Proteins are the source of nitrogen in the diet; thus, anorexia, combined with muscle breakdown and wastage, causes more nitrogen to be lost from the body than taken in, that is, a negative nitrogen balance.

Low carbohydrates and high fats will starve a tumour of its energy supply, but this regime may also increase the likelihood of cachexia. Fats become the tumour's secondary energy source, but that increases the production of toxic wastes from fat metabolism and inhibits corticosteroids, for example, cortisol, from the adrenal gland. Cortisol suppresses inflammation, so its reduced production raises the risk of increased inflammatory processes throughout the body. Fats used for energy may also increase the production of the protein **GDF15 (growth differentiation factor 15)**, which binds to the **GFRAL** (GDNF family receptor alpha-like) receptor in the brainstem (see 'GDF15, chromosome 19', Addendum, p. 358). This system is involved in controlling body weight by suppressing appetite, energy use, and food intake during cell stress, and it becomes another factor leading to loss of appetite (anorexia).

The metabolic changes seen in cancer patients are a mix of increases and decreases.

Increases in all the following:

1. Gluconeogenesis and glucose usage
2. Insulin resistance

3. Blood levels of lactic acid
4. Adipose breakdown and glycerol turnover
5. Blood fatty acid levels (**hyperlipidaemia**)
6. Whole-body protein turnover and skeletal muscle breakdown
7. Basal metabolic rate (BMR)

Decreases in the following:

1. Building of skeletal muscle
2. Appetite (**anorexia**)
3. Glucose tolerance
4. Activity of **lipoprotein lipase**, an enzyme that breaks down the fats (i.e. triglycerides) that are combined with protein, a combination called **chylomicrons** in circulation, where failure to break down these fats results in further high blood fat level (hyperlipidaemia)

The body has seriously unwanted chemical activity in progress, and the patient does not want to eat. They are also likely to have adverse psychological changes and may have lost the will to live.

Feeding may not always help, and certain feeding regimes, like **total parenteral feeding** (**TPN**), may sometimes exacerbate the problem. It is not just a lack of food; it is the inability of the body chemistry to handle that food. Each case must be assessed individually to determine the way forward. **Parenteral feeding** (or **total parenteral nutrition**, **TPN**) is the delivery of nutrition directly into the bloodstream by the intravenous route. This is done to avoid the entire digestive system when normal or enteral feeding is not possible. Delivery of nutrition directly to the blood means that digestion will not happen, so the nutrients themselves must already be in the form of the end products of digestion. Thus, the fluids used must already have proteins reduced to amino acids, carbohydrates reduced to glucose, and so on, with no fibre, since fibre never reaches the blood. Intravenous TPN is mostly delivered via a **central venous catheter**, that is, an intravenous line established into a central vein rather than a peripheral vein, and often maintained by an electric infusion pump. It is demanding on both the patient and the carer and still carries a risk of complications.

Foods as a cause or prevention of cancer

Some foods are said to be a potential cause of cancer, mainly because they contain substances claimed to be **carcinogenic**. On the other hand, other foods are claimed to be protective, that is, they prevent cancer, again because they have certain ingredients. This is always a complex and controversial subject, because there are constant uncertainties, such as:

1. If a food substance causes cancers in laboratory rats, does it cause cancer in humans?
2. If a food ingredient is thought to be carcinogenic to humans, what, if any, is a dangerous dose?
3. Are there any other unknown substances, good or bad, in our food? Research is suggesting that there are plenty of both.
4. Does organic production or the genetic modification (GM) of food change its health status, for good or bad?
5. Does cooking, prolonged storage, or going beyond the 'use by' date change the health status of our food?

There are other questions like these that need to be answered before we know the whole story about the food we eat. Science is catching up with the problem. Some of the claims made so far often have significant scientific support

The good

- **Polyphenols** are a large class of compounds found particularly in tea and pomegranates. They include flavonoids, phenolic acids, stilbenes, and other polyphenols. **Phenolic acids** include *caffeic acid, gallic acid,* and *ferulic acid.* Found in tea, they have more powerful antioxidant activity than vitamin C, E, or A. Black (Indian) tea, the type mostly drunk in the UK, is a fully oxidised form of the same leaves as green (Chinese) tea and contains similar quantities of phenolic acids as green tea. **Stilbenes** are increasing in importance due to their potential health benefits. The best-known stilbene is **resveratrol**, found in grape skins and red wine. Resveratrol shows a number of good health benefits, including the potential for suppressing cancer cell growth, but there are not enough human studies to assess its effectiveness in people, the dosage required, and any potential side effects. Other polyphenols include **curcumin** (see 'Turmeric', p. 335). **Phloretin** in **apples** is a polyphenol that blocks cancer cell replication and reduces colorectal cancers. Some of the polyphenols partly control and stabilise the signalling pathways which malignant cells require for development and progression, notably the p53 gene pathway (see 'Chromosome 17', Addendum, p. 356). They also protect against cancer risk factors (Cháirez-Ramírez et al. 2021).
- **Flavonoids** (or **bioflavonoids**) are a large subgroup of polyphenols, some of which are antioxidants, and as such, they may have anti-cancer properties (Table 18.1). Examples under examination are **naringenin** (found in grapefruit), **isoflavones** (found in soya), **hesperetin** (found in oranges), and **quercetin** (found in garlic and onions). People who eat foods rich in flavonoids are said to have an overall lower risk of cancers and other health benefits (Schiller 2021).
- **Other flavonoids** are found in tea, and these also have antioxidant activity. These are **catechins**, which are simple flavonoids found mostly in green tea. There are more complex flavonoids, called **theaflavins** and **thearubigins**, found in black tea. Green tea is protective against many cancers, for example, green tea has **epigallocatechin gallate (EGCG)**, also known as **epigallocatechin-3-gallate**, which is **another catechin antioxidant**. It is also a **urokinase (uPA)** inhibitor. The enzyme uPA helps cancers invade tissues and form metastases. By inhibiting this enzyme, EGCG is helping prevent cancer cells from spreading.
- Eating five or more portions of fruit and vegetables per day cuts cancer risk by 20% (Anonymous 1998a), and this has become government policy. A 'portion' is recognised as 80 g (or 2.8 oz). Spinach and beans of all kinds are especially healthy and protective against cancer. Between 66 and 75% of all gastric cancers are preventable by appropriate diet (Anonymous 1998b).
- Green vegetables are particularly valuable in the diet for many reasons, including as a protection against cancers. A chemical called **allyl-isothiocyanate (AITC)**, which is a breakdown product of a compound called **sinigrin**, is released when green vegetables are chopped, chewed, or cooked. AITC gives green vegetables a bitter taste and is probably why children particularly do not like eating greens. The **brassica** family of vegetables, such as cabbage, broccoli, cauliflower, sprouts, and swede, appears to be an important source for AITC. Two or three portions of the brassica family per week in the diet are

TABLE 18.1 The flavonoids

Flavonoid	Notes
Anthocyanins	From elderberry, blackcurrants, blueberry, red grapes, and other fruits and berries. They are plant pigments, including cyanidin, malvidin, pelargonidin, delphinidin, and peonidin. Blueberry flavonoids are antioxidant, antibacterial, and anti-inflammatory.
Flavanols (flavan-3-ols)	From green tea, cocoa, and chocolate. They include silibinin, taxifolin, and pinobanksin.
Flavones	From citrus fruit peels, parsley, celery, and capsicum peppers. They include tangeretin, nobiletin, and tricetin.
Flavanones	From citrus fruits. They include hesperetin, naringenin, eriodictyol, and dihydroquercetin.
Isoflavones	From soybeans and other legumes. They include genistein, daidzein, and glycitin.
Flavonols	Includes kaempferol and myricetin. Quercetin is the most abundant flavonol in the diet (from onions, apples, berries, and broccoli). It is a powerful antioxidant.
Catechins	Found in tea (see 'Other flavonoids', p. 332).
Myricetin	Found mostly in parsley, this flavonoid kills skin and colon cancer cells.
Apigenin	It prevents tumour blood vessel formation (angiogenesis) and improves chemotherapy. Apigenin is found in many plant foods, notably parsley, celery, spinach, onions, oranges, tarragon, and basil.

now recommended, with the best cancer protection occurring if they are cooked in a little water and for the shortest time as possible. AITC blocks reproduction of colon cancer cells and can trigger **apoptosis** (programmed cell death) in malignant cells. Broccoli contains the compound **sulforaphane**, which has been shown to kill prostate cancer cells in the laboratory and is now also considered to reduce the risk of colon cancer. Cabbage releases **indole-3-carbinol**, which soothes inflammation and regenerates normal cells. For the best results, cabbage should not be overcooked to the point of being mushy. People who eat very few green vegetables have double the risk of cancer compared with those who eat them regularly, indicating the anti-cancer protective role for green vegetables is significant. A life-long habit of eating green vegetables regularly is a healthy lifestyle that should be established early in childhood.

- **Omega-3 fatty acids** found in fish, but especially salmon, inhibit various cancers as well as being protective against a range of other diseases. Walnuts are also a good source of omega-3 and antioxidants and are also protective against many diseases, including cancer (see 'Nuts', p. 334).
- Citrus fruit has a compound called **limonene**, found in the oil of citrus fruit peel, which reduces the risks of skin cancers. Orange or lemon juice consumed at least three times per week reduces the risk of digestive tract and respiratory tract cancers.
- **Anthocyanin** in blueberries protects the skin against the harmful effects of sunlight and boosts brain function. Blueberries are a fruit that contains five different types of anthocyanins. Onions, especially red onions, also contain anthocyanins, which cause cancer cells to die by apoptosis. Onions and garlic together become a powerful force against cancer development (see 'Garlic', p. 334).

- **Lycopene** is a phytochemical from tomatoes, particularly cooked tomatoes, as in tomato ketchup. It is protective against cancers, especially breast, ovarian, gastrointestinal, and colorectal cancers, and prostate cancer in men. Lycopene is also found in watermelons, cantaloupes, and papayas.
- **Yoghurt** protects against cancers by reducing the chemical activity that otherwise would lead to the formation of carcinogens.
- **Soya beans**, when digested, produce a substance called **equol**, and this blocks the production of the male hormone **dihydrotestosterone (DHT)**. DHT causes growth of the male reproductive tract, including the prostate gland, and so may be involved in the cause of prostate cancers. By blocking DHT, equol may have a protective role against prostate cancer, as suggested by the lower rates in Japan, where soya beans are eaten widely. Soya beans also contain **genistein**, a component that helps in breast development and appears to be protective against breast cancers. Eating soya products during adolescence reduces the risk of breast cancers later in life, and those women having a soya-rich diet appear to have a 60% less risk of developing large amounts of dense breast tissue, which could lead to cancer.
- The Chinese mushrooms called **shiitake** and **reishi** contain the chemical **lentinan**, which boosts the immune system, notably natural killer (NK) cells, to destroy tumour cells. Other mushrooms are also a healthy part of the diet and may provide some prevention against cancers.
- **Selenium**, being a major **antioxidant**, prevents cell damage caused by free radicals. Patients with cancers have been found to have lower than average blood levels of selenium, and therefore, selenium may protect against some cancers, especially those of the breast, lung, colon, and prostate gland. It may even slow down that part of the process of ageing caused by free radical damage. Selenium levels in plant foods are somewhat dependent on the selenium level in the soil. European wheat contains less selenium than American wheat for this reason, and therefore, bread, a staple diet component, is apparently less selenium-rich in Europe than it is in America (Rayman 1997).
- **Nuts** contain selenium and other nutrients, such as vitamin E and magnesium. The best nuts for anti-cancer nutrients are walnuts, Brazil nuts, almonds, and hazelnuts (see also 'Omega-3 fatty acids', p. 333). One ounce of nuts per day is a good habit to adopt to reduce cancer risk.
- **Garlic** contains an organosulfur compound called **allicin** and the flavonoid **quercetin** (see 'Flavonoids', p. 332). Allicin is a potent antioxidant, antimicrobial, anti-cancer, and neuroprotective agent. It inhibits tumour growth and causes cancer cells to die through apoptosis (Nadeem et al. 2022).
- **Trans-vaccenic acid (TVA)** is a fatty acid that may prove to be a useful anti-cancer protection because it activates the immune T cells to kill tumours cells. Raised TVA in the blood also improves patients' response to immunotherapy. TVA is found naturally in milk and beef. Unfortunately, high levels of red meat consumption are linked to greater risk of certain cancers, and it may be better to isolate TVA as a separate supplement (Lesté-Lasserre 2023).
- **Rosemary** is a herb that has protective properties against cancer. It reduces the level of cancer-causing **heterocyclic amines (HCAs)** in food, for example, meat cooked at high temperature. HCAs are mutagenic and carcinogenic. Rosemary is rich in **carnosol**, a **phytochemical** which reduces cancer growth by slowing cell replication and boosts immunity. It also contains **carnosic acid** and **rosmarinic acid**, both of which are anti-inflammatory and reduce cancer risk.

- **Turmeric** contains **curcumin** (see 'Polyphenols', p. 332), which appears to kill cancer cells in the laboratory. Although not yet known as a cancer treatment, the addition of a little turmeric to the diet may help reduce symptoms.
- **Thyme** is another herb which contains **terpenoids**, a group of phytochemicals which are antioxidants and anti-inflammatory.
- **Raspberries**, **strawberries**, **pomegranates**, and other fruits contain **ellagic acid**, a phytochemical that is an antioxidant and anti-inflammatory. It decreases cancer cell replication and protects brain function. Twenty ounces per day of these fruits will provide significant benefits.
- **Cinnamon** can help stop cancer metastases due to the chemicals **procyanidins** and **cinnamaldehyde**.

And the bad

- **Acrylamide**, a known cancer-causing chemical, has been found in significant quantities in starch-based foods cooked at high temperatures, that is, frying and baking, but *not* boiling, such as chips, crisps, and breakfast cereals (Starck 2002).
- An excess of 250 calories per day above that normally required in the diet during childhood increases the risk of cancer later in life by 20% (Frankel et al. 1998).
- Some food emulsifiers that are found in processed foods increase the risk of prostate and breast cancers. The **monoglyceride** and **diglyceride** of fatty acids (E471)[1] increase the risk of cancer by 15% overall. However, they increase the risk of breast cancer by 24%, and prostate cancer by 46%. **Carrageenan** (E407) increases the risk of breast cancer by 32%.

The preceding claims are based largely on scientific research, which indicates a trend, and more research is constantly underway to confirm these trends. The trends do suggest that a healthy diet provides far more beneficial chemicals for our health than harmful ones, and diet should be given much greater consideration in sickness and in health.

Symptomology: cancer-related fatigue (CRF)

Throughout the text, symptoms of specific cancers have been identified, but cancers generally cause a few noteworthy symptoms (see 'Symptomology: chronic pain', Chapter 15, p. 279).

'Cancer-related fatigue' affects more than 80% of cancer patients; it is often more noticeable on waking in the morning and gets worse over time as the disease progresses. It is a profound weakness, a 'washed-out' feeling which is seriously distressing to the patient. They struggle to complete the most basic functions of living, for example, moving, eating, washing, and dressing. It generates a state of irritability and frustration, muscle and joint stiffness, a loss of concentration, and a significant loss of motivation. The cause is twofold: the body is using a lot of energy to fight the cancer, and the tumour is using up a lot of energy to grow and spread. Add to this some degree of appetite loss (anorexia), nausea, and vomiting, as seen in some cancers, and there is no new energy arriving in the body. This clearly becomes a major problem. One further symptom that stems from this is weight loss, where the body is using its energy stores. This means, initially, loss of fat, followed later by muscle loss (muscle wasting). Overlaying this scenario is the presence of pain, plus the psychological problems of stress, anxiety, and depression, and the patient can quickly loose the will to continue.

A strategy for reducing cancer risk

The World Cancer Research Fund and the American Institute for Cancer Research carried out a major detailed analysis of cancer preventative research which was published in a report (World Cancer Research Fund/American Institute for Cancer Research 2007). This resulted in a report published two years later setting out a lifestyle strategy to minimise the risk of developing cancer (World Cancer Research Fund/American Institute for Cancer Research 2009). In this report, the lifestyle strategy of ten points is as follows:

1. Be as lean as possible, without becoming underweight.
2. Be physically active for at least 30 minutes per day.
3. Avoid sugar in drinks, and reduce consumption of energy-dense food. Particularly avoid processed food high in added sugar and/or fats or low in fibre.
4. Eat more vegetables of all kinds, plus fruits and wholegrains and pulses.
5. Reduce and limit eating red meats, and avoid processed meats.
6. Limit alcohol to two dinks for men, and one drink for women, per day. Try to go alcohol-free if possible.
7. Reduce salt in the diet by avoiding highly salty foods.
8. Do not take food supplements solely for the purpose of avoiding cancer.
9. Breastfeeding mothers should breastfeed without additional formula milk for up to six months.
10. Add to these, **do not smoke** or **chew tobacco** (Pecorino 2011).

Final word . . . space

The fight against cancer has been taken into space. The research being done on the International Space Station (ISS) has benefitted, and continues to benefit, our understanding of the malignant cell and its environment and the development of more effective therapies. The presence of microgravity provides unique conditions unavailable in earthbound laboratories. Examples are:

- 3D cancer cells grow larger than on the ground and demonstrate their complexity in more clarity when used from a 3D bioprinter. The bioink used in these orbiting printers is a thick mix of cells in a nutrient matrix.
- Protein crystals for drug discovery grow larger and more uniform in space.
- Discovery of cancer biomarkers.
- Improved cultivation of stem cells and organoids[2] for disease modelling.
- Test new therapies to see if they work well in microgravity.
- To see how cosmic radiation may affect cancer growth.
- The Cancer Moonshot initiative, which aims to prevent 4 million cancer deaths by 2047.

Key points

Diet

- The 'well-balanced diet' contains proteins, carbohydrates, fats, vitamins, minerals, fibre, and water.
- A *negative energy balance* is the consumption of less energy in food than is used in the cells, and the long-term effect is gradual loss of stored energy, with ensuing weight loss.
- Proteins are a source of nitrogen, in the form of amino acids.
- Glucose may be stored as glycogen or delivered to body cells everywhere, where it is used to form energy.
- Fats, in the form of triglycerides, are stored in the body as adipose tissue.
- Water and electrolytes (charged mineral particles) should be in balance, that is, gain equals loss.
- The *basal metabolic rate* (BMR) is described as the minimum rate of internal energy expenditure whilst awake but at rest.

Cancer

- Progressive cancer causes a loss of weight, anorexia (loss of appetite), and fluid and electrolyte imbalance.
- *Kwashiorkor* is a protein lack coupled with stress, as is likely to occur in cancer patients.
- *Cachexia* is a syndrome identified by muscle wasting, adipose atrophy, weakness, and a sense of hopelessness.
- A ten-point plan for cancer risk reduction involves diet, alcohol, exercise, and tobacco lifestyle choices.

Notes

1 *E numbers*, short for Europe numbers, is a list of food additives.
2 *Organoids* are artificially grown cell masses that resemble organs.

REFERENCES

Anatomy and physiology

Clancy, J. and McVicar, A. (1998) Homeostasis – The key concept to physiological control (neurophysiology of pain), *British Journal of Theatre Nursing*, 7(10): 19–27.

Devlin, T. M. (ed) (2010) *Textbook of Biochemistry with Clinical Correlations* (7th edn), Wiley-Liss (John Wiley & Sons, Inc), New York.

Garrett, R. and Grisham, C. (2023) *Biochemistry* (7th edn), Brooks/Cole, Belmont, USA and London, UK.

Germann, W. J. and Stanfield, C. L. (2016) *Principles of Human Physiology* (6th edn), Pearson Education, New Jersey.

Marieb, E. N. and Hoehn, K. (2022) *Human Anatomy and Physiology* (12th edn), Pearson, London.

Martini, F. H., Nath, J. and Bartholomew, E. (2023) *Fundamentals of Anatomy and Physiology* (12th edn), Pearson Education, New Jersey.

Cancer causes, detection, diagnosis, and staging

American Cancer Society (2023) www.cancer.org/cancer/types/kidney-cancer/detection-diagnosis-staging/staging.html (accessed October 2023).

American Society of Clinical Oncology (ASCO) (2023) *Cancer.Net*. www.cancer.net/cancer-types/bladder-cancer/stages-and-grades (accessed 6th October 2023).

Blows, W. T. (2002) X-ray examination, *Nursing Times, Diagnostic Procedures supplement*: 44–47.

Cancer Research UK (2023) https//www.cancerresearchuk.org/about-cancer/stages-types/stages (Revised January 2023; accessed 4th October 2023).

Coutts, A. (2002) Diagnostic investigations part 2: Computerised tomography, *Nursing Times*, 98(37): 41.

Murray, P. R., Rosenthal, K. and Pfaller, M. A. (2020) *Medical Microbiology* (9th edn), Elsevier, New York and London.

NIH/NCI (National Institute of Health/National Cancer Institute) (2021) www.cancer.gov/about-cancer/diagnosis-staging/diagnosis/tumor-markers-list (accessed 5th December, 2023; updated 11th May 2021).

Pearce, F. (1997) Devil in the diesel, *New Scientist*, 25th October, 4.

Wilson, C. (2024) Lab-grown mini-tumours could revolutionise cancer therapy, *New Scientist*, 262 (3487): 13.

Tumour biology and prevention

Anderson, N. M. and Simon, M. C. (2020) Tumor microenvironment, *Current Biology*, 30(16): R921–R925.

Frappier, L. (2023) Epstein-Barr virus is an agent of genomic instability, *Nature*, 616: 441–442. *News and Views*, 2003. https://doi.org/10.1038/d41586-023-00936-y (accessed 12th March 2024).

Gibbs, W. W. (2004) Untangling the roots of cancer, in the science of staying young, *Scientific American (Special Edition)*, 14(3): 60–69.

Kahn, F. (1999) Cosmic radiation: High altitudes may be bad for your health, *Financial Times*, 12th April. www.cdc.gov/niosh/topics/aircrew/cosmicionizingradiation.html (accessed 2nd July 2023).

Kingman, S. (2004) Smoking shortens life by a decade, concludes 50-year study, *Bulletin of the World Health Organization*, August, 82(8): 632–633. www.scielosp.org/pdf/bwho/2004.v82n8/632-633 (accessed 2nd July 2023).

Kumar, V., Abbas, A., Aster, J. C., Deyrup, A. T. and Das, A. (2022) *Robbins and Kumar Basic Pathology* (11th edn), Elsevier, Philadelphia.

McCance, K. L. and Heuther, S. E. (2019) *Pathophysiology: The Biological Basis for Disease in Adults and Children*, Elsevier, St Louis, MO.

Pecorino, L. (2021) *Molecular Biology of Cancer, Mechanisms, Targets and Therapeutics* (5th edn), Oxford University Press, Oxford.

Wallis, C. (2019) A ticking cancer time bomb, *Scientific American*, 1st October, 321(4): 22. https://doi.org/10.1038/scientificamerican1019-22 (accessed 2nd July 2023).

Weinberg, R. A. (1996) How cancer arises, in what you need to know about cancer, *Scientific American* (Special Issue), 275(3): 32–40.

World Cancer Research Fund/American Institute for Cancer Research (2009) *Policy and Action for Cancer Prevention*, American Institute for Cancer Research, Washington, DC.

Diet and nutrition

Anonymous (1998a) Health, the 5+ a day way, *World Cancer Research Fund, Newsletter (on Diet, Nutrition and Cancer)*, issue 33: 3.

Anonymous (1998b) Stomach cancer . . . Facts in focus, *World Cancer Research Fund, Newsletter (on Diet, Nutrition and Cancer)*, issue 30: 3.

Cháirez-Ramírez, M. H., de la Cruz-López, K. G. and García-Carrancá, A. (2021) Polyphenols as antitumor agents targeting key players in cancer-driving signaling pathways, *Frontiers in Pharmacology*, 12(2021). https://doi.org/10.3389/fphar.2021.710304 (accessed 9th December 2023).

Frankel, S., Gunnell, D., Peters, T., Maynard, M. and Smith, G. (1998) Childhood energy intake and adult mortality: The Boyd Orr cohort study, *British Medical Journal*, 316: 499–504.

Kanasuo, E., Siiskonen, H., Haimakainen, S., Komulainen, J. and Harvima, I. T. (2022) Regular use of vitamin D supplement is associated with fewer melanoma cases compared to non-use: A cross-sectional study in 498 adult subjects at risk of skin cancers, *Melanoma Research*. https://doi.org/10.1097/CMR.0000000000000870 (accessed 19th December 2023).

Lesté-Lasserre, C. (2023) Nutrient found in milk and beef shows anti-cancer promise, *New Scientist*, 260(3467): 17.

Nadeem, M. S., Kazmi, I., Ullah, I., Muhammed, K. and Anwar, F. (2022) Allicin, an antioxidant and neuroprotective agent, ameliorates cognitive impairment, *Antioxidants (Basel)*, 11(1): 87. https://doi.org/10.3390/antiox11010087 (accessed 19th April 2024).

Rayman, M. (1997) Dietary selenium: Time to act, *British Medical Journal*, 314: 387–388.

Schiller, R. (2021) *What Are Flavonoids? Flavonoids: Sources, Functions, and Benefits*. verywellhealth.com (accessed 9th December 2023).

Stallard, E. (2023) Could ultra-processed foods be harmful for us?, *BBC Panorama*. www.bbc.co.uk/news/health-65754290 (accessed 1st July 2023).

Starck, P. (2002) Cancer risk in french fries, bread, *Women in Action*, (1): 66–57. WIA20021_23CancerRisksInFrenchFries.pdf (isiswomen.org) (accessed 9th December 2023).

World Cancer Research Fund/American Institute for Cancer Research (2007) *Food, Nutrition, Physical Activity, and the Prevention of Cancer: A Global Perspective*, American Institute for Cancer Research, Washington, DC. www.dietandcancerreport.org/.

Genetics

Nussbaum, R. L., McInnes, R. R. and Huntington, F. W. (2015) *Thompson and Thompson Genetics in Medicine* (8th edn), Elsevier, London and Amsterdam.

Passarge, E. (2017) *Color Atlas of Genetics* (5th edn), Thieme, Stuttgart.

Specific cancers

Cancer Research UK (2020) www.cancerresearchuk.org/about-cancer/kidney-cancer/stages-types-grades (accessed October 2023).

Cancer Research UK (2022a) www.cancerresearchuk.org/about-cancer/prostate-cancer/stages/grades (May) (accessed 14th October 2023).

Cancer Research UK (2022b) www.cancerresearchuk.org/about-cancer/prostate-cancer/stages/tnm-staging (April) (accessed 14th October 2023).

Funakoshi, Y., Hata, N., Kuga, D., Hatae, R., Sangatsuda, Y., Fujioka, Y., Takigawa, K. and Mizoguchi, M. (2021) Pediatric glioma: An update of diagnosis, biology, and treatment, *Cancers (Basel)*, 13(4): 758. https://doi.org/10.3390/cancers13040758 (accessed 27th December 2023).

Louis, D. N., Perry, A., Wesseling, P., Brat, D. J., Cree, I. A., Figalella-Branger, D., Hawkins, C., Ng, H. K., Pfister, S. M., Reifenberger, G., Soffietti, R., von Deimling, A. and Ellison, D. W. (2021) The 2021 WHO classification of tumors of the central nervous system: A summary (5th edition), *Neuro-Oncology*, 23(8): 1231–1251. https://doi.org/10.1093/neuonc/noab106 (accessed 25th December 2023).

Rawla, P. and Barsouk, A. (2019) Epidemiology of gastric cancer: Global trends, risk factors and prevention, *Przeglad Gastroenterologiczny*, 14(1): 26–38.

Drug treatment

Bachran, C. and Leppla, S. H. (2016) Tumor targeting and drug delivery by anthrax toxin, *Toxins (Basil)*, 8(7): 197. https://doi.org/10.3390/toxins8070197 (accessed 19th December 2023).

British National Formulary (BNF) 86 (2023) British Medical Journal (BMJ) & Royal Pharmaceutical Press, London.

Madhusoodanan, J. (2024) Targeting cancer, sparing patients, *Scientific American*, 330(3): 38–41.

Other treatments

Chu, D.-T., Nguyen, T. T., Nguyen, L. B. T., Tran, D.-K., Jeong, J.-H., Pham, G. A., Thanh, V. V., Dang, T. T. and Dinh, T. C. (2020) Recent progress of stem therapy in cancer treatment: Molecular mechanisms and potential applications, *Cells*, 9(3): 563. https://doi.org/10.3390/cells9030563.

Conlon, K. C., Miljkovic, M. D. and Waldmann, T. A. (2019) Cytokines in the treatment of cancer, *Journal of Interferon and Cytokine Research*, 39(1): 6–21. https://doi.org/10.1089/jir.2018.0019.

Le Page, M. (2023) How cancer-fighting immune cells could be made safer and more powerful, *New Scientist*, 5th August, 259(3450): 13.

Matuszak, N., Suchorska, W. M., Milecki, P., Kruszyna-Mochalska, M., Misiarz, A., Pracz, J. and Malicki, J. (2022) FLASH radiotherapy: An emerging approach in radiation therapy, *Reports of Practical Oncology and Radiotherapy*, 27(2): 344–351. https://doi.org/10.5603/RPOR.a2022.0038 (accessed 2nd March 2024).

Parakh, S., Lee, S. T., Gan, H. K. and Scott, A. M. (2022) Radiolabeled antibodies for cancer imaging and therapy, *Cancers (Basel)*, 14(6): 1454. https://doi.org/10.3390/cancers14061454.

Pecorino, L. (2011) *Why Millions Survive Cancer*, Oxford University Press, Oxford.

Roberts, M. (2022) Cancer-killing virus shows promise in patients, *BBC Health News*. www.bbc.co.uk/news/health-62833581 (accessed 19th July 2023).

Sounni, N. E. and Noel, A. (2013) Targeting the tumor microenvironment for cancer therapy, *Clinical Chemistry*, 59(1): 85–93.

Tobias, J. and Hochhauser, D. (2014) *Cancer and Its Management* (7th edn), Wiley-Blackwell, NJ.

Pain

Baker, C. and Wong, D. (1987) Q.U.E.S.T.T.: A process of pain assessment in children, *Orthopaedic Nursing*, 6(1): 11–21.

Manchester Triage Group (1997) Pain assessment as part of the triage process, in Mackway-Jones, K. (ed) *Emergency Triage*, British Medical Journal Publishing Group, London.

Wood, H., Dickman, A., Star, A. and Boland, J. W. (2018) Updates in palliative care – Overview and recent advancements in the pharmacological management of cancer pain, *Clinical Medicine* (London), February, 18(1): 17–22. https://doi.org/10.7861/clinmedicine (accessed 18th January 2017).

Wood, S. (2002) Special focus: Pain, *Nursing Times*, 98(38): 41–44.

World Health Organization (1986) *Cancer Pain Relief*, Author, Geneva, Switzerland.

Mental health aspects of cancer

Blows, W. T. (2022) *The Biological Basis of Mental Health* (4th edn), Routledge, Abingdon, Oxon.

Symptomology and drug side effects

Blows, W. T. (2024) *The Biological Basis of Clinical Observations* (4th edn), Routledge, Abingdon.

ADDENDUM

The chromosomes and the major genes linked to cancer

There are hundreds of genes with links to cancer when mutated. The following are 158 important genes that affect the development of human cancers. Definitions of terms and disorders are at the end of the text.

Chromosome 1

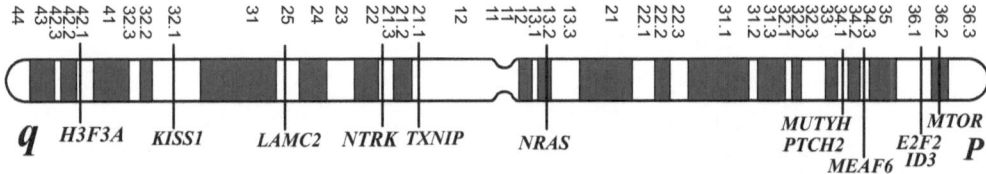

MUTYH (MutY DNA glycosylase) (1p34.1) encodes for a glycosylase enzyme required for DNA repair of point mutations involving adenine. Mutations are linked to gastric and colorectal cancers and Lynch syndrome (see 'Terms', p. 362).

NRAS (NRAS proto-oncogene GTPase) (1p13.2) (Figure 2.2) is part of the *RAS* family of genes, which also includes *HRAS* (chromosome 11) and *KRAS* (chromosome 12). This gene family produces proteins which are involved in cell signalling pathways for controlling cellular growth. Mutations of the *Ras* gene family are found in 20–30% of cancers generally, and up to 90% of pancreas, lung, and colon cancers. Mutations of *NRAS* (and the percentage of cases) are linked to head and neck cancers (2%), melanoma (17%), endometrial cancer (3%), colorectal cancer (4%), ovarian cancer (2%), and leukaemia (14%).

E2F2 (E2F transcription factor 2) (1p36.12) encodes for proteins which aid in the control of the cell cycle and activate other important genes. Mutations have been found in retinoblastomas, other retinal cancers, and maxillary sinus adenocarcinomas.

PTCH2 (patched 2) (1p34.1) encodes a protein which is one of the patched family of proteins involved in hedgehog signalling (see 'Terms', p. 362). This is a process that is important in embryonic development and tumour formation. Patched 1 and 2 are the proteins of the receptor for the hedgehog ligands. Mutations are associated with basal cell skin cancers (see also 'PTCH1, chromosome 9', p. 351).

LAMC2 (laminin subunit gamma 2) (1q25.3) encodes for a glycoprotein component of the basement membrane which is involved in cell adhesion and differentiation, cell migration, and cell signalling. Mutations are found in liver cancers.

NTRK (neurotrophic receptor tyrosine kinase 1) (1q21–q22) encodes for a neurotrophic tyrosine receptor involved in cell differentiation. Mutations are seen in thyroid cancers and ganglioneuromas.

H3F3A (H3.3 histone A) (1q42.12) encodes for one of two proteins that comprise histone H3.3. Histones are proteins around which DNA is wrapped within chromosomes (see 'Epigenetics', Chapter 2, p. 36). Mutations cause diffuse midline glioma (DMG) in the brain (see 'Paediatric-type diffuse low-grade and high-grade gliomas', Chapter 14, p. 260).

KISS1 (kisspeptin 1 metastasis suppressor) (1q32.1) is a tumour suppressor gene in melanoma and breast cancers (see 'Metastatic suppressors', Table 6.3, Chapter 6, p. 127).

TXNIP (thioredoxin-interacting protein) (1q21.1), also known as *VDUP1* gene (vitamin D up-regulating protein 1), is involved in cell stress response, cell cycle regulation, and tumour suppression. Low expression has been found in breast, liver, gastric, bladder, and lung cancers (see 'Metastatic suppressors', Table 6.3, Chapter 6, p. 127).

MEAF6 (MYST/Esa1-associated factor 6) (1p34.3) encodes for a nuclear-based transcription protein which is a component of the histone acetyltransferase complex. Mutations are seen in endometrial cancer.

ID3 (inhibitor of DNA binding 3) (1p36.12) encodes for a protein that is a transcriptional regulator that controls gene expression involved in cell activities, such as growth, differentiation, angiogenesis, and apoptosis. The ID3 protein increases anti-cancer activity in macrophages. Mutations are linked to Burkitt lymphoma, childhood lymphoma, and T cell acute lymphoblastic leukaemia.

MTOR (mechanistic target of rapamycin kinase) (1p36.22) encodes for a kinase central regulator of cell metabolism, growth, and survival. Mutations are found in many cancers, such as prostate, colorectal, kidney, ovarian, endometrial, cervical, and gastric cancers, and glioblastoma.

Chromosome 2

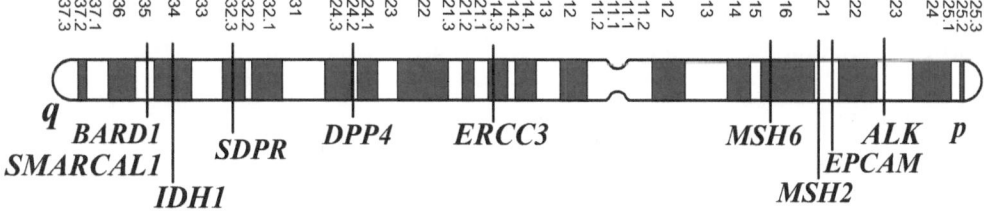

BARD1 (BRCA1-associated RING domain protein 1) (2q35) is a tumour suppressor gene that interacts with *BRCA1* during cell growth regulation. Mutations are linked to hereditary breast cancers.

SMARCAL1 (SWI/SNF-related, matrix-associated, actin-dependent regulator of chromatin, subfamily A Like 1) (2q35) encodes for a protein that remodels chromatin and is involved in

DNA damage repair and cell cycle progression. A deficiency of this protein increases the efficiency of anti-cancer therapy and reduces cancer resistance to chemotherapy. Drugs that target *SMARCAL1* activity, that is, *SMALCAL1* inhibitors, could be a useful therapeutic strategy.

EPCAM (epithelial cell adhesion molecule) (2p21) encodes for the epithelial cell adhesion protein, which sticks together epithelial cells, that is, cells that line body cavities. Mutations are linked to Lynch syndrome (see 'Terms', p. 362), colonic benign neoplasms, gastrointestinal carcinomas, plus inherited colorectal, pancreatic, endometrial, ovarian, and prostate cancers.

MSH2 (MutS homologue 2) (2p21–p16.3) is involved in mismatch DNA repair. Mutations are linked to Lynch syndrome (see 'Terms', p. 362); adenomas; small intestine and uterine cancers; sebaceous adenocarcinoma; inherited colorectal, endometrial, ovarian, gastric, pancreatic, and prostate cancers; and mismatch repair cancer syndrome.

MSH6 (MutS homologue 6) (2p16.3) encodes for a protein involved in DNA mismatch repair. Mutations are linked to Lynch syndrome (see 'Terms', p. 362); endometrial and small intestine cancers; adenomas; inherited pancreatic, colorectal, ovarian, gastric, and prostate cancers; and mismatch repair cancer syndrome.

DPP4 (dipeptidyl peptidase 4) (2q24.2) encodes for a protein which is one of a family of enzymes involved in glucose and insulin metabolism, as well as immune regulation in inflammation. Over-expression of the gene is linked to lung, liver, and other cancers.

IDH1 (isocitrate dehydrogenase (NADP (+)) 1) (2q34) encodes for the enzyme isocitrate dehydrogenase, which is involved in the conversion of isocitrate to 2-oxoglutarate in the tricarboxylic acid (Krebs) cycle. This cycle is the main energy-producing cycle within cells. This form of isocitrate dehydrogenase utilises NADP(+) as the main electron carrier. Mutations of this gene are found in cartilaginous cancers and myeloid leukaemia (see also 'Chromosome 15', p. 355).

ALK (ALK receptor tyrosine kinase) (2p23.2–p23.1) encodes for a tyrosine kinase receptor involved in brain development. Mutations are found in lymphomas, neuroblastoma, and lung cancer. It gets involved in fusion mutations with other genes, such as the *NPM1* gene on chromosome 5, to form the *ALK/NPM1* fusion.

SDPR (caveolae-associated protein 2) (2q32.3) is also known as cavin-2 gene. Caveolae are minute invaginations of the cell membrane that form specialised protein and lipid rafts. They are involved in cell signalling, lipid regulation, cell stress protection, and other functions, including reducing the factors leading to metastases (see 'Metastatic suppressors', Chapter 6, p. 127).

ERCC3 (ERCC excision repair 3, TFIIH core complex helicase subunit) (2q14.3) encodes for a helicase involved in nucleotide excision repair. Mutations are found in skin carcinoma and bladder, breast, ovarian, lung, prostate, colorectal, and gastric cancers.

Chromosome 3

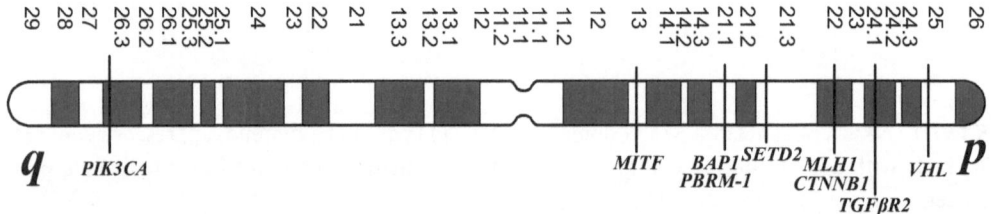

MLH1 (MutL homolog 1) (3p22.2) is involved in DNA mismatch repair. Mutations are linked to Lynch syndrome (see 'Terms', p. 362); sebaceous gland neoplasm; inherited pancreatic, colorectal, ovarian, gastric, and prostate cancers; and mismatch repair cancer syndrome.

CTNNB1 (catenin beta 1) (3p22.1) encodes for a protein that is part of the catenin complex involved in cell signalling and cell adhesion. Mutations are found in colorectal cancers, medulloblastomas, adenomas, and liver cancers.

TGFβR2 (transforming growth factor beta receptor 2) (3p24.1) encodes a protein which joins with others to form a transforming growth factor beta receptor that binds transforming growth factor beta. On binding, the complex controls other genes related to cell proliferation and stopping the cell cycle as required. Mutations can cause colorectal and oesophageal cancer and adenocarcinoma.

MITF (melanocyte-inducing transcription factor) (3p13) encodes for a protein that regulates melanocyte development. Mutations are involved in melanoma and other cancers.

BAP1 (BRCA1-associated protein 1) (3p21.1) encodes for a protein that binds to the protein derived from the gene *BRCA1* (see 'Chromosome 17', p. 356) and acts like a tumour suppressor. Mutations are found in kidney cancers, melanomas, mesothelioma, and meningiomas.

PIK3CA (phosphatidylinositol–4,5-bisphosphate 3-kinase catalytic subunit alpha) (3q26.32) encodes for the catalytic subunit of the enzyme phosphatidylinositol 3-kinase. It uses adenosine triphosphate (ATP) to phosphorylate lipid components of the cell membrane called phosphatidylinositols (Ptdins). Phosphorylation by this enzyme can result in various derivatives that are important for a range of cellular functions. Mutations are found in breast, cervical, and ovarian cancers, and hepatocellular carcinoma.

VHL (Von Hippel–Lindau tumour suppressor) (3p25.3) encodes for the protein called pVHL, which acts as a tumour suppressor. It is involved in ubiquitination (see 'Protac therapy', Chapter 17, p. 319) and degradation of transcription factor HIF (hypoxia-inducible factor), and it is also involved with cilia formation, cytokine signalling, and regulation of cell senescence. Mutations are found in non-papillary renal cell carcinoma (RCC) (see 'Renal cell carcinoma (RCC)', Chapter 10, p. 199), pheochromocytoma, lung, ovarian and gastric cancers.

PBRM-1 (polybromo 1) (3p21.1) encodes for a subunit of a complex involved in transcriptional activation and repression of specific genes. Mutations are found in non-papillary renal cell carcinoma (RCC), renal medullary carcinoma, endometrial carcinoma, and cholangiocarcinoma.

SETD2 (SET domain containing 2, histone lysine methyltransferase) (3p21.31) encodes for a tumour suppressor which also methylates histone H3 (see 'Epigenetics', Chapter 2, p. 36). Mutations are found in breast, prostate, ovarian, kidney, bladder, and endometrial cancers and acute leukaemia.

Chromosome 4

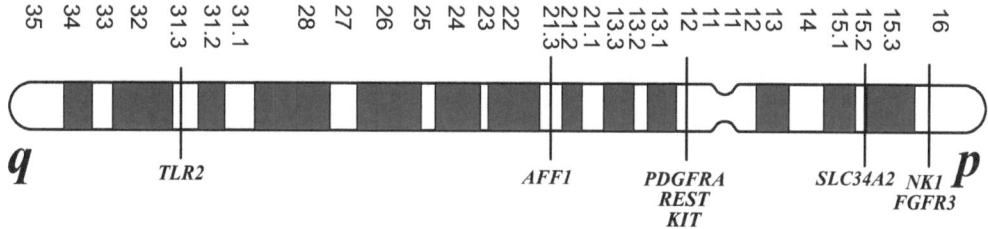

PDGFRA (platelet-derived growth factor receptor alpha) (4q12) encodes for a cell surface receptor to which platelet-derived growth factors bind and increase cell division and growth.

Mutations are found frequently in gastric stromal (connective tissue) cell tumours, chronic eosinophilic leukaemia, myeloid and lymphoid neoplasms, and malignant neurilemmoma (Schwannoma) (see 'Cranial and paraspinal nerve tumours', Chapter 14, p. 264).

REST (RE1-silencing transcription factor) (4q12) encodes for a transcription repressor factor which binds to DNA and silences neuronal gene transcription in non-neuronal cells. Mutations are linked to Wilms tumour (see 'Wilms tumour (nephroblastoma)', Chapter 10, p. 201).

NK1 (NK1 homeobox 1) (4p16.3) encodes for a protein that is a transcription factor essential for organ development. Mutations are linked to skin cancers.

KIT (KIT proto-oncogene, receptor tyrosine kinase) (4q12) encodes for a cell surface receptor protein important for blood cell production (haematopoiesis), formation of gametes, production of melanocytes, and several other functions. Mutations are found in a range of cancers.

AFF1 (ALF transcription elongator factor 1) (4q21.3–q22.1) encodes for a protein which is one of a family of proteins involved in regulating transcription elongation and chromatin remodelling. The family helps RNA polymerase II transcribe genes effectively. A translocation involving this gene with the *FLI1* gene (chromosome 11), that is, t(4;11)(q21;q23), is a causative factor in acute lymphoblastic leukaemia (see 'Leukaemia', Chapter 7, p. 133).

TLR2 (toll-like receptor 2) (4q31.3) encodes for the TLR2 protein, which is a member of the toll-like receptor family of cell surface receptors. It recognises many aspects of bacterial infection and activates innate immunity (see 'Innate (non-specific) immunity', Chapter 5, p. 78). It is linked to colorectal cancers but is also involved in the development of lung cancer staging (see 'Stages and treatment of lung cancer', Chapter 9, p. 189).

SLC34A2 (solute-carrier family 34, member 2) (4p15.2) encodes for sodium-dependent phosphate transport protein 2B, which is involved in transporting phosphate into cells. Mutations are found in some ovarian and breast cancers, and sometimes it fuses with *ROS1* gene in lung cancer (see 'Chromosome 6', p. 347).

FGFR3 (fibroblast growth factor receptor 3) (4p16.3) encodes for a cell surface receptor that binds fibroblast growth factor (FGF). When activated by the binding of FGF, the receptor is involved in a wide range of cellular functions, including proliferation, differentiation, bone development, and apoptosis. Mutations are found in multiple cancers, including bladder, breast, lung, colorectal, testicular, and cervical cancers, and multiple myeloma.

Chromosome 5

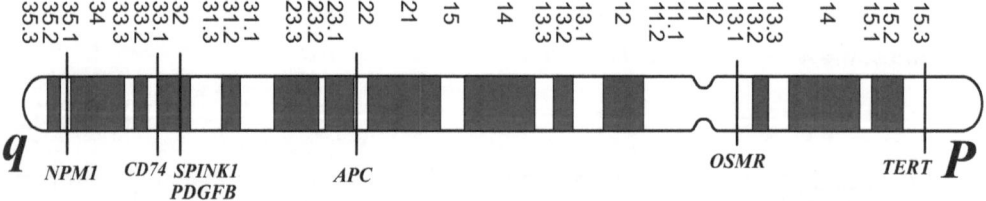

APC (adenomatous polyposis coli regulator of Wnt signalling pathway) (5q22.2) is a tumour suppressor gene encoding a protein that inhibits the Wnt pathway (see 'Terms', p. 362). Mutations are linked to gastric adenocarcinoma and intestinal **adenomatous polyposis coli (APC)** (see Table 8.5, Chapter 8, p. 167).

NPM1 (nucleophosmin 1) (5q35.1) is a gene that codes for a protein, **nucleophosmin**, which is found in the nucleolus and shuttles between the nucleolus and the cytoplasm. It has key roles in ribosome production, stability of the genome, progression of the cell around the cycle, and apoptosis. Mutations are sometimes found in acute myeloid leukaemia (AML) (see 'Leukaemia', Chapter 7, p. 133).

SPINK1 (serine peptidase inhibitor Kazal type 1) (5q32) encodes for a protein inhibitor of the enzyme trypsin from the pancreas. Mutations fail to inhibit trypsin within the pancreatic duct, causing pancreatitis, and are linked to inherited pancreatic cancer.

TERT (telomerase reverse transcriptase) (5p15.33) encodes for the enzyme protein telomerase that lengthens the telomere by adding the sequence TTAGGG (see 'Tissue invasion', 'Telomeres', Chapter 6, p. 123). Mutations are linked to melanoma and laryngeal cancer.

PDGFB (platelet-derived growth factor receptor beta) (5q32) encodes for a cell surface receptor that plays a vital role in embryonic development, cell growth, survival, and differentiation. Mutations are involved in meningiomas.

CD74 (cluster differentiation 74) (5q33.1) encodes for a protein that is a cell surface receptor associated with class II major histocompatibility complex (MHC) proteins. It is involved in antigen presentation as part of the immune response. Mutations are found in adenocarcinomas and lung cancers, where it fuses with *ROS1* gene to create an oncogene (see 'ROS1, chromosome 6', p. 348).

OSMR (oncostatin M receptor) (5p13.1) encodes for a type 1 cytokine cell surface receptor that binds OSM protein (see 'Chromosome 22', p. 359). Mutations are linked to pancreatic, ovarian, and bladder cancers, and glioblastoma (see also 'Kwashiorkor and cachexia', Chapter 18, p. 327).

Chromosome 6

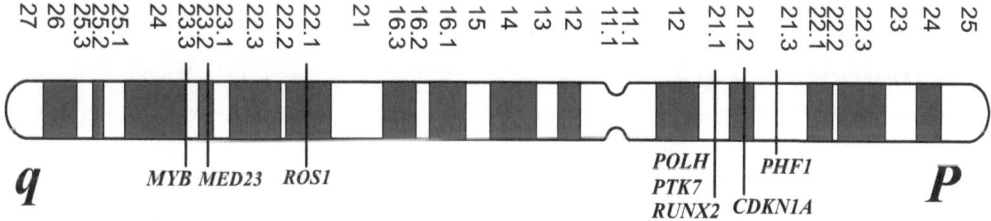

POLH (DNA polymerase eta) (6p21.1) encodes for a protein enzyme that repairs and copies specific DNA strands. Mutations of this gene are found in skin carcinomas.

PTK7 (protein tyrosine kinase 7) (6p21.1), also known as **CCK4** (colon carcinoma kinase 4), encodes a tyrosine kinase receptor component which is involved in signal transduction across the cell membrane. It is expressed in colon cancer, but not in the normal colon, so it may act as a marker for this disease.

RUNX2 (RUNX family transcription factor 2) (6p21.1) is a regulator of the production and function of osteoblasts, that is, bone-building cells, and therefore regulates bone development. Mutations can cause abnormal rapid osteoblast production due to gene over-expression, leading to primary bone cancer (osteosarcoma).

MYB (MYB proto-oncogene, transcription factor) (6q23.3) encodes for a transcription factor and regulator. It is important in haemopoiesis (blood cell formation). Mutations are linked to leukaemia, fibrosarcoma of bone, Burkitt lymphoma, and glioma.

CDKN1A (cyclin-dependent kinase inhibitor 1A) (6p21.2) encodes for a protein that inhibits cyclin-dependent kinase 2 and thus regulates cell cycle progression in G1 (see Figure 1.6, Chapter 1, p. 7). Mutations are linked to cancers of the tongue, thorax, and endocrine system.

ROS1 (ROS proto-oncogene 1, receptor tyrosine kinase) (6q22.1) encodes for a cell surface insulin receptor protein that activates tyrosine kinase. Mutations are fusions of *ROS1* with a range of other genes, notably *CD74* and *SLC34A2*. Such gene fusions drive tyrosine kinase consistently, causing rapid cell growth and replication. *ROS1* fusions are found in non-small-cell lung cancer (see 'Non-small-cell lung cancers (NSCLC)', Chapter 9, p. 187); gastric, ovarian, and colorectal cancers; and other tumours, for example, glioblastoma and melanoma.

MED23 (mediator complex subunit 23) (6q23.2) encodes for the cofactor required for SP1 transcriptional activation, subunit 3 (CRSP3), which is necessary for gene transcription. It also acts as a suppressor of metastases (see 'Metastatic suppressors', Table 6.3, Chapter 6, p. 127).

PHF1 (PHD finger protein 1) (6p21.32) encodes for a protein component of histone H3 complex (see 'Epigenetics', Chapter 2, p. 36). Mutations are seen in endometrial cancer.

Chromosome 7

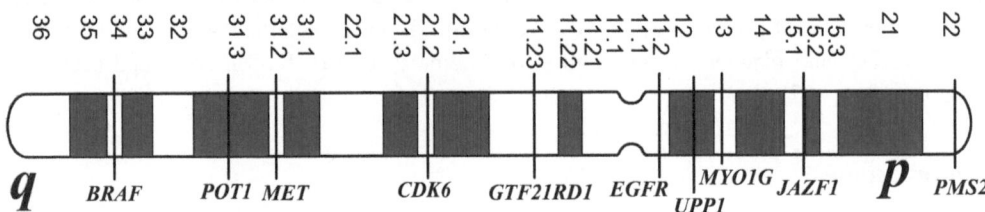

GTF21RD1 (GTF21 repeat domain containing 1) (7q11.23) promotes the cell cycle to progress by down-regulating the gene *TGFβR2* (see 'TGFβR2, chromosome 3', p. 345). Mutations are seen especially in colorectal cancers.

EGFR (erb-B1) (epidermal growth factor receptor) (7p11.2) is one of the growth factor receptor family of genes (*erb-B1*, *erb-B2*, *erb-B3*, and *erb-B4*) that code for cell surface receptors. These receptors bind growth hormones, that is, epidermal growth factors. Mutations are linked to lung cancer, adenocarcinomas, and biliary tract, oral, and vulva cancers.

PMS2 (PMS1 homolog 2) (7p22.1) is involved in DNA mismatch repair. Mutations are linked to Lynch syndrome (see 'Terms', p. 362); mismatch repair cancer syndrome; small intestinal cancer; inherited pancreatic, colorectal, gastric, and prostate cancers; and lymphoma.

CDK6 (cyclin-dependent kinase 6) (7q21.2), which encodes for a member of the serine/threonine protein family, forms a complex with CDK4 and cyclin D, which is important for the cell to progress around the cell cycle (Figure 2.28). Mutations have been linked to retinoblastoma, Kaposi's sarcoma (see 'Terms', p. 362), endometrial cancer, and squamous cell carcinoma.

BRAF (B-Raf proto-oncogene, serine/threonine kinase) (7q34) encodes for a protein that regulates cell growth and differentiation. Mutations promote cell growth and prevents apoptosis. One point mutation, called $BRAF^{V600E}$, involves replacing valine (*v*) with glutamic acid (*E*) at base sequence position 600. This mutation causes increased growth due to faster cell division and is found in melanomas, colorectal cancers, thyroid cancers, and various adenomas.

POT1 (protection of telomeres 1) (7q31.33) encodes for a protein involved in telomere maintenance (see 'Terms', p. 362). Mutations are found in melanomas and chronic leukaemia.

MET (MET proto-oncogene, receptor tyrosine kinase) (7q31.2) encodes for a receptor of the tyrosine kinase family with a role in cell survival, embryogenesis, and cell migration. Amplification mutations (see 'Mutation of genes, duplications', Chapter 2, p. 33) are seen in multiple cancers.

JAZF1 (JAZF zinc finger 1) (7p15.2–p15.1) encodes for a nuclear-based transcriptional repressor. Mutations are seen in endometrial and vaginal cancers.

UPP1 (uridine phosphorylase 1) (7p12.3) encodes for the enzyme **uridine phosphorylase**, which acts as a catalyst[1] for the reversible conversion of uridine and phosphate into the products uracil and alpha-D-ribose-1-phosphate. *Uracil* is a pyrimidine[2] that replaces thymine in RNA, and the uridine phosphorylase enzyme reaction allows cells to recover and reuse pyrimidine bases from RNA. Mutations are seen in gastric and colorectal cancers.

MYO1G (myosin 1G) (7p13) encodes for a myosin protein that is involved in T cell migration. Epigenetic errors are seen in smokers of Latino origin (see 'Tobacco smoking', Chapter 3, p. 48). Mutations are linked to breast, thyroid, cervical, and liver cancers, and childhood leukaemia.

Chromosome 8

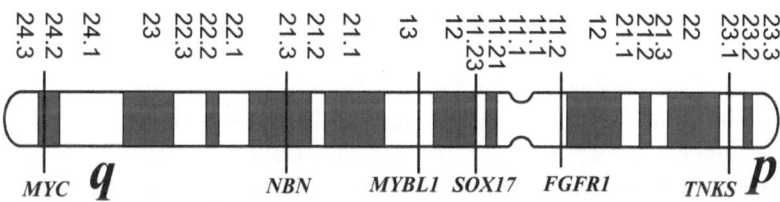

MYC (MYC proto-oncogene, BHLH transcription factor) (8q24.21) is a proto-oncogene that encodes for proteins that are transcription factors. *Transcription* is the process of producing an RNA copy of the DNA, that is, the first step for protein synthesis, and proteins from this gene regulate this process by binding to the DNA. They promote and accelerate transcription involved in cell cycle progression and apoptosis. Mutations create oncogenes, which can cause various forms of lymphoma, leukaemia, and melanoma.

NBN (nibrin) (8q21.3) is involved in DNA repair. Mutations are linked to acute lymphoblastic leukaemia and ovarian and breast cancers.

MYBL1 (MYB proto-oncogene like 1) (8q13.1) encodes for a transcription factor. It is a master regulator of sperm meiosis (sperm cell division). Mutations are found in cancers of the tonsils and adenoids, thalamus, and breast.

FGFR1 (fibroblast growth factor receptor 1) (8p11.23) is the first of the gene family (*FGFR1-4*) that encodes for fibroblast growth factor receptors. These are transmembranous cell surface receptors that bind fibroblast growth factors. On binding, the receptor activates the MAPK pathway, which is important for cell differentiation, proliferation, and migration during embryonic development. Mutations are linked to diffuse low-grade glioma with altered MAPK (see 'Diffuse low-grade glioma with altered MAPK', Chapter 14, p. 260).

TNKS (tankyrase) (8p23.1) encodes for the enzyme **tankyrase**, which is involved with gene transcription through activation of the **Wnt signalling pathway** (see Figure A1, Addendum, p. 363). Tankyrase is also involved in telomere maintenance (see 'Telomere and telomerase', Chapter 6, p. 124), DNA repair, and cellular metabolism. Mutations of *TNKS* are involved in the development and progression of lung, gastric, pancreatic, bladder, breast, and ovarian cancers, and glioblastomas.

SOX17 (SRY-box transcription factor 17) (8q11.23) encodes for a transcription factor that regulates embryonic development. Mutations are found in endometrial cancer, adenocarcinoma in situ, and hepatocellular carcinoma.

Chromosome 9

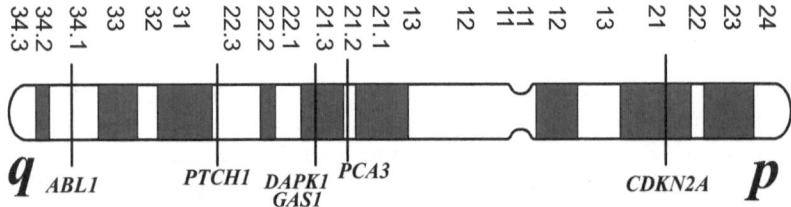

CDKN2A (cyclin-dependent kinase inhibitor 2A) (9p21.3) is a tumour suppressor gene that encodes for at least three proteins, two of which are inhibitors of CDK4 kinase (see 'CDK4, chromosome 12'). By inhibiting CDK4, they allow the protein pRB to function normally (see 'RB1, chromosome 13'). The third protein involves an *alternate open reading frame* (ARF), which stabilises the tumour suppression protein p53 (see 'TP53, chromosome 17', p. 356). It does this by interacting with the protein encoded by the gene *MDM2* (see 'MDM2, chromosome 12', p. 354), an enzyme which normally degrades p53. Some cancers over-express the *MDM2* gene and therefore render the p53 tumour suppression mechanism ineffectual. These three proteins (two CDK4 kinase inhibitors and ARF) are normally involved in cell cycle control by regulating the progression of the cell in G1. Mutations of *CDKN2A* are found in melanoma, pancreatic and oral cancers, and adenocarcinoma.

ABL1 (proto-oncogene 1, non-receptor tyrosine kinase) (9q34.12) encodes for a protein called **tyrosine kinase** which is important for activating a range of intracellular proteins. These proteins are part of the cell signalling system for growth. It is the deletion of the **SH3 domain** of the *ABL* gene, that is, the part which normally inhibits the tyrosine kinase function, that causes it to become an oncogene. The tyrosine kinase becomes increasingly produced and active in the cytoplasm, leading towards malignancy in that cell. The mutations are linked to chronic myeloid leukaemia. This genetic error frequently results from the *ABL* gene being involved in a translocation called the **Philadelphia chromosome** (or **Ph1**). The defect is a 9:22 translocation [t(9:22)], that is, parts of chromosomes 9 and 22 break off and swap places, so a short section of 9 attaches to 22, and part of 22 attaches to 9 (Figure 7.3, Chapter 7, p. 138). It is the addition of the *ABL* gene from chromosome 9 to part of the chromosome 22 known as the **BCR** (**break cluster region**) that creates the *ABL–BCR* combination. Chromosomes break more easily at specific sites. More than 150 breaking sites that can result in malignancy in cells are now known across all the 46 chromosomes. The resulting 9:22 *ABL–BCR* translocation is an oncogene found in 95% of patients with chronic myeloid leukaemia.

DAPK1 (death-associated protein kinase 1) (9q21.33) encodes for a protein kinase that facilitates tumour suppression and programmed cell death (apoptosis) (Figure 1.6, Chapter 1, p. 7). It is associated with cervical squamous carcinoma, pancreatic ductal adenocarcinoma, and bladder cancers.

PTCH1 (patched 1) (9q22.32) encodes for a protein which is one of the patched family of proteins involved in hedgehog signalling (see 'Terms', p. 362). This is a process that is important in embryonic development and tumour formation. Patched 1 and 2 are the proteins of the receptor for the hedgehog ligands. Mutations are associated with basal cell skin cancers (see also 'PTCH2, chromosome 1').

PCA3 (prostate cancer–associated 3) (9q21.2) codes for a long, non-coding stretch of RNA. The normal function of this RNA is not well understood, but it may regulate the expression of other genes involved in prostate development. This RNA is over-expressed in prostatic cancer cells and gets into the urine, where it acts as a biomarker for prostatic disease. Mutations are linked to prostate and ovarian cancers.

GAS1 (growth arrest specific 1) (9q21.33) protein has a role in suppressing cell growth by preventing the cell from entering the S phase when necessary. It plays the same role in tumour metastatic cell progression and must be down-regulated when metastases occur (see 'Metastatic suppressors', Table 6.3, Chapter 6, p. 127).

Chromosome 10

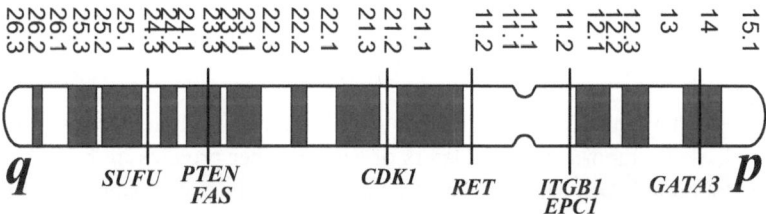

PTEN (phosphatase and tensin homolog) (10q23.31) is a tumour suppressor gene which helps regulate growth and survival of cells. Mutations are linked to prostate cancer and small-cell carcinoma; inherited breast, colorectal, and endometrial cancers; and melanoma.

ITGB1 (integrin subunit beta 1) (10p11.22) encodes for a beta subunit of integrin receptors which are involved in cell adhesion and multiple cell processes. Mutations are found in gall bladder and breast cancers, neuroblastomas, and sarcoma.

CDK1 (cyclin-dependent kinase 1) (10q21.2), which encodes for a member of the serine/threonine protein family, is important for the cell to progress into the mitosis (M) phase of the cell cycle (Figure 2.28). Mutations are seen in colorectal and breast cancers.

GATA3 (GATA binding protein 3) (10p14) encodes for a protein which is a member of the GATA transcription factor family. It has an important regulatory role in T cell and endothelial development. Mutations have been found in leukaemia and skin cancer.

SUFU (SUFU negative regulator of hedgehog signalling) (10q24.32) encodes for a protein involved in the hedgehog signalling pathway, which is vital for human development. Mutations are found in meningiomas, medulloblastomas, and basal cell carcinomas.

RET (RET proto-oncogene) (10q11.21) encodes for a member of the transmembranous tyrosine kinase receptor family involved in cell proliferation, differentiation, and migration. Mutations are found in thyroid adenomas and carcinomas and multiple endocrine neoplasia type 2 (see 'Multiple endocrine neoplasm (MEN)', Chapter 4, p. 76).

FAS (Fas cell surface death receptor) (10q23.31) encodes for a cell surface receptor which, if activated by the FasL ligand, causes programmed cell death (apoptosis) (see 'CD95', Chapter 5, p. 90). Mutations are linked to lung cancer.

EPC1 (enhancer of polycomb homolog 1) (10p11.22) encodes for a member of the histone acetyltransferase complex (see 'Epigenetics', Chapter 2, p. 36). Mutations are seen in adult T cell leukaemia/lymphoma.

Chromosome 11

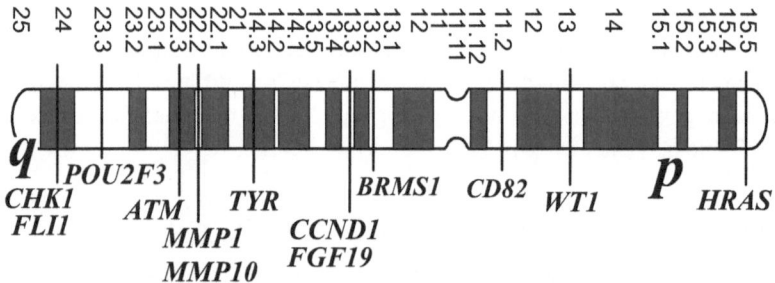

ATM (ATM serine/threonine kinase) (11q22.3) encodes for one of the proteins of the p13/p14 kinase family that are important as regulators of several other proteins in the cell cycle. *ATM* mutations are found in breast cancers; lymphomas; gliomas; inherited pancreatic, breast, ovarian, and prostate cancers; and leukaemia.

HRAS (HRas proto-oncogene, GTPase) (11p15.5) (Figure 2.2) is part of the *RAS* family of genes, which also includes *NRAS* (chromosome 1) and *KRAS* (chromosome 12). They encode for proteins involved in signalling pathways necessary for control of cell growth. *HRAS* mutations (and the percentage of cases) are linked to head and neck cancers (5%), melanomas (2%), and bladder cancers (7%), as well as some sarcomas and squamous cell carcinomas.

CHK1 (checkpoint kinase 1) (11q24.2) encodes for a protein of the serine/threonine kinase family. It halts the cell cycle in response to DNA damage. Mutations occur in Li–Fraumeni syndrome, retinoblastoma, and breast cancer.

WT1 (WT1 transcription factor) (11p13) is a transcription factor and tumour suppressor gene. It has an important function related to cell development and survival. Mutations are associated with some cases of Wilms tumour.

TYR (tyrosinase) (11q14.3) encodes for the enzyme tyrosinase, which carries out the first two stages of the conversion of tyrosine to melanin. Mutations are found in amelanotic melanoma.

CCND1 (cyclin D1) (11q13.3) encodes for a protein which is one of several cyclins involved in cell cycle regulation (Figure 2.4, Chapter 2, p. 31). Mutations are found in myelomas, leukaemia, lymphoma, and colorectal cancer.

FGF19 (fibroblast growth factor 19) (11q13.3) encodes for a member of the fibroblast growth factor family involved in wide-ranging cell division and cell survival activities. Mutations are found in melanomas.

MMP1 (matrix metallopeptidase 1) (11q22.2) and *MMP10* (matrix metallopeptidase 10) (11q22.2) encode for proteins which are members of the peptidase M10 enzyme family. These enzymes break down the surplus, unwanted extracellular matrix that forms during normal tissue development, such as embryonic development and tissue remodelling. Mutations are found in skin cancer.

POU2F3 (POU class 2 homeobox 3) (11q23.3) encodes for a protein transcription factor that regulates cell differentiation. It is mostly expressed in the epidermis of the skin, where is has a role in keratinocyte formation (Figure 13.1, Chapter 13, p. 242). Mutations are found in skin and cervical cancers.

FLI1 (Fli-1 proto-oncogene, ETS transcription factor) (11q24.3) encodes for a specific DNA transcription factor. Mutations are found in sarcomas, leukaemia, and lymphoma. A transloca-tion of *FLI1* with the gene *EWSR1* ('Chromosome 22', p. 360), that is, t(11;22)(q24:q12), results in Ewing sarcomas (see 'Ewing sarcoma', Chapter 14, p. 256) and various other tumours. An-other translocation of this gene with the gene *AFF1* ('Chromosome 4', p. 346), that is, t(4;11) (q21;q23), is recognised as a causative factor in acute lymphoblastic leukaemia.

BRMS1 (BRMS1 transcription repressor and anoikis regulator) (11q13.2) encodes for a breast cancer metastasis suppressor (BRMS) protein involved in suppressing breast cancer and melanoma metastases (see 'Metastatic suppressors', Table 6.3, Chapter 6, p. 127).

CD82 (cluster of differentiation 82 antigen) (11p11.2) (also called KAI1, kangai-1) encodes for a CD82 protein, a transmembranous glycoprotein which is a tumour suppressor protein. It is down-regulated in some cancers, notably prostate and bladder cancers, allowing progression of metastases (see 'Metastatic suppressors', Table 6.3, Chapter 6, p. 127).

Chromosome 12

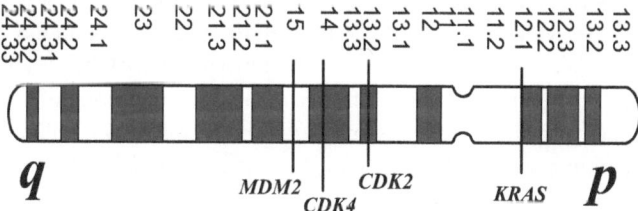

CDK4 (cyclin-dependant kinase 4) (12q14.1), which encodes for a member of the serine/threonine protein family which is important for the cell to progress from G1 of the cell cycle (Figure 1.6, Chapter 1, p. 7). Mutations of CDK4 have been found in melanoma, retinoblas-toma, liposarcoma, skin carcinomas and anaplastic astrocytoma.

KRAS (KRas proto-oncogene, GTPase) (12p12.1) is part of the *RAS* family of genes, which also includes *NRAS* ('Chromosome 1', p. 342) and *HRAS* ('Chromosome 11', p. 352). They encode for proteins involved in signalling pathways necessary for control of cell growth (see Figure 2.4, Chapter 2, p. 31). Mutations of KRAS (and the percentage of cases) are linked to the following cancers: colorectal (50%), pancreatic (88%), lung (32%), gall bladder (21%), endometrial (17%), ovarian (8%), urinary bladder (5%), and ameloblastoma (see 'Cancers of the mouth (oral cancers)', 'Ameloblastoma', Chapter 8, p. 155). This amounts to 10% of human cancers.

MDM2 (MDM2 proto-oncogene) (12q15) encodes for the enzyme **ligase**, which binds DNA strands together, rendering them ineffectual. The enzyme targets *TP53* (see 'TP53, chromosome 17'), but expression of the *MDM2* gene is regulated by the protein p53. Mutations of the *MDM2* gene are seen in a range of cancers where over-expression has allowed the cancer cell to escape p53 regulation.

CDK2 (cyclin-dependant kinase 2) (12q13.2), which encodes for a member of the serine/threonine protein family, is important for the cell to progress from G1 of the cell cycle (Figure 2.4). Mutations have been found in breast cancer.

Chromosome 13

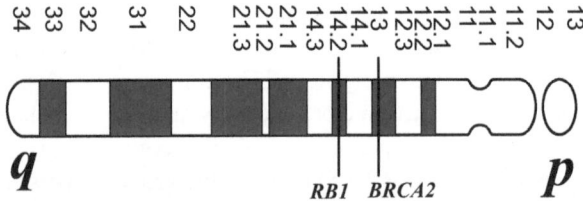

BRCA2 (breast cancer 2 DNA repair associated) (13q13.1) is a tumour suppressor gene that repairs and stabilises DNA. Mutations are found in inherited breast, pancreatic, prostate, fallopian tube, and ovarian cancers.

RB1 (retinoblastoma 1 transcriptional corepressor) (13q14.2) is a tumour suppressor gene that codes for the **pRb** protein, a powerful growth inhibitory molecule (Figure 2.28). The pRB protein halts the cell in G_1 of the cell cycle (Figure 1.6, Chapter 1, p. 7), and this controls any further growth. The pRB protein binds and blocks the function of transcription factors of the E2F protein family, the function of which is essential for the cell to progress around the cycle. This loss of E2F protein function in G_1 causes blockage of further progression of the cell. The protein pRB is, itself, switched on (activated) or switched off (deactivated) by the action of other proteins. Mutation of the *RB1* gene is seen in an eye tumour called **retinoblastoma**, but also in cancers of the lung, bladder, and pituitary gland, in osteogenic sarcoma, and in adenocarcinomas.

Chromosome 14

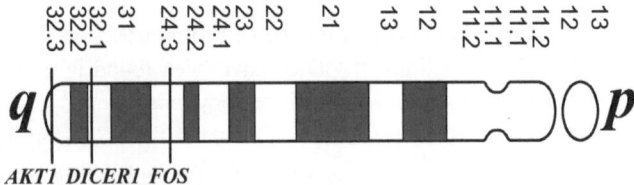

AKT1 (AKT serine/threonine kinase 1) (14q32.33) encodes for one of the serine/threonine kinase protein families, which are involved in a range of cell signalling pathways leading to control of cellular growth, survival, and metabolism. Mutations are found in breast, ovarian, and colorectal cancers; adenocarcinomas; and meningiomas.

FOS (FOS proto-oncogene, AP-1 transcription factor subunit) (14q24.3) is one of the four *FOS* gene families (*FOS*, *FOSB*, *FOSL1*, and *FOSL2*) which encode for proteins which work in conjunction with *JUN* gene proteins to create the transcription factor AP-1. This is a regulator of cell proliferation and transformation. Mutations are found in osteoblastoma and liver cancer.

DICER1 (Dicer 1, ribonuclease III) (14q32.13) encodes for a double-stranded (ds) RNA that acts as an endoribonuclease, an enzyme required for cutting up RNA and post-transcriptional gene silencing, that is, switching off gene expression. Mutations are found primarily in pulmonary blastomas, benign nephroma, and Sertoli–Leydig cell tumours (see 'Testicular cancer', 'Sex cord–stromal tumours', Chapter 12, p. 238). In addition, *DICER1* mutations are also found in approximately 25 disorders seen in other organ systems.

Chromosome 15

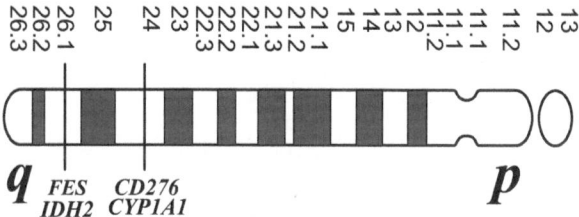

CD276 (CD276 molecule) (15q24.1) encodes for an immunoglobulin protein which regulates T cell immune response. Mutations are found in neuroblastoma and craniopharyngioma.

FES (FES proto-oncogene, tyrosine kinase) (15q26.1) encodes for a tyrosine kinase that is involved in the production of the cell cytoskeleton, microtubules, and cell attachments. Mutations are associated with soft connective tissue and bone sarcoma, and myeloid leukaemia.

IDH2 (isocitrate dehydrogenase (NADP (+)) 2) (15q26.1) encodes for the enzyme isocitrate dehydrogenase, which is involved in the conversion of isocitrate to 2-oxoglutarate in the tricarboxylic acid (Krebs) cycle. This cycle is the main energy-producing cycle within cells. This form of isocitrate dehydrogenase utilises NADP(+) as the main electron carrier. Mutations of this gene are found in cartilaginous cancers and myeloid leukaemia (see also 'Chromosome 2', p. 343).

CYP1A1 (cytochrome P450 family 1, subfamily A, member 1) (15q24.1) encodes for a cytochrome P450 enzyme involved in synthesis of cholesterol and other lipids and the catabolism of drugs. Mutations are seen in oral cancers.

Chromosome 16

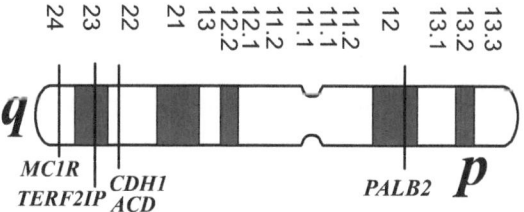

CDH1 (cadherin 1) (16q22.1) is involved in cell-to-cell adhesion and cellular mobility and has an invasive suppressor function. Mutations are found in endometrial, ovarian, gastric, tongue, and breast cancers.

PALB2 (partner and localiser of BACA2) (16p12.2) is a tumour suppressor gene, the protein of which works closely with, and localises, the BACA2 protein. Mutations are found in ovarian, fallopian tube, breast, prostate, and pancreatic cancers, and in Lynch syndrome (see 'Terms', p. 362).

MC1R (melanocortin 1 receptor) (16q24.3) encodes for a receptor protein that bonds melanocyte-stimulating hormone (MSH). Mutations are found in melanomas and skin cancers.

ACD (ACD shelterin complex subunit and telomerase recruitment factor) (16q22.1) encodes for one of six proteins which maintain telomere function (see 'Terms', p. 362). Mutations are found in melanomas.

TERF2IP (TERF2-interacting protein) (16q23.1) encodes for a protein which is part of a complex of proteins that regulate telomeric length and protection (see 'Terms', p. 362). Mutations are found in melanomas and astrocytomas.

Chromosome 17

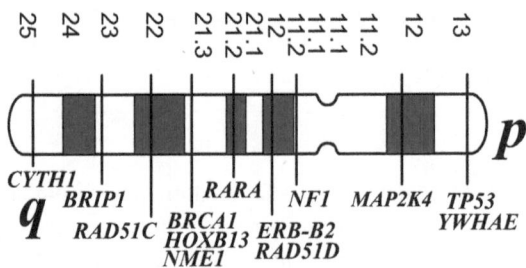

TP53 (tumour protein P53) (17p13.1) is a tumour suppressor gene that codes for the protein p53. This has some control over monitoring DNA for its integrity and initiates repair as required (Figure 2.4). Mutations are found in 50–70% of cancers, especially breast, cervical, colorectal, oral, skin, lung, oesophagus, bladder, ovarian, liver, pancreas, and bone cancers. About 30% of leukaemia, sarcoma, testicular cancer, and melanoma have *TP53* mutations, and it occurs in B cell lymphomas and Li–Fraumeni syndrome (see 'Terms', p. 362).

BRCA1 (breast cancer 1 DNA repair associated) (17q21.31) is a tumour suppressor gene that repairs and stabilises DNA. Mutations are found in breast, ovarian, fallopian tube, prostate, and pancreatic cancers, and in Lynch syndrome (see 'Terms', p. 362).

BRIP1 (BRCA1-interacting helicase 1) (17q23.2) encodes for the *BRIP1* protein, which joins with *BRCA1* protein to carry out an important double-stranded DNA break repair function. Mutations are found in breast and ovarian cancer.

NF1 (neurofibromin 1) (17q1 1.2) is a tumour suppressor gene, the protein product of which reduces *RAS* gene activity. Mutations are seen in neurofibroma, acoustic neuroma, leukaemia, breast cancer, and optic nerve neoplasm.

RAD51C (RAD51 paralog C) (17q22) encodes for a protein that is involved in DNA repair. Mutations are found in breast, ovarian, and fallopian tube cancer, and in Lynch syndrome (see 'Terms', p. 362).

RAD51D (RAD51 paralog D) (17q12) encodes for a protein that is involved in DNA repair. Mutations are found in breast, ovarian, and gastric cancers, and Lynch syndrome (see 'Terms', p. 362).

HOXB13 (homeobox B13) (17q21.32) is a transcription factor, that is, one of several proteins that regulate cellular development. Mutations are involved in prostate, pancreas, and small-cell cancers, and in spinal cord and myxopapillary ependymomas.

ERB-B2 (ERB-B2 receptor tyrosine kinase 2) (17q12) encodes for part of the receptor for binding epidermal growth factor. Mutations are found in ovarian, gastric, and lung cancers; gliomas; and breast carcinomas. The gene is often over-expressed due to amplification (Figure 2.6D, Chapter 2, p. 34) in 20–30% of invasive breast carcinomas.

RARA (retinoic acid receptor alpha) (17q21.2) encodes a receptor protein for the metabolite of vitamin A called **retinoic acid**. This regulates gene transcription and expression. RARA translocations are linked to acute myelocytic leukaemia (AML) (see 'Acute myelocytic (or myeloblastic) leukaemia (AML)', Chapter 7, p. 136).

NME1 (NME/NM23 nucleoside diphosphate kinase 1) (17q21.33) encodes for a protein involved in cellular development, differentiation, proliferation, signal transduction, and gene expression. This gene is down-regulated in metastatic cells (see 'Metastatic suppressors', Table 6.3, Chapter 6, p. 127). Mutations are found in aggressive neuroblastomas, breast ductal cancers, large-cell lung cancers, and other tumours.

MAP2K4 (mitogen-activated protein kinase, kinase 4; also called MKK4) (17p12) encodes for a protein which is a member of the mitogen-activated protein kinase (MAPK) family. It is involved in cellular differentiation, proliferation, transcription regulation, and development. Mutations are seen in lung and pancreatic cancers. MAP2K4 acts as a metastatic suppressor through several mechanisms (see 'Metastatic suppressors', Table 6.3, Chapter 6, p. 127).

YWHAE (tyrosine 3-monooxygenase/tryptophan 5-monooxygenase activation protein epsilon) (17p13.3) encodes for a protein involved in a diverse number of cell transduction signalling pathways. Mutations are seen in endometrial and renal sarcomas.

CYTH1 (cytohesin 1) (17q25.3) encodes for a protein which is highly expressed in NK cells and peripheral T cells. It is involved in the movement of substances within the cell and across the cell membranes. Epigenetic errors cause cancers in African American smokers (see 'Tobacco smoking', Chapter 3, p. 48). Mutations are linked to breast, ovarian, and pancreatic cancers, and leukaemia.

Chromosome 18

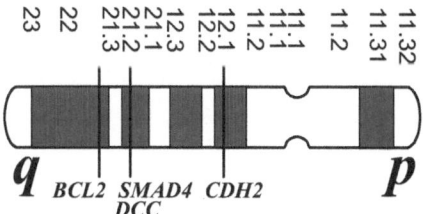

BCL2 (B cell lymphoma 2 apoptosis regulator) (18q21.33) encodes a protein that suppresses apoptosis (see 'Terms', p. 362). Over-expression of this gene is caused by a translocation between chromosomes 14 and 18, that is, t(14;18), found in B cell lymphomas. The result is inadequate apoptosis, allowing too many abnormal B cells to survive, which then form the lymphoma.

SMAD4 (SMAD family member 4) (18q21.2) encodes for a signal transduction protein involved in the transforming growth factor beta (TGFβ) cell signalling pathway. Mutations are found in pancreatic and bile duct cancers, adenomas, and adenocarcinomas.

CDH2 (cadherin 2) (18q12.1) is involved in cell-to-cell adhesion and neurological, bone, and cartilage development. Mutations occur in bladder cancers.

DCC (deleted in colon cancer netrin 1 receptor) (18q21.2) encodes for a membrane receptor that binds the protein netrin-1. This protein is involved in neuronal guidance during the development of the nervous system. *DCC* is also thought to act as a tumour suppressor gene, although this is somewhat controversial. Normally, there should be two copies of this gene (called **alleles**), one from each parent. Loss of *heterozygosity*, that is, deletion of one copy of this gene, is seen in several cancers, including colon cancer.

Chromosome 19

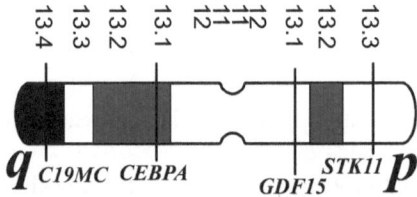

STK11 (serine/threonine protein kinase 11) (19p13.3) is a tumour suppressor gene that helps control growth and apoptosis (see 'Terms', p. 362). Mutations are linked to lung, gastric, ovarian, breast, endometrial, cervical, colorectal, and pancreatic cancers, and melanoma. Loss of this gene is seen in Peutz–Jeghers syndrome (see Table 8.5, Chapter 8, p. 167).

C19MC (*MIR520G* microRNA 520g) (19q13.4) is a DNA region that contains a cluster of microRNA genes that regulate the expression of other genes involved with cell proliferation, differentiation, and apoptosis. The region is linked to some cancers, for example, brain cancer (see 'Medulloepithelioma', Chapter 14, p. 261).

CEBPA (CCAAT enhancer binding protein alpha) (19q13.11) codes for a protein that, in conjunction with beta and gamma proteins, binds to the CCAAT portion of DNA and is important in cell cycle regulation. Mutations are found in some cases of acute myeloid leukaemia (AML).

GDF15 (growth differentiation factor 15) (19p13.11) encodes for one of the transforming growth factor beta (TGF-Beta) family of proteins. It binds to the GFRAL (GDNF family receptor alpha like) receptor which is in the brainstem. The GDF15 growth factor is involved in the regulation of food intake, energy use, and body weight in response to cell metabolic and toxic stresses. Mutations are linked to colorectal, pancreatic, lung, prostate, breast, and gastric cancers.

Chromosome 20

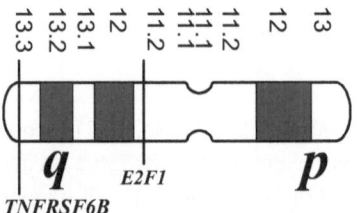

TNFRSF6B (TNF receptor superfamily member 6b) (20q13.33) encodes for a tumour necrosis factor that protects the cell against apoptosis (see 'Terms', p. 362). Mutations are seen in pancreatic cancers, and over-expression of this gene is found in gastrointestinal tumours.

E2F1 (E2F transcription factor 1) (20q11.22) encodes for proteins which aid in the control of the cell cycle and activates other important genes. Mutations have been found in lung and bladder cancers, squamous cell carcinomas, and retinoblastomas.

Chromosome 21

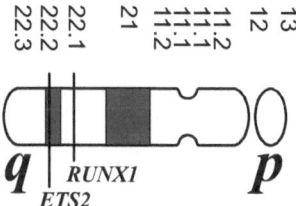

ETS2 (ETS proto-oncogene 2, transcription factor) (21q22.2) encodes for a transcription factor which is involved in cell development and apoptosis (see 'Terms', p. 362). Mutations are seen in leukaemia, endometrial carcinoma, and choriocarcinoma (see 'Terms', p. 362).

RUNX1 (RUNX family transcription factor 1) (21q22.12) encodes for a protein transcription factor that binds to a number of gene promotor sequences. In combination with the protein CBFB (core-binding factor), it stabilises blood cell formation and differentiation into myeloid and lymphoid cell lines. Mutations are found in some acute myeloid leukaemia (AML).

Chromosome 22

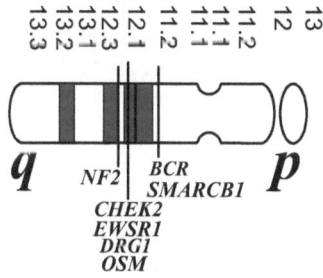

CHEK2 (checkpoint kinase 2) (22q12.1) is a tumour suppressor gene involved in DNA repair. With p53, it restricts progression of the cell cycle in G1. Mutations are linked to prostate, breast, and colorectal cancer, and osteogenic sarcoma.

BCR (break cluster region activator of RhoGEF and GTPase) (22q11.23) encodes for a protein that is involved in the activity of the enzyme GTPase (Figure 2.2, Chapter 2, p. 28). It can produce a reciprocal translocation with the *ABL* gene to form the *BCR–ABL* Philadelphia chromosome, an oncogene involved in chronic myeloid leukaemia (CML) ('ABL gene, Chromosome 9', p. 350) (see 'Chronic myeloid leukaemia', Chapter 7, p. 137).

SMARCB1 (SWI/SNF-related, matrix-associated, actin-dependent regulator of chromatin, subfamily B, member 1) (22q11.23) encodes for a protein that is one part of a complex required to allow more efficient transcription of target genes. Mutations are linked to kidney rhabdoid tumours (see 'Rhabdoid tumour of the kidney (RTK)', Chapter 10, p. 202) and meningiomas.

EWSR1 (EWS RNA-binding protein 1) (22q12.2) encodes for a protein involved in many cell processes, notably gene expression, RNA processing, and cell signalling. A translocation of *EWSR1* with the gene *FLI1* gene ('Chromosome 11', p. 353), that is, t(11;22)(q24:q12), results in Ewing sarcomas (see 'Ewing sarcoma', Chapter 14, p. 256) and various other tumours.

NF2 (NF2, moesin-ezrin-radixin like (MERLIN) tumour suppressor) (22q12.2) encodes for protein similar to the ezrin, radixin, moesin family of proteins that bind cytoskeleton components to the cell membrane. This protein is involved in the regulation of contact inhibition[3] of growth and cell-to-cell adhesion. Mutations are found in vestibular schwannomas, acoustic neuromas, meningiomas, and nerve sheath tumours.

DRG1 (developmentally regulated GTP binding protein 1) (22q12.2) encodes for a protein involved in microtubule and mitotic spindle assembly. It also acts as a metastatic suppressor in prostate, breast, and colon cancers by interfering with several cancer cell signalling pathways (see 'Metastatic suppressors', Table 6.3, Chapter 6, p. 256).

OSM (oncostatin M) (22q12.2) encodes for a cytokine, leukaemia inhibitory factor, and growth factor, which is often secreted by tumours. Mutations are found in Kaposi's sarcoma (see 'Vascular tumours', 'Kaposi's sarcoma', Chapter 13, p. 250).

Chromosome X

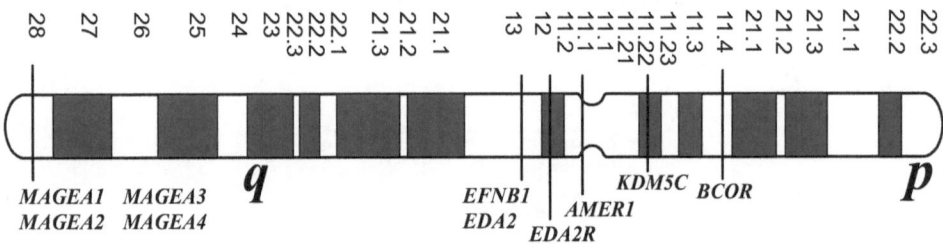

MAGEA1 (MAGE family, member A1), **MAGEA2** (MAGE family, member A2), **MAGEA3** (MAGE family, member A3), and **MAGEA4** (MAGE family, member A4) (Xq28) is a gene cluster at Xq28 which encodes for proteins which may regulate transcription and embryonic development. Mutations of *MAGEA1* have been found in testicular cancer, melanoma, and squamous cell carcinoma. Mutations of *MAGEA2* have been found in melanoma and squamous cell carcinoma. Mutations of *MAGEA3* have been found in testicular and oesophageal cancer, melanoma, and squamous cell carcinoma. Mutation of *MAGEA4* have been found in testicular cancer, melanoma, and squamous cell carcinoma.

EFNB1 (ephrin B1) (Xq13.1) encodes for a cell surface protein involved in cell adhesion and the development and maintenance of the nervous system. Mutations are involved in pancreatic and gastric cancers and squamous cell carcinoma of the head and neck.

AMER1 (alias *WTX*) (APC membrane recruitment protein 1) (Xq11.1) encodes for a protein that is involved in the Wnt signalling pathway (see 'Terms', p. 362). Mutations of this gene are seen in Wilms tumour (see 'Wilms tumour (nephroblastoma)', Chapter 10, p. 201) and colorectal cancer.

BCOR (BCL6 corepressor) (Xp11.4) encodes for a protein which suppresses unnecessary gene transcription. Mutations are linked to acute myeloid leukaemia and kidney clear cell sarcoma.

EDA2 (ectodysplasin A2) (Xq13.1) encodes for a tumour necrosis factor/cytokine that is involved with epithelial–mesenchymal signalling during development of ectodermal organs, such as the skin, sweat glands, and tooth enamel. It is the ligand for the EDA2R receptor. Mutations are linked to lung and colorectal cancers and osteogenic sarcoma (see also 'Kwashiorkor and cachexia', Chapter 18, p. 327).

EDA2R (ectodysplasin A2 receptor) (Xq12) encodes for the receptor for EDA2 protein. Mutations are linked to prostate, pancreas, ovarian, and renal cancers (see also 'Kwashiorkor and cachexia', Chapter 18, p. 327).

KDM5C (lysine demethylase 5C) (Xp11.22) encodes for a histone demethylation protein which is also a transcription repression factor for neurogenic genes. Mutations are found in multiple myeloma, plasma cell neoplasia, chromophobe renal cell carcinoma, and renal cell cancer (non-papillary).

Chromosome Y

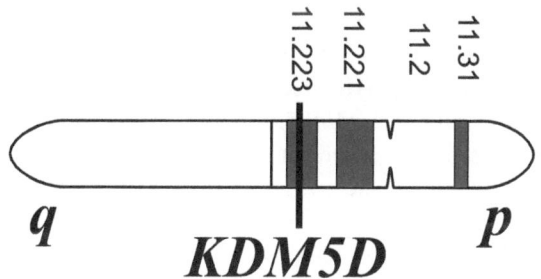

KDM5D (lysine demethylase 5D) (Yq11.223) encodes for an enzyme that demethylates, that is, removes methyl groups (CH_3), from certain histones (see 'Epigenetics', 'DNA methylation', Chapter 2, p. 36). Mutations are found in prostate, bladder, head and neck, gastric, lung, and colorectal cancers and squamous cell carcinomas. In colorectal cancers, this upregulated gene, driven by mutations of the *KRAS* gene ('Chromosome 12', p. 353), appears to loosen cell adhesion (see 'Cell adhesion molecules (CAMs)', Chapter 6, p. 114) and promote metastases and mortality. Deleting the gene increases tight junctions (see 'Other cell-to-cell junctions', Chapter 6, p. 117) and promotes cancer killing by T cells. In contrast, the absence of the gene, that is, in older men who have naturally lost the Y chromosome due to the aging process, appears to make bladder cancers more aggressive. More work is needed to clarify this dichotomy. The presence or absence of this gene may be one reason that some cancers are worse in men than in women.

Terms

The following terms have been used in the preceding text:

- *Ameloblastoma* is a rare benign tumour of the jaw. It starts in the tooth enamel and is aggressive, developing into a large tumour that may grow into the jawbone.

- *Anaplastic astrocytoma* is a rare malignant brain tumour developing from astrocytes.
- *Apoptosis*, or *programmed cell death*, is a natural process of cellular changes resulting in the death of a cell. This happens when cells are produced in excess to body needs, as in embryological development, or as a result of DNA damage which cannot be repaired occurring during the cell cycle.
- *Choriocarcinoma* is a rapidly growing cancer of the uterus.
- *Gene locus* (pl. *loci*) is the address on the chromosome where the gene is found. For example, in the case of *TP53*, the locus is 17p13.1, where *17* is the chromosome number; *p* means the short arm of the chromosome, that is, above the centromere; and *13.1* is the location counted away from the centromere. In other examples, the letter *q* means the long arm of the chromosome, that is, below the centromere.
- *Kaposi's sarcoma* is a rare form of tumour that affects the skin and mouth. Various forms are known; some affect a limited area, and others are more widely spread. It is caused by the human herpesvirus 8 (HHV-8), also known as Kaposi's sarcoma–associated herpesvirus (KSHV).
- *Li–Fraumeni syndrome* is an inherited *TP53* mutation that increases the risk of developing leukaemia, breast and bone cancers, and soft tissue sarcomas.
- *Lynch syndrome* is an inherited disorder involving mutations in genes *MLH1*, *MSH2*, *MSH6*, *PMS2*, and *EPCAM,* causing errors in DNA mismatch repair. It is also known as **hereditary non-polyposis colorectal cancer (HNPCC)** (Table 8.5, Chapter 8, p. 167).
- *Mismatch repair cancer syndrome* (MMRCS) is a rare childhood cancer syndrome involving four major new growths: blood, colorectal, central nervous system, and intestinal polyps. It may also involve other malignancies. It is of autosomal recessive inheritance (see 'Gene inheritance', Chapter 2, p. 30).
- *Myxopapillary ependymomas* are slow-growing tumours of the supportive tissue within the central nervous system.
- *Neurilemmoma* (schwannoma) is a tumour of the myelin sheath, which covers neuronal fibres (axons) and is originally formed by Schwann cells. It is usually benign but can become malignant.
- *Neurofibrosarcoma* is a malignant peripheral nerve sheath (myelin sheath) tumour.
- *Osteogenic sarcoma* (osteosarcoma) is the commonest form of primary bone tumour. *Primary* means it is an original tumour, not caused by metastases.
- *Retinoblastoma* is a rare form of eye cancer that usually begins in early childhood.
- *Squamous cell carcinoma* is a cancer of the flat surface cells (squamous cells) of the skin epidermis.
- *Hedgehog signalling* is an essential signalling mechanism for embryonic development and cellular differentiation. In adults, it is required to aid stem cell differentiation in tissues that require regular replacement.
- *Telomere* is a sequence of repetitive DNA bases at the end of the chromosome that protect the chromosome from damage and shorten after each cellular mitotic replication (see 'Tissue invasion: telomeres', Chapter 6, p. 124).
- *Wnt* (Wingless and Int-1) *pathway* is a cell signalling pathway for the control of gene transcription (Figure A1).

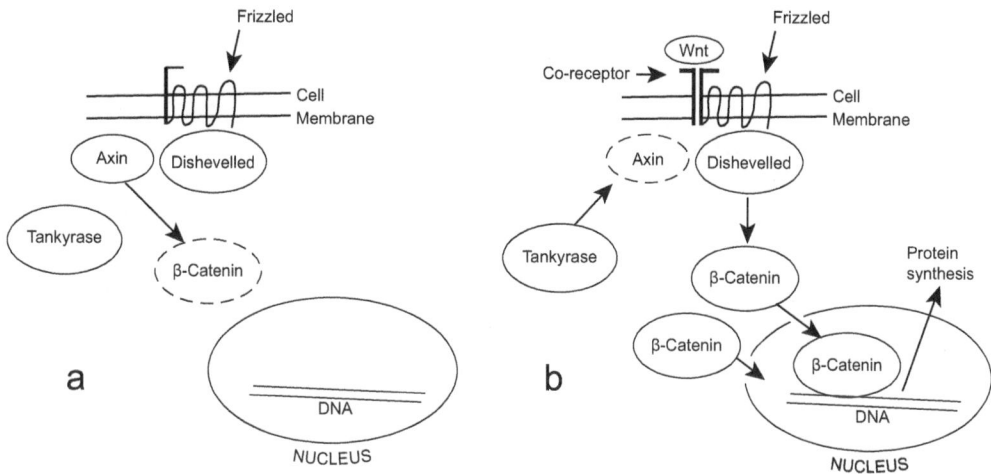

FIGURE A1 Simplified view of the canonical Wnt (Wingless and Int-1) signalling pathway: (a) In the absence of Wnt, the protein Axin, along with other proteins, degrade (broken line) β-catenin, which then becomes unavailable for entering the nucleus. (b) When the Wnt protein binds to the frizzled receptor and a co-receptor on the cell membrane, the signal is passed to the dishevelled protein on the inner surface of the cell membrane. Tankyrase protein then interacts with multiple proteins, notably Axin, which is then degraded, allowing β-catenin to increase and enter the nucleus, where it triggers gene expression, leading to protein synthesis.

Notes

1 Catalysts, as with all enzymes, facilitate and promote a chemical reaction without themselves being chemically changed.
2 See Figure 16.6, Chapter 16, p. 300.
3 *Contact inhibition* means that when cells make contact with each other, they automatically stop growing.

GENETIC INDEX

Genes, chromosomes, genetic syndromes and diseases

INDEX